Infection Prevention and Control in Healthcare, Part I: Facility Planning

Editors

KEITH S. KAYE
SORABH DHAR

INFECTIOUS DISEASE CLINICS OF NORTH AMERICA

www.id.theclinics.com

Consulting Editor
HELEN W. BOUCHER

September 2021 • Volume 35 • Number 3

ELSEVIER

1600 John F. Kennedy Boulevard • Suite 1800 • Philadelphia, Pennsylvania, 19103-2899.
http://www.theclinics.com

INFECTIOUS DISEASE CLINICS OF NORTH AMERICA Volume 35, Number 3
September 2021 ISSN 0891–5520, ISBN-13: 978-0-323-83516-9

Editor: Kerry Holland
Developmental Editor: Jessica Nicole B. Cañaberal

Photocopying

Single photocopies of single articles may be made for personal use as allowed by national copyright laws. Permission of the Publisher and payment of a fee is required for all other photocopying, including multiple or systematic copying, copying for advertising or promotional purposes, resale, and all forms of document delivery. Special rates are available for educational institutions that wish to make photocopies for non-profit educational classroom use. For information on how to seek permission visit www.elsevier.com/permissions or call: (+44) 1865 843830 (UK)/(+1) 215 239 3804 (USA).

Derivative Works

Subscribers may reproduce tables of contents or prepare lists of articles including abstracts for internal circulation within their institutions. Permission of the Publisher is required for resale or distribution outside the institution. Permission of the Publisher is required for all other derivative works, including compilations and translations (please consult www.elsevier.com/permissions).

Electronic Storage or Usage

Permission of the Publisher is required to store or use electronically any material contained in this periodical, including any article or part of an article (please consult www.elsevier.com/permissions). Except as outlined above, no part of this publication may be reproduced, stored in a retrieval system or transmitted in any form or by any means, electronic, mechanical, photocopying, recording or otherwise, without prior written permission of the Publisher.

Notice

No responsibility is assumed by the Publisher for any injury and/or damage to persons or property as a matter of products liability, negligence or otherwise, or from any use or operation of any methods, products, instructions or ideas contained in the material herein. Because of rapid advances in the medical sciences, in particular, independent verification of diagnoses and drug dosages should be made.

Although all advertising material is expected to conform to ethical (medical) standards, inclusion in this publication does not constitute a guarantee or endorsement of the quality or value of such product or of the claims made of it by its manufacturer.

Infectious Disease Clinics of North America (ISSN 0891–5520) is published in March, June, September, and December by Elsevier Inc., 360 Park Avenue South, New York, NY 10010-1710. Periodicals postage paid at New York, NY and additional mailing offices. Subscription prices are $347.00 per year for US individuals, $922.00 per year for US institutions, $100.00 per year for US students, $396.00 per year for Canadian individuals, $973.00 per year for Canadian institutions, $432.00 per year for international individuals, $973.00 per year for international institutions, $100.00 per year for Canadian students, and $200.00 per year for international students. To receive student rate, orders must be accompanied by name of affiliated institution, date of term, and the *signature* of program/residency coordinator on institution letterhead. Orders will be billed at individual rate until proof of status is received. Foreign air speed delivery is included in all *Clinics* subscription prices. All prices are subject to change without notice. **POSTMASTER:** Send address changes to *Infectious Disease Clinics of North America*, Elsevier Health Sciences Division, Subcription Customer Service, 3251 Riverport Lane, Maryland Heights, MO 63043. **Customer Service: 1-800-654-2452 (US). From outside of the US and Canada, call 1-314-447-8871. Fax: 1-314-447-8029. E-mail: JournalsCustomerService-usa@elsevier.com (print support) or JournalsOnlineSupport-usa@elsevier.com (online support).**

Infectious Disease Clinics of North America is also published in Spanish by Editorial Inter-Médica, Junin 917, 1er A 1113, Buenos Aires, Argentina.

Reprints. For copies of 100 or more, of articles in this publication, please contact the Commercial Reprints Department, Elsevier Inc., 360 Park Avenue South, New York, New York 10010-1710. Tel. 212-633-3874, Fax: 212-633-3820, E-mail: reprints@elsevier.com.

Infectious Disease Clinics of North America is covered in *MEDLINE/PubMed (Index Medicus), Current Contents/ Clinical Medicine, Science Citation Alert, SCISEARCH,* and *Research Alert.*

Contributors

CONSULTING EDITOR

HELEN W. BOUCHER, MD, FIDSA, FACP
Director, Infectious Diseases Fellowship Program, Division of Geographic Medicine and Infectious Diseases, Tufts Medical Center, Associate Professor of Medicine, Tufts University School of Medicine, Boston, Massachusetts

EDITORS

KEITH S. KAYE, MD, MPH
Professor of Medicine, Division of Infectious Diseases, University of Michigan, University of Michigan Medical School, Professor of Internal Medicine, Director of Research, Division of Infectious Diseases, University of Michigan Health, Ann Arbor, Michigan

SORABH DHAR, MD
Associate Professor of Medicine, Division of Infectious Diseases, Wayne State University, School of Medicine, Director of Infection Prevention, Hospital Epidemiology and Antimicrobial Stewardship, John D. Dingell VA Medical Center, Detroit, Michigan

AUTHORS

OWEN R. ALBIN, MD
Division of Infectious Diseases, Department of Internal Medicine, Michigan Medicine, Ann Arbor, Michigan

MEREDITH AMBROSE, MHA
National Infectious Diseases Service, Specialty Care Services, Veterans Health Administration, Department of Veterans Affairs (VA), Washington, DC

JOHN M. BOYCE, MD
J.M. Boyce Consulting, LLC, Middletown, Connecticut

PHILIP C. CARLING, MD
Professor of Clinical Medicine, Department of Infectious Diseases, Boston University School of Medicine, Director of Infectious Diseases, Carney Hospital, Boston, Massachusetts

MARCO CASSONE, MD, PhD
Division of Geriatric and Palliative Medicine, University of Michigan Medical School, Ann Arbor, Michigan

SORABH DHAR, MD
Associate Professor of Medicine, Division of Infectious Diseases, Wayne State University, School of Medicine, Director of Infection Prevention, Hospital Epidemiology and Antimicrobial Stewardship, John D. Dingell VA Medical Center, Detroit, Michigan

MICHELLE FLOOD, RN, MSN, CIC, FAPIC
Department of Infection Prevention and Control, Ascension St. John Hospital, Grosse Pointe Woods, Michigan

SHANTINI D. GAMAGE, PhD, MPH
National Infectious Diseases Service, Specialty Care Services, Veterans Health Administration, Department of Veterans Affairs (VA), Washington, DC; Division of Infectious Diseases, Department of Internal Medicine, University of Cincinnati College of Medicine, Cincinnati, Ohio

KEITH S. KAYE, MD, MPH
Professor of Medicine, Division of Infectious Diseases, University of Michigan, University of Michigan Medical School, Professor of Internal Medicine, Director of Research, Division of Infectious Diseases, University of Michigan Health, Ann Arbor, Michigan

STEPHEN M. KRALOVIC, MD, MPH
National Infectious Diseases Service, Specialty Care Services, Veterans Health Administration, Department of Veterans Affairs (VA), Washington, DC; Division of Infectious Diseases, Department of Internal Medicine, University of Cincinnati College of Medicine, Cincinnati VA Medical Center, Cincinnati, Ohio

KERRY L. LAPLANTE, PharmD
Infectious Diseases Research Program, Center of Innovation in Long-Term Support Services, Providence Veterans Affairs Medical Center, Department of Health Services Policy and Practice, Center for Gerontology and Health Care Research, Brown University School of Public Health, Division of Infectious Diseases, Warren Alpert Medical School of Brown University, Providence, Rhode Island; College of Pharmacy, University of Rhode Island, Kingston, Rhode Island

WILLIAM LEBAR, MS
Manager, Clinical Microbiology Laboratory, Department of Pathology, University of Michigan Medical School, Ann Arbor, Michigan

PAUL LEPHART, PhD, D(ABMM)
Associate Director, Clinical Microbiology Laboratory, Assistant Professor of Pathology, Department of Pathology, University of Michigan Medical School, Ann Arbor, Michigan

MICHAEL Y. LIN, MD, MPH
Associate Professor, Division of Infectious Diseases, Department of Medicine, Rush University Medical Center, Chicago, Illinois

GINA MAKI, DO
Senior Staff, Division of Infectious Diseases, Henry Ford Hospital, Detroit, Michigan

LONA MODY, MD, MSc
Division of Geriatric and Palliative Medicine, University of Michigan Medical School, Geriatrics Research, Education and Clinical Center, Veterans Affairs Ann Arbor Healthcare System

ANA MONTOYA, MD, MPH, CMD
Division of Geriatric and Palliative Medicine, University of Michigan Medical School, Ann Arbor, Michigan

JEROD L. NAGEL, PharmD
Department of Pharmacy, Michigan Medicine, University of Michigan College of Pharmacy, Ann Arbor, Michigan

DUANE NEWTON, PhD, D(ABMM), FIDSA
Partner, NaviDx Consulting, Adjunct Professor, Department of Pathology, University of Michigan Medical School, Ann Arbor, Michigan

RUSSELL N. OLMSTED, MPH, CIC, FAPIC
Director of Infection Prevention Management, Integrated Clinical Services (ICS), Trinity Health, Livonia, Michigan

TRISH M. PERL, MD, MSc
Division of Infectious Diseases and Geographic Medicine, Jay Sanford Professor of Medicine and Infectious Diseases, Chief of Infectious Diseases and Geographic Medicine, UT Southwestern Medical Center, Dallas, Texas

JASON M. POGUE, PharmD
Department of Clinical Pharmacy, University of Michigan College of Pharmacy, Ann Arbor, Michigan

GARY A. ROSELLE, MD
National Infectious Diseases Service, Specialty Care Services, Veterans Health Administration, Department of Veterans Affairs (VA), Washington, DC; Division of Infectious Diseases, Department of Internal Medicine, University of Cincinnati College of Medicine, Cincinnati VA Medical Center, Cincinnati, Ohio

WILLIAM A. RUTALA, PhD, MPH
Professor, Division of Infectious Diseases, University of North Carolina School of Medicine, Chapel Hill, North Carolina

AVNISH L. SANDHU, DO
Assistant Professor of Medicine, Division of Infectious Diseases, Wayne State University, School of Medicine, Detroit, Michigan

ERICA S. SHENOY, MD, PhD
Associate Professor of Medicine, Infection Control Unit, Division of Infectious Diseases, Massachusetts General Hospital, Harvard Medical School, Boston, Massachusetts

GEETA SOOD, MD, MSc
Division of Infectious Diseases, Assistant Professor of Medicine and Hospital Epidemiologist, Johns Hopkins School of Medicine, Johns Hopkins Bayview Medical Center, Baltimore, Maryland

LISA STURM, MPH, CIC, FAPIC
Ascension Healthcare, Infection Prevention, St Louis, Missouri

WILLIAM E. TRICK, MD
Professor, Department of Medicine, Rush University Medical Center and Director, Health Research and Solutions, Cook County Health, Chicago, Illinois

AMANDA VALYKO, MPH, CIC, FAPIC
Director, Department of Infection Prevention and Epidemiology, University of Michigan Health, Ann Arbor, Michigan

LARAINE WASHER, MD, FACP
Clinical Associate Professor, Division of Infectious Diseases, Hospital Epidemiologist, Department of Infection Prevention and Epidemiology, University of Michigan Health, Ann Arbor, Michigan

DAVID J. WEBER, MD, MPH
Sanders Distinguished Professor of Medicine, Pediatrics and Epidemiology, UNC School of Medicine, Gillings School of Global Public Health, Division of Infectious Disease, The University of North Carolina at Chapel Hill, Department of Hospital Epidemiology, UNC Medical Center, University of North Carolina Health Care System, Chapel Hill, North Carolina

MARCUS ZERVOS, MD
Head, Division of Infectious Diseases, Henry Ford Hospital, Professor of Medicine and Assistant Dean of Global Affairs, Wayne State University, Detroit, Michigan

SHIWEI ZHOU, MD
Division of Infectious Diseases, Department of Internal Medicine, Michigan Medicine, Ann Arbor, Michigan

Contents

Successful Infection Prevention Programs (IPPs) consist of a multidisciplinary team led by a hospital epidemiologist and managed by infection preventionists. Knowledge of the economics of health care–associated infections (HAIs) and the ability to make a business plan is now essential to the success of programs. Prevention of HAIs is the core function of IPPs with impact on patient outcomes, quality of care, and cost savings for hospitals. This article discusses the structure and responsibilities of an IPP, the regulatory pressures and opportunities that these programs face, and how to build and manage a successful program.

Hand hygiene by health care personnel is an important measure for preventing health care–associated infections, but adherence rates and technique remain suboptimal. Alcohol-based hand rubs are the preferred method of hand hygiene in most clinical scenarios, are more effective and better tolerated than handwashing, and their use has facilitated improved adherence rates. Obtaining accurate estimates of hand hygiene adherence rates using direct observations of personnel is challenging. Combining automated hand hygiene monitoring systems with direct observations is a promising strategy, and is likely to yield the best estimates of adherence. Greater attention to hand hygiene technique is needed.

All invasive procedures involve contact by a medical device or surgical instrument with a patient's sterile tissue or mucous membranes. The level of disinfection is dependent on the intended use of the object: critical, semi-critical, or noncritical. New issues and practices can affect the risk of infection associated with devices and surfaces. Endoscopes continue to represent a nosocomial hazard. The contaminated surface environment in hospital rooms is important in the transmission of health care–associated pathogens. Thoroughness of cleaning must be monitored and no-touch room decontamination technology should be used. In general, emerging pathogens are susceptible to currently available disinfectants.

Recent research has significantly clarified the impact of optimizing patient-zone environmental hygiene. New insights into the environmental microbial epidemiology of many hospital-associated pathogens, especially Clostridioides difficile, have clarified and quantified the role of ongoing occult pathogen transmission from the near-patient environment. The recent development of safe, broadly effective surface chemical disinfectants has led to new opportunities to broadly enhance environmental hygiene in all health care settings. The Centers for Disease Control and Prevention has recently developed a detailed guidance to assist all health care settings in implementing optimized programs to mitigate health care-associated pathogen transmission from the near-patient surfaces.

Outbreaks and pseudo-outbreaks in health care settings are complex and should be evaluated systematically using epidemiologic and molecular tools. Outbreaks result from failures of infection prevention practices, inadequate staffing, and undertrained or overcommitted health care personnel. Contaminated hands, equipment, supplies, water, ventilation systems, and environment may also contribute. Neonatal intensive care, endoscopy, oncology, and transplant units are areas at particular risk. Procedures, such as bronchoscopy and endoscopy, are sources of infection when cleaning and disinfection processes are inadequate. New types of equipment can be introduced and lead to contamination or equipment and medications can be contaminated at the manufacturing source.

Health care facility water systems have been associated with the transmission of opportunistic premise plumbing pathogens such as Legionella and nontuberculous mycobacteria. These pathogens can enter a building's water system in low numbers and then proliferate when conditions are conducive to their growth. Patients and residents in health care facilities are often at heightened risk for opportunistic infections, and cases and outbreaks in the literature highlight the importance of routine water management programs and occasions for intervention to prevent additional cases. A multidisciplinary proactive approach to water safety is critical for sustained prevention of health care–associated water-related infections.

The built environment has been integral to response to the global pandemic of severe acute respiratory syndrome coronavirus-2 (SARS-CoV-2). In particular, engineering controls to mitigate risk of exposure to SARS-CoV-2 and other newly emergent respiratory pathogens in the future will be important. Anticipating emergence from this pandemic, or at least adaptation given increasing administration of effective vaccines, and the safety of patients, personnel, and others in health care facilities remain the core goals. This article summarizes known risks and highlights prevention strategies for daily care as well as response to emergent infectious diseases and this parapandemic phase.

An effective occupational health program is a key aspect of preventing exposure to infectious agents and subsequent infection, as well as evaluation and management of postexposure prophylaxis and infections in health care personnel (HCP) by educating HCP regarding proper handling of sharps, early identification and isolation of potentially infectious patients, implementation of standard and transmission-based precautions, and offering counseling of HCP regarding nonroutine prophylaxis. Occupational health services (OHS) must also apply standardized processes for determining when exposures have occurred and providing appropriate management, and provide immediate availability of a medical evaluation following a nonprotected exposure to an infectious disease.

Health care personnel (HCP) are at risk of exposure to infectious agents depending on their job duties and other factors. Risks include percutaneous exposure to blood-borne pathogens via sharp injuries (eg, human immunodeficiency virus, hepatitis B virus, hepatitis C virus); exposure by direct contact, droplet, or airborne transmission of pathogens through direct patient care (eg, pertussis, invasive meningococcus infections, tuberculosis); and through indirect contact transmission related to the contaminated health care environment (eg, Clostridioides difficile). Occupational health programs must effectively identify and respond to potential exposures and provide guidance to HCP on postexposure prophylaxis.

Computer informatics have the potential to improve infection control outcomes in surveillance, prevention, and public health. Surveillance activities include surveillance of infections, device use, and facility/ward outbreak detection and investigation. Prevention activities include awareness of multidrug-resistant organism carriage on admission, identification of high-risk individuals or populations, reducing device use, and antimicrobial stewardship. Enhanced communication with public health and other health care facilities across networks includes automated electronic communicable disease reporting, syndromic surveillance, and regional outbreak detection. Computerized public health networks may represent the next major evolution in infection control. This article reviews the use of informatics for infection control.

Shiwei Zhou, Jerod L. Nagel, Keith S. Kaye, Kerry L. LaPlante, Owen R. Albin, and Jason M. Pogue

Antibiotic overuse and misuse has contributed to rising rates of multidrug-resistant organisms and Clostridioides difficile. Decreasing antibiotic misuse has become a national public health priority. This review outlines the goals of antimicrobial stewardship, essential members of the program, implementation strategies, approaches to measuring the program's impact, and steps needed to build a program. Highlighted is the alliance between antimicrobial stewardship programs and infection prevention programs in their efforts to improve antibiotic use, improve diagnostic stewardship for C difficile and asymptomatic bacteriuria, and decrease health care–associated infections and the spread of multidrug-resistant organisms.

Paul Lephart, William LeBar, and Duane Newton

A great clinical microbiology laboratory supporting a great infection prevention program requires focusing on the following services: rapid and accurate identification of pathogens associated with health care–associated infections; asymptomatic surveillance for health care–acquired pathogens before infections arise; routine use of broad and flexible antimicrobial susceptibility testing to direct optimal therapy; implementation of epidemiologic tracking tools to identify outbreaks; development of clear result communication with interpretative comments for clinicians. These goals are best realized in a collaborative relationship with the infection prevention program so that both can benefit from the shared priorities of providing the best patient care.

Lisa Sturm, Michelle Flood, Ana Montoya, Lona Mody, and Marco Cassone

Patients increasingly receive care from a large spectrum of different settings, placing them at risk for exposure to pathogens by many different sources. Each health care environment has its own specific challenges, and thus infection control programs must be tailored to each specific setting. High-turnover outpatient settings may require additional considerations, such as establishing patient triage and follow-up protocols, and broadened cleaning and disinfection procedures. In nursing homes, infection control programs should focus on surveillance for infections and antimicrobial resistance, outbreak investigation and control plan for epidemics, isolation precautions, hand hygiene, staff education, and employee and resident health programs.

Gina Maki and Marcus Zervos

Health care–associated infections (HAIs) account for many morbidity and mortality worldwide, with disproportionate adverse effects in low- and middle-income countries (LMIC). Many factors contribute to the impact in LMIC, including lack of infrastructure, inconsistent surveillance, deficiency in trained personnel and infection control programs, and poverty-related factors. Therefore, optimal approaches must be tailored for LMIC and balance effectiveness and cost in the control of HAIs.

INFECTIOUS DISEASE CLINICS
OF NORTH AMERICA

Preface

Infection Prevention and Control in Health Care, Part 1: Facility Planning and Management

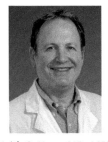 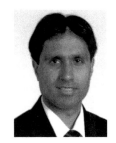

Keith S. Kaye, MD, MPH   Sorabh Dhar, MD
Editors

The field of Infection Prevention and Control has once again been thrust into the spotlight with the global COVID-19 pandemic. It has transcended from its original focus of occupational health and hospital infection control and is now implicit in the daily activities of every individual on this planet. What has become apparent is that the core Infection Prevention concepts used within hospitals are just as applicable in the community to prevent spread of infections within public spaces, as well as within a person's home. The effectiveness of these core principles and practices has been demonstrated, but there remains a need for additional high-quality data to understand the transmission of infections in various settings, clarify the optimal preventative practices, and identify barriers to their practical implementation.

While individual textbooks, articles, and other resources are available to address specific questions and issues pertaining to Infection Prevention and Control, this issue (as well as the subsequent one) of the *Infectious Diseases Clinics of North America* serves as an inclusive, relatively concise and focused primer on Infection Control. This issue focuses on facility planning and infrastructure necessary to support a comprehensive, effective infection prevention program. A multitude of topics are covered, including hand hygiene, environmental hygiene, sterilization and disinfection, water safety, occupational health, informatics, construction, outbreak investigation, the clinical microbiology laboratory, antimicrobial stewardship, and infection prevention in alternative and resource limited settings. It is intended to serve as a useful reference and primer for infection prevention and control, particularly with regards to facility planning and infrastructure.

We would like to thank the authors who have contributed valuable time and effort to this issue. We hope that you will enjoy it and find it to be a valuable resource for helping

Infect Dis Clin N Am 35 (2021) xiii–xiv
https://doi.org/10.1016/j.idc.2021.04.002
0891-5520/21/© 2021 Published by Elsevier Inc.

id.theclinics.com

to build and sustain a successful and impactful Infection Prevention and Control program.

Keith S. Kaye, MD, MPH
University of Michigan Medical School
5510A MSRB 1, SPC 5680
1150 West Medical Center Drive
Ann Arbor, MI 48109-5680, USA

Sorabh Dhar, MD
Harper University Hospital
5 Hudson
3990 John R Street
Detroit, MI 48201, USA

E-mail addresses:
keithka@med.umich.edu (K.S. Kaye)
sdhar@med.wayne.edu (S. Dhar)

Strategies for Effective Infection Prevention Programs: Structures, Processes, and Funding

Sorabh Dhar, MD[a,b,]*, Avnish L. Sandhu, DO[a],
Amanda Valyko, MPH, CIC, FAPIC[c], Keith S. Kaye, MD, MPH[d],
Laraine Washer, MD, FACP[e,f]

KEYWORDS

- Infection prevention • Infection control • Hospital epidemiology
- Hospital-acquired infections

KEY POINTS

- Infection Prevention and Epidemiology Programs are responsible for monitoring and preventing health care–associated infections (HAIs) in hospitals and ambulatory care settings.
- Infection Prevention Programs (IPPs) have been shaped by a complex landscape of pandemic, health care safety, regulatory, reporting, and payment requirements.
- The Infection Prevention Committee is a multidisciplinary team led by a hospital epidemiologist, managed by infection preventionists, and includes both clinical and nonclinical members who meet routinely to review data, develop and update policies, and meet local and national requirements.
- Knowledge of the structure of infection control programs, the ability to make a business case/economic model, and navigate an everchanging medico-social landscape are essential competencies of a successful program.

[a] Division of Infectious Diseases, Wayne State University, Harper University Hospital, 5 Hudson, 3990 John R, Detroit, MI 48201, USA; [b] Department of Hospital Epidemiology and Infection Prevention, John D. Dingell VA Medical Center, Detroit, MI, USA; [c] Department of Infection Prevention and Epidemiology, Michigan Medicine, 300 North Ingalls – NIB8B02, Ann Arbor, MI 48109-5479, USA; [d] Division of Infectious Diseases, University of Michigan, University of Michigan Medical School, 5510A MSRB 1, SPC 5680, 1150 West Medical Center Drive, Ann Arbor, MI 48109-5680, USA; [e] Department of Infection Prevention and Epidemiology, Michigan Medicine, F4151 University Hospital South, 1500 East Medical Center Drive, SPC 5226, Ann Arbor, MI 48109-5226, USA; [f] Division of Infectious Diseases, University of Michigan, Ann Arbor, MI, USA
* Corresponding author. Harper University Hospital, 5 Hudson, 3990 John R, Detroit, MI 48201.
E-mail address: sdhar@med.wayne.edu

Infect Dis Clin N Am 35 (2021) 531–551
https://doi.org/10.1016/j.idc.2021.04.001
0891-5520/21/© 2021 Elsevier Inc. All rights reserved.
id.theclinics.com

OVERVIEW

Infection control is defined as the discipline responsible for preventing health care–associated infections (HAIs). Over the past decades, "infection control" has grown from a largely anonymous field, to a highly visible, multidisciplinary field of incredible importance with regard to the safety of patients and health care workers, regulation and accreditation of health care facilities, and finances. There has been an increasing focus on prevention rather than control of HAIs. Individuals working in infection control have seen their titles change from "infection control practitioner" to "infection control professional" and most recently to "infection preventionist," emphasizing their critical role in protecting patients. The scope of Infection Prevention Programs (IPPs) spans multiple disciplines including medicine, surgery, nursing, occupational health, microbiology, pharmacy, sterilization and disinfection, emergency preparedness, and information technology. Infection prevention efforts were once focused mostly on inpatient acute care but have now expanded to outpatient clinics, ambulatory surgery centers, physician practices, and long-term care facilities.[1] Programs are shaped by the needs of the health care setting and risks of the population as well as increasing demands from external stakeholders to provide transparency to the consumer: the patient. These external stakeholders include government and regulatory agencies, professional organizations, industry, media, and payers of health care (**Fig. 1**).[2] The Coronavirus Disease 2019 (COVID-19) pandemic has highlighted the critical role of IPPs, as well as their strengths and limitations to meet this challenge, and will shape prevention activities for the foreseeable future.

This article discusses the structure and responsibilities of an IPP, the regulatory pressures and opportunities that these programs face, and how to build and manage a successful program.

EMERGENCE AND DEVELOPMENT OF REGULATION AND REQUIREMENTS OF INFECTION PREVENTION AND CONTROL

There were an estimated 687,000 HAIs in US acute-care hospitals in 2015, of which 72,000 died during their hospitalizations. On any given day, 1 in 31 hospital patients has at least 1 HAI.[3] Three percent of hospitalized patients in a 2015 multistate Centers for Disease Control and Prevention survey had 1 or more HAI.[4] The most common types of HAIs in this study were pneumonia (26.2%), gastrointestinal infection (25.7%), surgical site infection (SSI) (23.8%), bloodstream infection (14.9%), and urinary tract infection (9.5%). Total annual costs resulting from HAIs in the United States have been estimated at $9.8 billion in 2009.[5] Estimated average additional costs for specific HAIs per patients are $13,793 for catheter-associated urinary tract infections (CAUTI); $48,108 for central-line associated bloodstream infections (CLABSI); $28,219 for SSIs; $47,238 for ventilator-associated pneumonia; and $17,260 for *Clostridioides difficile* infections (CDIs).[6] Estimates of excess mortality (relative risk of death) for these HAIs are 1.5, 2.72, 3.32, 1.48, and 1.6, respectively.[6] Approximately 55% to 75% of HAIs are preventable, translating into potential savings of $5.5 billion along with improved patient outcomes. As a result, HAI prevention is a national priority resulting in a significant evolution of infection prevention and control programs.[7]

The prevention of HAIs gained public attention when several studies demonstrated that HAIs are avoidable. These studies have helped to shape current prevention initiatives. The Institute of Medicine's 1999 report "To Err is Human: Building a Safer Healthcare System" and the subsequent 2003 report "Transforming Healthcare Quality" focused on HAI prevention as a priority area for national action.[8] Subsequently, national organizations have advocated for or required HAI prevention and reduction

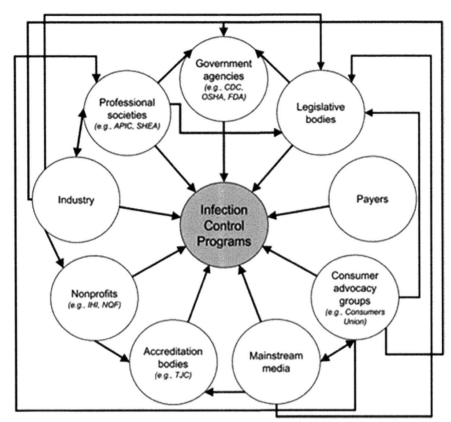

Fig. 1. The changing landscape of infection control. External entities that influence priorities of IPPs and other stakeholders are diagrammed. FDA, US Food and Drug Administration; NQF, National Quality Forum; OSHA, Occupational Safety and Health Administration. (*From* Edmond M, Eickhoff TC. Who is steering the ship? External influences on infection control programs. Clin Infect Dis. 2008 Jun 1;46(11):1746-50; *with permission.*)

initiatives, including the Institute for Healthcare Improvement (IHI) and the Agency for Healthcare Research and Quality (AHRQ).[9,10] In 2008 ,the US Department of Health and Human Services released its national action plan to prevent HAIs, which provided a road map for the reduction of CLABSIs, CAUTIs, SSIs, and CDI in various health care settings.[7] This national action plan was updated in April 2013 and provides a detailed account of the progress that has been made in HAI reduction and highlights further opportunities.[1] In 2018, an additional component to the plan focusing on antibiotic stewardship was added.[11] Such initiatives have successfully solicited hospital administration to participate in their campaigns and to invest resources to reduce HAIs.

Health care reform acts in the first decade of this century (such as the Deficit Reduction Act of 2005 and the Affordable Care Act of 2010) and categorization of HAIs as preventable, have led to a paradigm shift in the reporting and reimbursement related to these infections. In 2011, with an increasing need for transparency for both consumers and stakeholders, the Centers for Medicare and Medicaid Services (CMS) required reporting of hospital-specific HAI data by using the preexisting Centers for Disease Control and Prevention's (CDC's) National Healthcare Safety Network (NHSN) for hospitals to qualify for full reimbursement. As of federal fiscal year (FFY)

2021, data being reported from acute-care hospitals include CLABSIs and CAUTIs in adult and pediatric critical care units, medical units, surgical units, and medical/surgical units; SSI (following inpatient colon and abdominal hysterectomy surgery), LabID events (methicillin-resistant *Staphylococcus aureus* [MRSA] bacteremia and CDI) and health care worker influenza immunization.[12] These reporting requirements encompass inpatient and outpatient facilities, acute care and long-term acute care, as well as specialized centers (such as outpatient hemodialysis, cancer facilities, inpatient psychiatry, ambulatory surgery, and inpatient rehabilitation).[12,13] These data are used as metrics by CMS to determine hospital payments under Value-Based Purchasing (VBP) and Hospital-Acquired Condition (HAC) programs. Data used by CMS to determine hospital payments are publicly available to consumers.[14,15] In addition to federal requirements for mandatory reporting, individual states have initiated state-specific requirements, which in some cases exceed those of the federal government.

Similarly, accreditation organizations such as The Joint Commission (TJC) have been influential in guiding the course of infection prevention. TJC has issued various sentinel event alerts, standards, and patient safety goals that hospitals must meet to become accredited and eligible for Medicare reimbursement.[16] In 2004, these recommendations became a part of the National Patient Safety Goals,[17] which were further broadened by 2012 to include a focus on reducing the risks associated with multidrug-resistant organisms (MDROs), CLABSIs, SSIs, and CAUTIs.[18] These National Patient Safety Goals, regulations, and standards have helped guide the development, scope, policies, and willingness of hospital leadership to fund and support IPPs.[19]

As a result of these changes in reporting and reimbursement, there has been significant pressure to achieve "zero rates" of HAIs. From 2018 to 2019, the CDC's HAI Progress Report describes significant reductions in the rates of CLABSIs (7%), CAUTIs (8%), and hospital-onset *C difficile* infection (18%). There was no significant change in hospital-onset MRSA bacteremia or SSIs.[20] Although not all HAIs are preventable, the Association for Professionals in Infection Control and Epidemiology (APIC) and other experts agree that a primary goal of infection prevention should be the elimination of all preventable infections. The focus should be on "getting to zero" HAIs by optimizing processes pertaining to the prevention of HAIs. Increased use of invasive devices (central lines and indwelling urinary catheter) during the COVID-19 pandemic posed a significant challenge in reducing HAIs. Increased CAUTI and CLABSI rates were observed when comparing HAI rates 6 months before the COVID-19 pandemic and during the pandemic; in 1 center an 83% higher CAUTI rate and 65% higher CLABSI rate was observed during the COVID-19 pandemic.[21]

In the face of the COVID-19 pandemic, the importance of infection prevention has never been greater. The same principles apply to prevention of the spread of severe acute respiratory syndrome coronavirus 2 in the hospital as to HAIs. With the high transmission potential of the virus and a dearth of effective therapies, preventing spread of this deadly virus has reemphasized how important infection prevention is and how impactful it can be.[22]

INFECTION PREVENTION AND CONTROL PROGRAM
Mission, Vision, and Values

There are 3 foundational concepts to all programs: mission statement, vision, and core values. The mission statement reflects the primary goals of the organization or needs to be addressed by infection prevention. The vision statement describes future goals for the organizations. Last, a core value statement describes "how" the program functions on a daily basis and serves as the blueprint for the program. A typical mission statement may be: *"Our facility maintains an organized, effective hospital-wide program designed to systematically identify and reduce the risk of acquiring and transmitting infections among patients, visitors, and healthcare workers."* A program's vision or goal may be that no patient in the critical care unit will acquire a CLABSI. A core value might be the following: The IHI CLABSI bundle[9] will be implemented and compliance with all bundle elements will be monitored and reported to the appropriate stakeholders.

The reporting structure for the program must be transparent with sharing of key metrics with hospital leadership and to frontline staff. This ensures continued support and funding for ongoing prevention efforts and fosters teamwork to embed infection prevention practices in daily care.[23] Hospital organizational charts can clarify reporting and flow of information to stakeholders, and ensure that IPPs have input during key decisions impacting areas that relate to prevention of infections (such as construction, purchasing of new medical equipment, or changes in cleaning products) (**Fig. 2**).

Infection Prevention and Control Committee

The organization's governing body typically delegates authority and responsibility for the infection prevention program to the infection prevention and control committee (IPCC), often via a formal infection control hospital authority statement. The IPCC is the central decision and policymaking body whose primary purpose is to advocate for infection prevention and control[24] and has the authority to take immediate action in the event that patient, visitor, or health care worker safety is endangered because of infection risk. In most health care organizations, the IPCC is designated as a "medical staff" committee or a "quality" committee and has reporting obligations to both the hospital leadership and medical staff. The committee is chaired by the hospital epidemiologist or another physician who has knowledge and interest in infection prevention. Specific membership requirements and responsibilities are often delineated in the organization's bylaws.

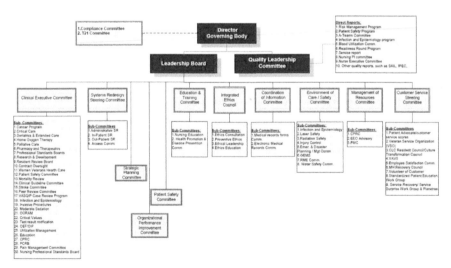

Fig. 2. Example of hospital organizational chart. In this example, the infection control committee is a subcommittee to the Clinical Executive Committee and of the Environment of Care/Safety committee. It also presents direct reports to the Quality Leadership Committee to ensure that key stakeholders are updated on infection prevention metrics and initiatives.

The IPCC is multidisciplinary, with representation from a variety of specialties and services. At a minimum, membership should include personnel from infection prevention, administration, nursing, medical staff, microbiology, occupational health, surgical services, central sterilization, environmental health/safety management services, and antimicrobial stewardship. Members should represent the continuum of care (ambulatory, acute-care hospital, homecare) and the populations (adult, pediatric, obstetrics, general care, intensive care) served by the organization. Other staff members are asked to provide input as needed. The IPCC should meet on a regular basis (ie, monthly) as determined by the complexity and needs of the facility with a predetermined time; meetings may occur in person or remotely depending on circumstances.

Core members of the IPCC include the administrative director of infection prevention or designated IP, the physician epidemiologist/chair, a data analyst, and administrative assistant. This core group ensures that surveillance data and activities are accurate and presented to the committee, reviews compliance with regulatory standards related to infection prevention, and oversees HAI prevention activities. Before the IPCC meeting, the core group develops agenda items and achieves consensus among team members on proposed recommendations. A meeting agenda is circulated to IPCC members before the meeting with action and/or approval items. It is imperative that complete and accurate minutes of the committee's discussion, actions and recommendations be recorded for each meeting and reported to all appropriate stakeholders, based on the organizational infrastructure. These minutes are necessary for "ownership" of projects and monitoring progress. All IPCC minutes should be marked as "peer review and/or confidential." **Box 1** summarizes the responsibilities of the IPCC members.

KEY MEMBERS OF THE INFECTION PREVENTION TEAM AND/OR PROGRAM

The key leaders of a successful IPP are the hospital epidemiologist (HE) and the administrative director. A strong partnership is imperative to a successful program.

Box 1
Primary responsibilities for infection prevention/control committee

1. Identify strategies designed to reduce or eliminate risk of acquiring a hospital-acquired and/or health care–associated infection

2. Review findings related to hospital-acquired and health care–associated infections

3. Review findings related to outbreak investigations

4. Review relevant infection prevention and control guidelines

5. Review findings related to monitoring of antibiotic resistant organisms (infection and/or colonization)

6. Make recommendations and take action based on findings from activities described previously

7. Address issues related to emerging and reemerging communicable diseases

8. Make recommendations for new procedures, policies, and/or activities as appropriate

9. Participate in the review and revision of the infection prevention/control risk assessment and program as warranted to improve outcomes

10. Approve all hospital-wide infection prevention/control policies

11. Review elements of the occupational health program that impact infection prevention policies or procedures

12. Approve an annual report of committee activities

Hospital Physician Epidemiologist or Medical Director of Infection Prevention

HEs are typically physicians, often specializing in infectious diseases, with expertise in the field of infection prevention and act as a watchman for the modern health system.[25–27] They provide clinical oversight for infection control in larger health care facilities. Some hospitals, such as smaller community hospitals, might not have a trained HE or infectious diseases physician, so other members of the medical staff (eg, the hospital pathologist) might serve this role. Medical staff leadership is essential to achieve infection prevention goals and objectives. **Box 2** summarizes the major responsibilities of the HE.

The physicians assuming the role of HE have preferably received training from senior epidemiologists in longstanding programs; however, frequently physicians might find themselves in this position without training, out of necessity. Contrary to infection preventionists (IPs), there is no formal certification process for the HE. The Society for Healthcare Epidemiology (SHEA) has published guidance to highlight the skills necessary for physicians who run effective IPPs. The roles of the HE are many and might include that of an epidemiologist, subject-matter expert, quality and performance improvement leader, regulatory/public health liaison, health care administrator, clinician educator, outcomes assessment evaluator, and researcher. The HE must be skilled at verbal and written communications to advance the goals of the IPP. These diverse areas highlight the multifaceted components and the increasing needs, demands, and complexities of IPPs, and represent the core competencies that are vital in this demanding field.[25]

Administrative Director

The administrative director is an experienced IP leader who has attained certification in infection prevention and control (CIC) and is responsible for oversight of the IPP,

---

Box 2
Primary responsibilities of the hospital physician epidemiologist or medical director of infection prevention

- Provide medical and technical advice and support within the department, as well as within the health care facility

- In collaboration with the administrative director, establish long-term and short-term goals for the department

- Provide clinical expertise in regard to health care–associated infections, emerging communicable diseases, postexposure management, isolation precaution(s), as well as construction and environmental issues/concerns

- Oversee development of programs designed to prevent and/or reduce the transmission of epidemiologically important microorganisms within the facility (ie, antibiotic resistant organisms) and/or other projects with which the department may be involved

- Participate in and oversee analysis of surveillance findings and development of interventional strategies

- Assist with preparation of data and policy revisions for presentation to the infection prevention and control committee (IPCC)

- Serve as the liaison between the infection prevention department, other members of the medical staff, and often with external agencies (state health departments, free press)

- Represent infection prevention in quality meetings and efforts

- Communicate infection control/prevention data to the IPCC, members of the medical staff, quality of care team(s), and other internal committees/teams as appropriate

including direct supervision of team members. Administrative directors possess the skillset of proficient to expert IP according to APIC's competency model.[28] **Box 3** lists the primary responsibilities of administrative directors.

Infection Preventionist

IPs carry out the daily activities of an IPP. Responsibilities include rounding, education, quality improvement with respect to HAIs, surveillance, exposure investigations, and policy revision. Based on the size and complexity of the facility, this individual may perform additional key functions, such as occupational health and nursing education. IPs predominately have backgrounds in nursing, medical technology, microbiology, and/or public health.[29] Certification in infection prevention demonstrates competency and most programs require that an IP obtain certification within 2 years of beginning infection prevention practice. Clinical experience, managerial experience, and good communication skills are also prerequisites. Daily responsibilities are multifaceted and require strong organizational skills. **Box 4** lists some of the major responsibilities of IPs in the hospital. IPs must also have the ability to lead and manage a multitude of diverse health care workers. Being familiar with different leadership and management styles and applying them to specific situations is essential to implementing change. The APIC competency[30,31] model is a comprehensive tool for defining the scope and expectations for different levels of IPs and provides growth tiers for the team members.

Data Programmer and Analyst

Data programmers and analysts are essential for the development and maintenance of databases used in infection prevention. These individuals collaborate with the infection prevention department regarding database structure, organization of data related to infection prevention activities, and preparing visual presentation of that data (eg, graphs, tables). These persons should be able to manipulate existing databases or the electronic medical records to retrieve baseline data that are necessary to define a problem, set baseline benchmarks, and collect outcomes data. They are critical in

---

Box 3
Primary responsibilities of administrative directors

- Responsible for the oversight of departmental operations, coordination and supervision of team members
- Coordinates the work of the infection prevention team across the health system
- In conjunction with hospital epidemiologist, develops and implements short and long-range goals and objectives designed to assess and review the prevention and control of health care–associated infections
- Oversees the creation, implementation and timely revision of all related policies
- Ensures compliance with applicable institution, state and federal regulations and policies related to infection prevention
- In conjunction with hospital epidemiologist, develops and oversee the Annual Risk Assessment and Surveillance Plan
- Ensure readiness/preparedness for novel pathogens
- Along with hospital epidemiologist, represent infection prevention at institutional committees

---

Box 4
Primary responsibilities of the infection preventionists

- Application of epidemiologic principles in the performance of surveillance activities, including data collection and analysis as directed by the infection prevention/control plan and risk assessment

- Assist with product evaluation

- Develop and present educational programs designed for employee and patient education

- Consult with internal and external customers on issues related to infection prevention

- Review hospital and department specific IP policies and procedures

- Conduct outbreak investigations

- Conduct infection control risk assessment for all construction activities

- Report IP surveillance findings to the IPCC, hospital leadership, specific hospital departments and committees, public health department (local and state and referring/receiving health care facilities as appropriate)

- Assist other departments by serving as a resource for continuous compliance with federal/state (eg, Occupational Safety and Health Administration) and accreditation (eg, The Joint Commission) standards as they pertain to infection prevention and control activities

---

distributing hospital data to the appropriate committees or hospital leaders and ensuring a rapid and consistent submission of data to national databases (such as NHSN).

Administrative Assistant

Effective administrative assistants possess the essential qualities needed to enhance the effectiveness and productivity of IPPs. They are highly skilled in organizing and scheduling appointments and/or meetings for the HE, administrative director, IPs, and other team members. These individuals serve as the "gatekeeper" and organizer for the infection prevention department to assist in eliminating unnecessary interruptions and unscheduled appointments.

Environmental Health Specialist

An embedded environmental health specialist (EHS) or access to one, can ensure a focus on critical work related to the environment of care such as execution of a water management plan and subject-matter expertise with air handling. The EHS can also provide consultations for potential environmental factors contributing to an outbreak.

STRATEGIES FOR A SUCCESSFUL INFECTION PREVENTION PROGRAM
Meeting Management

Meetings consume an enormous amount of human resources, and when executed suboptimally, do not achieve desired goals. The IPCC is only one of many multidisciplinary groups whose activities involve infection prevention. IPs can facilitate efficient, effective meetings by using key strategies. **Box 5** list various strategies for conducting effective and efficient meetings.

Infection Prevention Staffing

Staffing for infection prevention is an ongoing challenge for most programs. However, there is a lack of strong recommendations from recognized experts in the field, such

---

Box 5
Strategies for conducting effective, efficient meetings

1. Be prepared
   All items included on the agenda should be reviewed in advance. Surveillance data should be evaluated for accuracy and completeness and presented in a visual, easy-to-understand format. Items requiring approval should be distributed in advance.

2. Have an agenda
   The agenda should be distributed before the meeting. Most institutions distribute the agenda no less than 1 week before the meeting to give members an opportunity to review and be prepared to discuss issues.

3. Start and end on time
   This simple concept demonstrates respect for members' time and work schedule. When meetings do not begin and end on time members become disengaged and often times will stop attending.

4. Meet only when necessary
   Base your frequency of meetings on your facility's activities and needs. Meeting schedules vary from monthly to quarterly. Selecting the appropriate frequency will also help with number 2 (starting and ending on time). Some individual states have included a specific requirement for the frequency of IPCC meetings. Be sure that you are aware of what your state requirements are and that your schedule is in compliance.

5. Include all issues and solicit input relevant to all committee members
   Members want to be part of the team and when they do not feel included, they will be less likely to offer new ideas and input.

6. Stay on target
   Stick to the agenda items as outlined. Some facilities actually time the agenda with an estimated allotment for each discussion or activity. Issues that cannot be resolved or generate more discussion than anticipated can be tabled or deferred until the next meeting.

7. Capture action items
   The Joint Commission will expect to see closure to action items. The minutes should reflect approval, rejection, or deferral of action items and the supporting rationale.

8. Get feedback
   An effective way of improving the flow and productivity of meeting is to request feedback from the members. It is generally more successful if this is included as an agenda item and feedback is solicited immediately after the meeting. Feedback also can be obtained through written or verbal communication after the meeting.

9. A secret "ninth" key
   Having the meeting at mealtime will typically improve attendance, and providing food is an inexpensive way to demonstrate appreciation for the committee members' time.

---

as the CDC. In the early 1970s, the CDC's SENIC project (Study on the Efficacy of Nosocomial Infection Control) recommended that hospitals have at least 1 full-time equivalent (FTE) infection control professional for every 250 occupied beds.[32] Later in the 1990s, participation in the National Nosocomial Infections Surveillance System required 1 infection control professional FTE for the first 100 beds and then 1 FTE for each additional 250 beds.[33] In 2002, APIC initiated the DELPHI project on staffing, which considered not only the number of occupied beds but also the scope of the program, complexity of the health care organization, patient characteristics, and the unique needs of the facility, and recommended a ratio of 0.8 to 1.0 IPs per 100 occupied beds.[34] A recent study aimed to identify a systematic approach that would quantify IP work, not just in the inpatient setting, but also incorporating the complexity of ambulatory care, home care, and long-term care.[35] This study identified a staffing model of 1 IP per 69 beds when ambulatory, home, or long-term care were included in the IP duties.

Despite various recommendations and need for increased IP staffing, many organizations have understaffed programs. As the scope and complexity of IPPs have increased, the traditional ratios used to estimate IP staffing needs do not provide adequate estimates of necessary resources. Alternative staffing ratios have been proposed. For example, one proposal counts an intensive care unit bed as the equivalent of 2 acute-care beds (ACBs), and a long-term care bed as one-half an ACB; and counts a hemodialysis facility as the equivalent of 50 ACBs, and an ambulatory clinic the equivalent of 10 ACBs.[36] These adjusted calculations may more accurately capture workload and should be factored into business models when developing or expanding programs. Although not substitutes for trained IPs, adjuncts such as electronic surveillance systems, unit-based nurse liaisons, and nurse advisors can help to facilitate the work of IPs and should also be factored into staffing calculations and needs. Unfortunately, the increased demands on IPs has not led to a proportional increase in infection control staffing, with reports indicating that only 18% of programs have received increased support following the implementation of the CMS Inpatient Prospective Payment System.[37]

Budget

Budget preparation is an essential component of any efficient program. IPs may have total responsibility for budget preparation or may be responsible for providing input. Chief executive officers will often use budget variances as the financial metric for the IPP. Basic components of any budget include labor, capital, and miscellaneous expenses. Elements of each are described in **Box 6**. The cost of HAIs has become an integral component of financial planning for organizations. Decreased reimbursement and nonpayment for certain conditions have forced hospital administration to confront the financial impact of HAIs.

Box 6
Budget: major components

Labor expenses:
　Includes staffing expenses for IPs, clerical support, data entry/analyst support, hospital epidemiologist or IPCC physician chair support. Consideration also should be given to the labor expenses required in the event that an outbreak investigation would be necessary as well as supporting internship programs to introduce students to the field of infection preventions and mentoring them.

Capital expenses:
　Most organizations have a minimum cost that items must incur before qualifying as a capital expense. These are "big ticket" items and requests requiring capital expenses should be well thought out and have supportive rationale.

Other Expenses:
　All other expenses fall into this category and typically include education, travel, journals, professional memberships, rewards and recognition, and so on. Travel and participation in professional organizations are often critical for recruitment and retention. Additional considerations should be given to budgeting for surveillance cultures as part of an outbreak investigation or routine surveillance that might be done as part of a water management program.

Surveillance

Infection surveillance data are used to establish baseline rates for comparison, to measure the success of interventions, to identify opportunities for improvement, and to meet public reporting mandates. Surveillance is therefore a core component of all successful IPPs.[38] The 2015 APIC MegaSurvey reported that surveillance and investigation accounted for 25.4% of infection prevention efforts.[39] **Table 1** lists the percentage of time spent on each work task as reported by IPs.

The type of surveillance activities conducted will be influenced by the following:

- Organizational demographics
  - Critical access center versus community hospital versus academic medical center
  - Ambulatory care versus acute-care hospital versus post-acute care
  - Adult versus pediatric
  - Independent facility versus part of health system
- Community demographics (urban or rural)
- Types of procedures and services provided
- Annual infection prevention risk assessment
- Annual infection prevention plan and goals

There are various types of surveillance methodologies. Concurrent surveillance conducted while the patient is still in the hospital is preferred to retrospective surveillance. Retrospective surveillance should be used only when patients are discharged before all pertinent data can be obtained.[40] Hospital-wide or whole house surveillance provides data on all organisms and infections throughout the facility and is now typically conducted for many device-related infections and CDI. Rates should be reported separately for specific HAIs and stratified by service and/or department. In contrast to hospital-wide surveillance, targeted surveillance is conducted only in a particular type of unit or area where high-risk and/or high-volume activities occur with regard to HAI. For example, rather than identifying every infection in the hospital, targeted surveillance to detect device-related infections only in critical care areas or burn units and/or hematology wards may be performed. In most facilities, SSI surveillance is not performed for all surgical procedures but is targeted to high-risk or volume services and for those procedures in which data are required by regulatory agencies and in which national benchmarks are available.[41] A combination strategy incorporating

Table 1		
Self-reported time spent on typical activity by infection preventionists		
	%	**Standard Deviation**
Surveillance/investigation	25.4	15.9
Prevention/control transmission	15.6	8.7
Identification of infection	14.2	10.6
Management/communication	12.2	10.9
Education/research	10.3	8.4
Environment	9.5	6.5
Cleaning/sterilization	8.7	7.2
Employee/occupational health	8	10.3

From Landers T, Davis J, Crist K, Malik C. APIC MegaSurvey: Methodology and overview. *Am J Infect Control.* 2017;45(6):584–588; *with permission.*

both targeted and modified hospital-wide surveillance is used by many programs to monitor targeted events in defined populations while also monitoring selected events housewide.[42]

CDC and TJC recommend infection surveillance be focused on high-risk, high-volume activities. Surveillance priorities should include the following: device-associated infections (CLABSIs, CAUTIs, and ventilator-associated events [VAEs]), infections associated with procedures (SSIs), and infections related to epidemiologically important microorganisms (MDROs).

Standardized definitions such as NHSN HAI surveillance definitions must be applied consistently to ensure reproducibility and allow accurate comparisons between different facilities.[43] Surveillance involves review of many data sources such as laboratory, radiology, and pathology reports; admissions/discharge records; pharmacy databases; patient charts; and vital signs records. Often, effective surveillance requires the application of clinical criteria to laboratory-based surveillance data. Automated surveillance technologies allow for a paperless method of analyzing, documenting, categorizing, and uploading HAI data into national databases.

HAI data are usually presented as rates; however, NHSN has shifted to Standardized Infection Ratios (SIRs) for reporting HAIs. The SIR compares the actual number of HAIs with the predicted number based on the baseline US experience.[44] When calculating infection rates, it is important to select the most appropriate and accurate denominator. Whenever possible, the denominator should reflect the "exposure risk," that is, number of surgical procedures, number of device days, or number of patient days on a given unit or in the hospital.

Examples of numerators, denominators, and rate calculation are shown as follows:

- Device-Associated Infections: rate of infections per 1000 device days
  (number of device-associated infections/number of device days) $\times$ 1000
- Surgical Site Infections: rate of SSIs per 100 procedures
  (number of SSIs/number of surgical procedures) $\times$ 100
- Multidrug-Resistant Organism Infections: rate of infection per 1000 patient days
  (number of infections/number of patient days) $\times$ 1000
- SIR = Observed HAIs/Expected HAIs

Other surveillance methodologies include the use of "active surveillance" (AS) for certain populations and/or pathogens.[45] AS proactively identifies asymptomatically colonized patients. Specimens for culture or molecular testing are obtained from the body sites that serve as common reservoirs for a specific organism, that is, nares for MRSA or perirectal area for vancomycin-resistant enterococci or carbapenem-resistant Enterobacteriaceae. Samples are generally obtained on high-risk patients at the time of admission to the facility or before surgery. AS may be repeated on a routine basis (typically weekly) during hospitalization, until a positive result is recovered, or the patient is discharged. AS may provide opportunity for interventions such as enacting contact isolation. AS data should be trended and reported to the IPCC and to hospital departments or units and be used to inform prevention efforts.

It is recommended that IPPs participate in external validation programs if available within their states and intermittently perform internal validation for agreement among IPs within the same program. Validation should be conducted for both numerators and denominators.[46] Much can be learned with validation exercises. Validation efforts in 23 states found that hospitals had a pooled error rate of 4.4% in CLABSI reporting (82.9% sensitivity, 98.5% specificity, positive predictive value 94.1%, negative predictive value 95.0%).[47] Reviews by 1 state health department found that CLABSIs were underreported by up to 50%[48] and SSIs after colectomy were underreported by

34%.[49] CAUTI underreporting to NHSN has also been a concern.[50] Reasons for misclassification were due to misinterpretation of the NHSN definitions, applying clinical over surveillance definitions and variations in case-finding methods.

IPs should consult with the HE if clinical judgment is needed to appropriately interpret patient data. However, IPs must strictly apply surveillance definitions even if they conflict with the clinical diagnosis. Given the increased focus on HAIs and their financial implications, IPs should work routinely with HEs to identify areas for process improvement to reduce risk for HAIs such as CLABSIs, CAUTIs, and SSIs.

Automated surveillance technologies have become an essential part of the infection prevention and control activities.[51] Automated surveillance can be defined as the process of obtaining useful information for infection prevention surveillance from hospital databases through the systematic application of medical informatics and computer science technologies.[51] These automated technologies can be developed by hospital data programmers or purchased through third-party vendors, including the makers of electronic medical records. Automated surveillance can increase ability of IP programs to conduct broader surveillance programs, to rapidly identify HAIs and trends in infections and importantly, facilitate surveillance efforts for IPs. Automated surveillance can decrease IP effort spent on surveillance by up to 61%, which allows IPs to reallocate their efforts and spend less time entering and mining data and more time rounding, educating, analyzing, and implementing programs.[52] Rapid evolution of information technology has promise to continue to improve efficiency, standardization and reliability of surveillance data.[53] However, technologies are not yet sufficient to be fully automated for most surveillance indications.[54]

Outbreak Investigation

Outbreaks of both infectious and noninfectious adverse events can occur in any health care setting and pose a threat to patient safety. An outbreak is defined as an increased occurrence of a disease and/or infection above the usual or expected frequency. In some cases, even a single case may constitute an outbreak (eg, smallpox). Outbreaks are usually identified when there is an increase in rates or numbers of infections from the "endemic" infection rate, which is defined as the usual or expected occurrence of a disease and/or infection. An endemic infection rate represents a baseline or background rate, which may fluctuate slightly from month to month.[55]

The ultimate goal of any outbreak investigation is to identify factors contributing to the outbreak and to stop or reduce the risk for further occurrences.[55] One of the key components for investigating an outbreak is developing a case definition, which details specific criteria for identifying a case. Initially this may be a broad definition that is refined as the investigation proceeds and a specific agent or diagnosis is confirmed. This topic is covered in greater detail in the article "Outbreaks in Health Care Settings," elsewhere in this issue.

Quality Improvement: Role of the Infection Preventionist

Measuring quality of care and reporting the findings is not a new concept. Florence Nightingale collected mortality data and related it to the lack of sanitary conditions.[56] In the early twentieth century, Dr Ernest Codman proposed to his surgeon colleagues that they measure their SSI rates and disclose them to the public.[57] Performance improvement encompasses all of the systems, projects, and team activities an organization implements to achieve its goals. These goals include the prevention of HAIs for patients, visitors, and staff.[30]

Using a multidisciplinary team approach, systems should be designed to monitor processes as well as outcomes. Direct patient care staff should be included as partners and team members and be provided with training regarding quality concepts and team-building skills. IPPs should design systems and processes to ensure timely feedback of infection prevention data to all disciplines as appropriate. Feedback should include outcome measures, infection rates, and process measures, such as compliance with hand hygiene or compliance with the central-line insertion bundle. Surveillance activities and feedback of data provide value only when findings are used as a mechanism to raise awareness among health care workers and to improve the quality of care that is provided to patients.

Pandemic Preparedness

IPPs play critical roles in preparing and leading health systems through epidemics, pandemics, and other novel infectious hazards. Programs have recently gained experience during the previous 2009 H1N1 influenza pandemic and Ebola preparedness efforts. This role has again been placed front and center in the COVID-19 pandemic. Successful IPPs must be well-integrated into health systems emergency management operations and be versed in the incident response framework. IPPs must maintain clear and open relationships with local and regional public health departments. Relationships with key partners, such as hospital leadership, communications experts, supply chain experts, clinical leadership, information technologists, and others developed during pandemic planning pay dividends during crisis. IPPs should develop and practice skills in crisis and emergency risk communication.[58–60]

ECONOMICS AND BUSINESS PLAN

Society clearly benefits from a reduced incidence of HAIs and transmission of MDROs within health care institutions. Unfortunately, there are currently no direct reimbursement programs related to hospital-based infection prevention and control. Hospitals are required by regulatory bodies to have an IPP, but the funding is often based on their administrators' subjective discretions. Therefore, for IPPs to achieve desirable goals, one critical role of HEs and the administrative IP director is to convince administrators of the beneficial impact of investing in infection control activities, and demonstrate that these activities will ultimately lead to improved patient care and reduced hospital costs.[61] IPPs have been demonstrated to be cost-effective.[62] In 1 report, IPPs were demonstrated to be more cost-effective than many other commonly applied health care practices, such as Pap-smear screening to prevent cervical cancer, mammography screening to prevent breast cancer, and cholesterol screening programs in high-risk populations.[63] Because IPPs are typically categorized as cost centers and not as revenue generators, they are often identified as potential areas for budget cuts.[64] In fact, many IPPs have faced downsizing in recent years.[61,65,66] This downsizing has occurred during a period in which the roles and responsibilities of IPPs have continuously and rapidly increased.

To obtain adequate funding from hospital leadership, IPPs need to construct a business case and to demonstrate the cost-effectiveness of an intervention. Guidelines published by SHEA provide guidance regarding constructing a business case for infection control that can assist hospital epidemiologists in justifying and expanding their programs.[61] These guidelines also provide references and tools to assist IPPs in developing a business plan to support a specific intervention.[61] In addition, there are multiple published economic analyses that can be used to support business cases for infection control interventions and practices.[61–64,67–79] Using data such as published costs of HAIs and MDROs are key ingredients to justifying interventions. Although published costs and cost-effectiveness analyses have limitations regarding applicability and generalizability, HEs and IPs can still use these analyses to make persuasive cases for hospital support. The hospital VBP and HAC programs have tied HAIs directly to CMS reimbursement. Thus, VBP and HACs should be used as components of business plans for IPPs.

Preparation of a successful business plan takes planning and when possible input from financial professionals. It is important to make an honest assessment of the infection control situation at your institution. Most HEs and IPs want to increase the resources available for infection control activities, but it is important to avoid overestimating potential benefits and the rapidity with which benefits might be achieved or underestimating staff costs and efforts required for success.[61] Overestimation of efficacy in an initial analysis may provide resources in the short term, but will undermine efforts and necessary trust for success in the long term.[61] The SHEA guidelines outline a 9-step approach for completing a business case analysis, so that all crucial components can be assessed and included.[61] Some key components include identifying the right audience and stakeholders to support and approve a business proposal and meeting with key leaders and administrators early in the process of developing a business plan to get feedback and input to effectively frame the business case before a formal presentation.

In the era of limited resources, IPPs and infection prevention initiatives are subject to continuous threats of budget reductions. HEs should be familiar with the basics involved with preparing a business case and try to establish relationships with financial experts and administrators who can provide advice and assist in business case preparation. Although most infection control professionals do not have formal economic or business training, fiscal analysis and responsibility has become a critical part of hospital epidemiology. The role of effective business plans and cost justifications will continue to grow in importance for IPPs. Despite limitations, the medical literature provides economic data that can assist the HEs and IPs in constructing a business plan for establishing and maintaining an infection control program.

SUMMARY

In summary, this is an exciting but challenging time for infection prevention and control. The past 2 decades have witnessed changes in the way that HAIs are viewed: from passive acceptance to the stout view of preventability, leading to policy changes, transparency, and increased collaboration among various agencies at federal and state levels.[80,81] IPPs remain in the crossfire of regulatory bodies, and payers such as TJC and CMS, manifested by increasing regulatory requirements and hospital efforts to meet the elusive goals of "Zero Infections." The recent COVID-19 pandemic has thrust infection prevention even further into the spotlight and has created unpredictable and changing challenges and opportunities. As such, these programs have a unique opportunity to impact and reshape the way that health care is delivered, and to create a safer environment for patients and health care workers.

CLINICS CARE POINTS

- IPPs have seen much evolution in terms of scope of activities and complexity since their inception in the 1970s.
- Successful programs consist of a multidisciplinary team led by an HE and managed by IPs.
- Staffing of IPPs remains a challenge; however, several models may assist in defining need.
- Knowledge of the economics of HAIs and the ability to make a business plan is now essential to the success of programs.

- Prevention of HAIs is the core function of IPPs with impact on patient outcomes, quality of care, and cost savings for hospitals.

DISCLOSURE

The authors have nothing to disclose.

REFERENCES

1. National action plan to prevent health-care associated infections: road map to elimination April 2013. Available at: http://health.gov/hcq/prevent-hai-action-plan.asp. Accessed January 11, 2021.
2. Edmond M, Eickhoff TC. Who is steering the ship? External influences on infection control programs. Clin Infect Dis 2008;46(11):1746–50.
3. Center for Disease Control and Prevention. Healthcare associated infections - data portal. 2020. Available at: https://www.cdc.gov/hai/data/portal/index.html. Accessed March 18, 2021.
4. Magill SS, O'Leary E, Janelle SJ, et al. Changes in prevalence of health care-associated infections in U.S. hospitals. N Engl J Med 2018;379(18):1732–44.
5. Zimlichman E, Henderson D, Tamir O, et al. Health care-associated infections: a meta-analysis of costs and financial impact on the US health care system. JAMA Intern Med 2013;173(22):2039–46.
6. Agency for Healthcare Research and Quality (AHRQ). Estimating the additional hospital inpatient cost and mortality associated with selected hospital acquired conditions. 2017. Available at: https://www.ahrq.gov/hai/pfp/haccost2017.html. Accessed January 14, 2021.
7. Yokoe DS, Anderson DJ, Berenholtz SM, et al. A compendium of strategies to prevent healthcare-associated infections in acute care hospitals: 2014 updates. Infect Control Hosp Epidemiol 2014;35(8):967–77.
8. Yokoe DS, Mermel LA, Anderson DJ, et al. A compendium of strategies to prevent healthcare-associated infections in acute care hospitals. Infect Control Hosp Epidemiol 2008;29(Suppl 1):S12–21.
9. Institute for Healthcare Improvement (IHI). Healthcare-associated infections. Available at: http://www.ihi.org/Topics/HAI/Pages/default.aspx. Accessed January 12,2021.
10. Agency for Healthcare Research and Quality. AHRQ's healthcare-associated infections program. Available at: https://www.ahrq.gov/hai/index.html. Accessed January 12, 2021.
11. U.S. Department of Health and Human Services (HHS). National action plan to prevent health care-associated infections: road map to elimination. Phase four: coordination among federal partners to leverage HAI prevention and antibiotic stewardship. 2018. Available at: https://health.gov/sites/default/files/2019-09/National_Action_Plan_to_Prevent_HAIs_Phase_IV_2018.pdf. Accessed March 18, 2021.
12. Centers for Disease Control (CDC). Healthcare facility HAI reporting requirements to CMS via NHSN– current or proposed requirements. 2019. Available at: https://www.cdc.gov/nhsn/pdfs/cms/cms-reporting-requirements.pdf. Accessed January 12, 2021.

13. Healthcare facility HAI reporting requirements to CMS via NHSN– current or proposed requirements. Available at: http://www.cdc.gov/nhsn/pdfs/cms/cms-reporting-requirements.pdf. Accessed April 9, 2021.

14. Centers for Medicare and Medicaid Services. Medicare.gov: Hospital Compare. Available at: http://www.medicare.gov/hospitalcompare/search.html. Accessed April 9, 2021.

15. Medicare.gov. Find & compare nursing homes, hospitals & other providers near you. Available at: https://www.medicare.gov/care-compare/. Accessed January 12, 2021.

16. Sydnor ER, Perl TM. Hospital epidemiology and infection control in acute-care settings. Clin Microbiol Rev 2011;24(1):141–73.

17. 2004 National patient safety goals. 2004. Available at: http://www.jointcommission.org/PatientSafety/NationalPatientSafetyGoals/2004_npsgs.htm. Accessed May 31, 2006.

18. Hospital accreditation program: 2009 national patient safety goals. In: Reduce the risk of healthcare associated infections: the Joint Commission. 2009. p. 11–7.

19. The Joint Commission. Hospital: 2021 national patient safety goals. 2021. Available at: https://www.jointcommission.org/standards/national-patient-safety-goals/hospital-national-patient-safety-goals/. Accessed January 12, 2021.

20. Centers for Disease Control (CDC). 2019 National and State Healthcare-Associated Infections Progress Report. Available at: https://www.cdc.gov/hai/pdfs/progress-report/2019-Progress-Report-Executive-Summary-H.pdf. Accessed March 19, 2021.

21. Knepper BC, Wallace K, Young H. 95. CAUTI and CLABSI in hospitalized COVID-19 patients. Open Forum Infect Dis 2020;7(Supplement_1):S178.

22. Campbell K. The art of infection prevention. Nature 2020;586:s53–4.

23. Hale R, Powell T, Drey NS, et al. Working practices and success of infection prevention and control teams: a scoping study. J Hosp Infect 2015;89(2):77–81.

24. Holmes K, McCarty J, Steinfeld S. Infection prevention and control programs. 2021. Available at: https://text.apic.org/toc/overview-of-infection-prevention-programs/infection-prevention-and-control-programs. Accessed March 19, 2021.

25. Kaye KS, Anderson DJ, Cook E, et al. Guidance for infection prevention and healthcare epidemiology programs: healthcare epidemiologist skills and competencies. Infect Control Hosp Epidemiol 2015;36(4):369–80.

26. Doll M, Hewlett AL, Bearman G. Infection prevention in the hospital from past to present: evolving roles and shifting priorities. Curr Infect Dis Rep 2016;18(5):16.

27. Morgan DJ, Deloney VM, Bartlett A, et al. The expanding role of the hospital epidemiologist in 2014: a survey of the Society for Hospital Epidemiology of America (SHEA) Research Network. Infect Control Hosp Epidemiol 2015;36(5):605–8.

28. Association for Professionals in Infection Control and Epidemiology (APIC). CIC Certification. Available at: https://apic.org/education-and-events/certification/. Accessed January 15, 2021.

29. Friedman C. Infection prevention and control programs. APIC text of infection control and epidemiology. 2014. Available at: https://text.apic.org/toc/overview-of-infection-prevention-programs/infection-prevention-and-control-programs. Accessed January 30, 2021.

30. Murphy DM, Hanchett M, Olmsted RN, et al. Competency in infection prevention: a conceptual approach to guide current and future practice. Am J Infect Control 2012;40(4):296–303.

31. Billings C, Bernard H, Caffery L, et al. Advancing the profession: an updated future-oriented competency model for professional development in infection prevention and control. Am J Infect Control 2019;47(6):602–14.

32. Haley RW, Quade D, Freeman HE, et al. The SENIC Project. Study on the efficacy of nosocomial infection control (SENIC Project). Summary of study design. Am J Epidemiol 1980;111(5):472–85.

33. Stone PW, Dick A, Pogorzelska M, et al. Staffing and structure of infection prevention and control programs. Am J Infect Control 2009;37(5):351–7.

34. Friedman C. Infection prevention and control programs. In: Carrico R, editor. APIC text of infection control and epidemiology, Vol 1, 3rd ed. Washington, DC: APIC; 2009.

35. Bartles R, Dickson A, Babade O. A systematic approach to quantifying infection prevention staffing and coverage needs. Am J Infect Control 2018;46(5):487–91.

36. Gase KA, Babcock HM. Is accounting for acute care beds enough? A proposal for measuring infection prevention personnel resources. Am J Infect Control 2015;43(2):165–6.

37. Septimus E, Yokoe DS, Weinstein RA, et al. Maintaining the momentum of change: the role of the 2014 updates to the compendium in preventing healthcare-associated infections. Infect Control Hosp Epidemiol 2014;35(Suppl 2):S6–9.

38. Storr J, Twyman A, Zingg W, et al. Core components for effective infection prevention and control programmes: new WHO evidence-based recommendations. Antimicrob Resist Infect Control 2017;6:6.

39. Landers T, Davis J, Crist K, et al. APIC MegaSurvey: methodology and overview. Am J Infect Control 2017;45(6):584–8.

40. Center for Disease Control and Prevention (2021). National Health and Safety Network (NHSN) Patient Safety Manual. Available at: https://www.cdc.gov/nhsn/pdfs/pscmanual/pcsmanual_current.pdf. Available at: January 11, 2021.

41. Anderson DJ, Perl TM. Basics of surgical site infection: surveillance and prevention. In: Lautenbach E, Shuman EK, Han JH, et al, editors. Practical healthcare epidemiology. 4 ed. Cambridge: Cambridge University Press; 2018. p. 147–61.

42. Arias KM. Surveillance. APIC text of infection control and epidemiology. 2014. Available at: https://text.apic.org/toc/epidemiology-surveillance-performance-and-patient-safety-measures/surveillance. Accessed January 30,2021.

43. Center for Disease Control and Prevention. National Health and Safety Network (NHSN) patient safety manual. 2021. Available at: https://www.cdc.gov/nhsn/pdfs/pscmanual/pcsmanual_current.pdf. Accessed January 11, 2021.

44. Centers for Disease Control and Prevention. National Health and Safety Network (NHSN) SIR. 2021. Available at: https://www.cdc.gov/nhsn/pdfs/ps-analysis-resources/nhsn-sir-guide.pdf. Accessed January 11, 2021.

45. Calfee DP, Salgado CD, Milstone AM, et al. Strategies to prevent methicillin-resistant *Staphylococcus aureus* transmission and infection in acute care hospitals: 2014 update. Infect Control Hosp Epidemiol 2014;35(7):772–96.

46. Centers for Disease Control and Prevention. National Health and Safety Network (NHSN) Data Validation. 2021. Available at: https://www.cdc.gov/nhsn/validation/index.html. Accessed January 11, 2021.

47. Bagchi S, Watkins J, Pollock DA, et al. State health department validations of central line-associated bloodstream infection events reported via the National Healthcare Safety Network. Am J Infect Control 2018;46(11):1290–5.

48. Backman LA, Melchreit R, Rodriguez R. Validation of the surveillance and reporting of central line-associated bloodstream infection data to a state health department. Am J Infect Control 2010;38(10):832–8.

49. Backman LA, Carusillo E, D'Aquila LN, et al. Validation of surgical site infection surveillance data in colon procedures reported to the Connecticut Department of Public Health. Am J Infect Control 2017;45(6):690–1.

50. Bagchi S, Watkins J, Norrick B, et al. Accuracy of catheter-associated urinary tract infections reported to the National Healthcare Safety Network, January 2010 through July 2018. Am J Infect Control 2020;48(2):207–11.

51. Greene L, Cain, TA, Khoury, R. APIC position paper: the importance of surveillance technologies in the prevention of healthcare-associated infections 2009. Available at: http://www.apic.org/Resource_/TinyMceFileManager/Advocacy-PDFs/Surveillance_Technologies_position_paper_2009-5_29_09.pdf. Accessed May 29, 2009.

52. Grota PG, Stone PW, Jordan S, et al. Electronic surveillance systems in infection prevention: organizational support, program characteristics, and user satisfaction. Am J Infect Control 2010;38(7):509–14.

53. Sips ME, Bonten MJM, van Mourik MSM. Automated surveillance of healthcare-associated infections: state of the art. Curr Opin Infect Dis 2017;30(4):425–31.

54. Streefkerk HRA, Verkooijen RP, Bramer WM, et al. Electronically assisted surveillance systems of healthcare-associated infections: a systematic review. Euro Surveill 2020;25(2):1900321.

55. Campbell EA, Eichhorn CL. Outbreak investigations. In: APIC text of infection control and epidemiology. 2020. Available at: https://text.apic.org/toc/epidemiology-surveillance-performance-and-patient-safety-measures/outbreak-investigations. Accessed January 11, 2021.

56. McDonald L. Florence Nightingale and the early origins of evidence-based nursing. Evid Based Nurs 2001;4(3):68–9.

57. Shahian DM, Edwards FH, Jacobs JP, et al. Public reporting of cardiac surgery performance: Part 1–history, rationale, consequences. Ann Thorac Surg 2011;92(3 Suppl):S2–11.

58. Banach DB, Johnston BL, Al-Zubeidi D, et al. Outbreak response and incident management: SHEA guidance and resources for healthcare epidemiologists in United States acute-care hospitals. Infect Control Hosp Epidemiol 2017;38(12):1393–419.

59. Center for Disease Control and Prevention. Crisis and emergency risk communication. 2018. Available at: https://emergency.cdc.gov/cerc/. Accessed January 11, 2021.

60. Tumpey AJ, Daigle D, Nowak G. Communicating during an outbreak or public health investigation. The CDC Field Epidemiology Manual. Available at: https://www.cdc.gov/eis/field-epi-manual/chapters/Communicating-Investigation.html. Accessed January 11, 2021.

61. Perencevich EN, Stone PW, Wright SB, et al. Raising standards while watching the bottom line: making a business case for infection control. Infect Control Hosp Epidemiol 2007;28(10):1121–33.

62. Dick AW, Perencevich EN, Pogorzelska-Maziarz M, et al. A decade of investment in infection prevention: a cost-effectiveness analysis. Am J Infect Control 2015;43(1):4–9.

63. Maragakis LL, Perencevich EN, Cosgrove SE. Clinical and economic burden of antimicrobial resistance. Expert Rev Anti Infect Ther 2008;6(5):751–63.

64. Murphy DM. From expert data collectors to interventionists: changing the focus for infection control professionals. Am J Infect Control 2002;30(2):120–32.

65. Burke JP. Infection control - a problem for patient safety. N Engl J Med 2003; 348(7):651–6.

66. Calfee DP, Farr BM. Infection control and cost control in the era of managed care. Infect Control Hosp Epidemiol 2002;23(7):407–10.

67. Graves N, Halton K, Lairson D. Economics and preventing hospital-acquired infection: broadening the perspective. Infect Control Hosp Epidemiol 2007; 28(2):178–84.

68. Perencevich EN, Thom KA. Commentary: preventing *Clostridium difficile*-associated disease: is it time to pay the piper? Infect Control Hosp Epidemiol 2008; 29(9):829–31.

69. Anderson DJ, Kirkland KB, Kaye KS, et al. Underresourced hospital infection control and prevention programs: penny wise, pound foolish? Infect Control Hosp Epidemiol 2007;28(7):767–73.

70. Kaye KS. The financial impact of antibiotic resistance. In: Soule BM, Weber S, editors. What every health care executive should know: the cost of antibiotic resistance. IL: Oakbrook Terrace; 2009. p. 29–42.

71. Ju MH, Ko CY, Hall BL, et al. A comparison of 2 surgical site infection monitoring systems. JAMA Surg 2015;150(1):51–7.

72. Lee KK, Berenholtz SM, Hobson DB, et al. Building a business case for colorectal surgery quality improvement. Dis Colon Rectum 2013;56(11):1298–303.

73. van Limburg M, Wentzel J, Sanderman R, et al. Business modeling to implement an eHealth portal for infection control: a reflection on co-creation with stakeholders. JMIR Res Protoc 2015;4(3):e104.

74. Branch-Elliman W, Wright SB, Howell MD. Determining the ideal strategy for ventilator-associated pneumonia prevention. Cost-benefit analysis. Am J Respir Crit Care Med 2015;192(1):57–63.

75. Gidengil CA, Gay C, Huang SS, et al. Cost-effectiveness of strategies to prevent methicillin-resistant *Staphylococcus aureus* transmission and infection in an intensive care unit. Infect Control Hosp Epidemiol 2015;36(1):17–27.

76. Goldsack JC, DeRitter C, Power M, et al. Clinical, patient experience and cost impacts of performing active surveillance on known methicillin-resistant *Staphylococcus aureus* positive patients admitted to medical-surgical units. Am J Infect Control 2014;42(10):1039–43.

77. Kollef MH. Ventilator-associated pneumonia prevention. Is it worth it? Am J Respir Crit Care Med 2015;192(1):5–7.

78. McKinnell JA, Bartsch SM, Lee BY, et al. Cost-benefit analysis from the hospital perspective of universal active screening followed by contact precautions for methicillin-resistant *Staphylococcus aureus* carriers. Infect Control Hosp Epidemiol 2015;36(1):2–13.

79. Murthy A, De Angelis G, Pittet D, et al. Cost-effectiveness of universal MRSA screening on admission to surgery. Clin Microbiol Infect 2010;16(12):1747–53.

80. Srinivasan A, Craig M, Cardo D. The power of policy change, federal collaboration, and state coordination in healthcare-associated infection prevention. Clin Infect Dis 2012;55(3):426–31.

81. U.S. Department of Health and Human Services (HHS). National action plan to prevent health care-associated infections: road map to elimination. 2020. Available at: https://health.gov/our-work/health-care-quality/health-care-associated-infections/national-hai-action-plan. Accessed January 14, 2021.

Hand Hygiene, an Update

John M. Boyce, MD

KEYWORDS

- Hand hygiene • Handwashing • Compliance • Monitoring • Infection prevention
- Cross-transmission • Healthcare-associated infections

KEY POINTS

- Hand hygiene by health care personnel is one of the most important measures for preventing health care–associated infections, but adherence rates and hand hygiene technique remain suboptimal.
- Alcohol-based hand rubs are the preferred method of hand hygiene in most clinical scenarios, are more effective and better tolerated than handwashing, and facilitate improved hand hygiene.
- Obtaining accurate estimates of hand hygiene adherence rates is challenging, and combining automated monitoring systems with direct observation is a promising strategy.

BACKGROUND

Soap has been used for washing the hands and body since its cleansing properties were recognized by ancient Egyptian and Greek civilizations, and handwashing has been promoted for religious reasons for many years.[1] In the mid-1800s, the role of hand hygiene in the prevention of health care–associated infections (HAIs) (ie, puerperal fever) was first recognized by Oliver Wendell Holmes and by Ignaz Philip Semmelweis, who is considered to be the father hand hygiene.[2,3] In the early 1960s, Mortimer and colleagues[4] conducted a prospective-controlled trial that demonstrated that infants who were cared for by nurses who did not wash their hands after touching an index infant colonized with *Staphylococcus aureus* acquired the organism significantly more often and more rapidly than did infants cared for by nurses who washed their hands with hexachlorophene soap between contact with infants.[2]

Before 2002, handwashing by health care personnel (HCP) in the United States was performed almost exclusively using either non-antimicrobial or antimicrobial soap. Evaluation of alcohol-based hand rubs (ABHRs) as an alternative to soap and water handwashing began as early in the late 1970s, with their adoption in some European hospitals during the next 20 years.[5–7] However, the Centers for Disease Control and Prevention (CDC) guidelines on environmental control and handwashing published in 1985 recommended that alcohol-containing solutions only be used for hand hygiene

J.M. Boyce Consulting, LLC, 62 Sonoma Lane, Middletown, CT 06457, USA
E-mail address: jmboyce69@gmail.com

Infect Dis Clin N Am 35 (2021) 553–573
https://doi.org/10.1016/j.idc.2021.04.003
0891-5520/21/© 2021 Elsevier Inc. All rights reserved.

id.theclinics.com

in emergency settings where sinks were not available.[2] In the period 1997 to 2000, seminal publications by European investigators demonstrated the advantages of ABHRs,[6–9] which stimulated greater interest in their adoption in the United States.

GUIDELINE DEVELOPMENT

In 2002, the HICPAC/SHEA/APIC/IDSA Guideline for Hand Hygiene in Healthcare Settings was published.[2] One of the major changes in the guideline was the recommendation that ABHRs be used as the preferred method of hand hygiene in most clinical scenarios (**Box 1**).[2] The recommendations were based on persistently poor handwashing compliance by HCP over a period of decades, and the advantages that ABHRs have over washing hands with soap and water. With input of more than 100 experts, the updated and more comprehensive World Health Organization (WHO) Guidelines on Hand Hygiene in Health Care were published in final form in 2009.[3] The WHO guideline also recommended ABHRs as the preferred method of hand hygiene.[3] The 2014 Society for Healthcare Epidemiology of America (SHEA)/Infectious Diseases Society of America (IDSA) Practice Recommendations on hand hygiene provide a concise set of updated recommendations, compared with the CDC and WHO guidelines, and identify areas requiring additional research.[10]

Box 1
Centers for Disease Control and Prevention indications for hand hygiene

A. When hands are visibly dirty or contaminated with proteinaceous material or visibly soiled with blood or other body fluids, wash hands with either a non-antimicrobial soap and water or an antimicrobial soap and water

B. If hands are not visibly soiled, use ABHRs for routinely decontaminating hands in all other clinical situations described as follows. Alternatively, wash hands with an antimicrobial soap and water in all clinical situations described as follows.

C. Decontaminate hands before having direct contact with patients

D. Decontaminate hands before donning sterile gloves when inserting a central intravascular catheter

E. Decontaminate hands before inserting indwelling urinary catheters, peripheral vascular catheters, or other invasive devices that do not require a surgical procedure

F. Decontaminate hands after contact with a patient's intact skin (eg, when taking a pulse or blood pressure, and lifting a patient)

G. Decontaminate hands after contact with body fluids or excretions, mucous membranes, nonintact skin, and wound dressings if hands are not visibly soiled

H. Decontaminate hands if moving from a contaminated body site to a clean body site during patient care

I. Decontaminate hands after contact with inanimate objects (including medical equipment) in the immediate vicinity of the patient

J. Decontaminate hands after removing gloves

K. Before eating and after using the restroom, wash hands with a non-antimicrobial soap and water or with an antimicrobial soap and water

From Boyce JM, Pittet D. Guideline for Hand Hygiene in Healthcare Settings. Recommendations of the Healthcare Infection Control Practices Advisory Committee and the HICPAC/SHEA/APIC/IDSA Hand Hygiene Task Force. Society for Healthcare Epidemiology of America/Association for Professionals in Infection Control/Infectious Diseases Society of America. MMWR Recomm Rep 2002;51 (RR-16):1-45.

The guidelines in **Box 1** and a recently published book dedicated to hand hygiene provide a wealth of information regarding the many facets of hand hygiene.[2,3,11] The purpose of this article was to review briefly the basic concepts of hand hygiene and to emphasize recent studies that add to our understanding of hand hygiene. Common hand hygiene terms are defined in **Table 1**.

MICROBIOME OF HANDS

Two types of microorganisms comprise the normal flora of hands: transient flora and resident flora.[3] Transient flora, which are often acquired by HCP during contact with patients or environmental surfaces, colonize the superficial layers of the skin. They represent the microorganisms most commonly associated with HAIs, and are easier to remove from the skin by using an ABHR or washing hands. Common examples of transient flora include methicillin-resistant *S aureus* (MRSA), vancomycin-resistant enterococci, and multidrug-resistant gram-negative bacteria. Resident flora colonize the deeper layers of the skin, are less likely to cause infections, and are more resistant to removal. Early studies using standard culture-based methods revealed total bacterial counts ranging from 3.9×10^4 to 4.6×10^5 colony-forming units (CFU)/cm^2.[3] Cultures of fingertips using agar plate methods have yielded counts ranging from 0 to 300 CFU.[3] A recent study of 50 healthy women found an average of 5.85 log_{10} CFU (range 4.42–7.36) aerobic bacteria per hand, and an average of 6.12 log_{10} CFU of anaerobic bacteria per hand.[12]

Newer 16 S ribosomal RNA (rRNA) gene sequencing methods can identify microorganisms that are not detected using standard culture-based methods. As a result, culture-based methods significantly underestimate the diversity of bacterial

Table 1 Definition of terms	
Term	Definition
Plain soap	Detergent that does not contain antimicrobial agents, or contains such agents solely as preservatives
Antimicrobial soap	Detergent containing an antimicrobial agent in concentrations sufficient to inactivate or temporarily suppress the growth of microorganisms
ABHR (Alcohol-based hand sanitizer)	Alcohol-containing preparation (liquid, gel, foam) formulated for application to the hands for reducing the number of viable microorganisms on the hands
Hand hygiene	A general term that applies to either handwashing or application of an ABHR
Handwashing	Washing hands with either plain soap or antimicrobial soap, followed by rinsing with water and drying hands
Hand antisepsis	Application of either an ABHR or washing hands with an antimicrobial soap
Surgical scrub or surgical hand rub	Hand antisepsis performed preoperatively by surgical personnel to eliminate transient flora and reduce resident hand flora

Adapted from Refs.[2,3]

communities on the hands.[12] One study cited by Edmonds-Wilson and colleagues[13] used 16 S rRNA sequencing methods and found an average of more than 150 bacterial species on the palms. Staphylococcaceae, Corynebacteriaceae, Propionibacteriaceae, and Streptococcaceae have been identified on the hands in most studies.[13] Viruses and fungi account for less than 20% of the hand microbiome.

Of interest, a study using 16 S rRNA sequencing of samples obtained before and after hand hygiene revealed (1) that the sampling methods could affect the results, (2) ABHR had no more effect on microbiome diversity than rinsing with water, and (3) skin hydration was a major variable affecting bacterial abundance and community composition.[12] Use of ABHR temporarily reduces the number of microbiota on the hands, without producing significant long-term changes in the hand microbiome.[12,14] Additional studies of the effects of different hand hygiene products should include a variety of HCP (nurses, physicians, and other personnel) involved in patient care in various health care settings.

ROLE OF HANDS IN TRANSMISSION OF PATHOGENS

Transmission of health care–associated pathogens from one patient to another requires that the following sequence of events occur.[2]

1. Organisms present on the patient's skin or on an environmental surface must be transferred to the hands of a health care worker
2. Organisms must be capable of remaining viable for at least several minutes on the health care worker's hands
3. Hand hygiene technique is inadequate, or hand hygiene is performed with an inappropriate agent, or is omitted entirely
4. Contaminated hands of the health care worker must come in direct contact with another patient, or with an inanimate object that will come in direct contact with a patient

A patient's skin is frequently colonized with a variety of health care–associated pathogens, including multidrug-resistant organisms (MDROs),[15] and is the most common source of transient contamination of the hands of HCP. Environmental surfaces in patient rooms are also often contaminated with MDROs.[15,16] HCP frequently touch the skin of patients, potentially contaminated environmental surfaces near the patient, and their own body and clothing. For example, a study in which intensive care unit (ICU) personnel wore a head-mounted camera revealed that they had hand (or glove) contact with a surface an average of once every 4.2 seconds.[17] As a result, HCP frequently contaminate their hands with health care–associated pathogens.[2] Hands of HCP may also become contaminated with gram-negative bacteria dispersed from contaminated sinks.[18] A recent systematic review and meta-analysis revealed that the pooled prevalence of MDRO contamination of HCP hands ranged from 4% to 9%, with considerable variation for MRSA, vancomycin-resistant enterococci, and gram-negative bacteria, depending on the geographic area, method of sampling hands, and health care setting.[19] One study found that 5.5% to 6.5% of S aureus could be transferred from a heavily contaminated dry surface biofilm to the hands following a single touch, with subsequent transfer to other surfaces that were touched.[20] Although little is known about how many bacteria must be present on hands in order for cross-transmission to occur, Bellissimo-Rodrigues and colleagues[21] found that individuals whose hands were contaminated with more than 1 $\log_{10}$ Escherichia coli could transmit the organism to the hands of another person if their hands were in contact for 1 minute. Additional studies of the level of hand contamination required for cross-transmission to occur are needed, and research using innovative surrogate markers such as viral DNA or silica nanoparticles are warranted to gain a better understanding of transmission patterns.[22,23]

INDICATIONS FOR HAND HYGIENE

Hand hygiene guidelines published by the CDC and WHO, and SHEA/IDSA practice recommendations on hand hygiene have specified the clinical situations in which hand hygiene is indicated (see **Box 1**). Furthermore, the WHO guideline introduced the concept of "My 5 Moments for Hand Hygiene" (M5M)[3]:

- Moment 1: Before touching a patient
- Moment 2: Before a clean/aseptic procedure
- Moment 3: After a body fluid exposure risk
- Moment 4: After touching a patient
- Moment 5: After touching patient surroundings

This concept was designed to aid in educating HCP about when to perform hand hygiene and to provide a framework for monitoring hand hygiene compliance.

HAND HYGIENE PRODUCTS
Alcohol-Based Hand Rubs

Compared with handwashing with soap and water, ABHRs have the following advantages[6,7]:

- More effective than soap and water in reducing viable organisms on the hands.
- Excellent activity against a broad range of pathogens (except spores), with somewhat less activity against some nonenveloped viruses
- Require much less time than washing hands with soap and water, rinsing, and drying
- Cause less skin irritation and dryness than frequent use of soap and water
- Unlike handwashing sinks, can be made available at the bedside and in many other locations
- Have been associated with improved compliance with hand hygiene

Product format
ABHR products are available in several formats, including liquids (with consistency similar to water), gels, and foams. All product formats are appropriate for use in health care settings, because product format does not significantly affect antimicrobial efficacy.[24,25] Liquid products with higher alcohol concentrations dry faster, but tend to drip more onto clothing or floors. Currently, alcohol-based wipes are not recommended for HCP hand hygiene in health care settings.[2,3,26]

Formulation issues
The concentration of alcohol in ABHRs does not significantly affect efficacy, as evidenced by the fact that some products formulated with 70% ethanol are more efficacious than products with higher ethanol concentrations.[27] This can be explained by the manner in which products are formulated, and the types of other constituents included. Not surprisingly, the greater the volume of product applied to the hands, the longer hands must be rubbed together before they feel dry (dry-time).[24,25,28] The major factor affecting antimicrobial efficacy is the dry-time, with longer dry-times leading to greater efficacy.[28]

The antimicrobial efficacy of ABHRs depends on other factors as well, including the test methods used, the alcohol tested, the presence of other constituents (product formulation), and the volume applied.[24,25,27-29] For example, one in vivo study that applied 2 mL of 11 different products to hands found that mean log_{10} reductions after a single application varied from 2.48 to 3.58.[27] In another study that applied a volume more typically delivered by dispensers (1.1 mL) to hands, the mean log_{10} reduction after a single application was 2.85.[30] Although the CDC and WHO hand hygiene guidelines recommended using a product with persistent or sustained activity for surgical hand antisepsis, the WHO 2016 Guideline on Prevention of Surgical Site Infections did not make a recommendation on whether or not products for surgical hand antisepsis need to have sustained activity.[31] Of note, recent studies have confirmed the efficacy of ABHRs against severe acute respiratory syndrome coronavirus 2.[32,33]

Safety of alcohol-based hand rubs

ABHRs are safe and effective when used as directed. Adverse events related to ingestion by in-patients have rarely been reported. Restricting access to ABHRs by patients with psychiatric or dementia problems seems prudent, and is commonly practiced in health care facilities. Depending on the facility, this may be accomplished by placing dispensers in areas not accessible to patients, or by providing personnel with pocket bottles. Because some nurses may perform hand hygiene with ABHRs more than 100 times per 12-hour shift,[34] the Food and Drug Administration (FDA) has mandated that industry conduct a "maximum-use trial" to confirm the safety of very frequent use of ABHRs. During the Coronavirus Disease 2019 (COVID-19) pandemic, worldwide shortages of ABHRs resulted in production of ABHRs by some distilleries and by companies that did not follow good manufacturing processes. Episodes of methanol toxicity related to poorly formulated products produced outside the United States have been reported,[35] and resulted in the FDA issuing warnings to avoid some products produced in Mexico.

Delivery systems

ABHRs are made available in manual and touch-free wall-mounted dispensers, freestanding pump bottles, and pocket bottles. Although some HCP have expressed concern about contaminating their hands by touching manual wall-mounted dispensers or pocket bottles, there is no evidence that touching such items has resulted in transmission of pathogens. Any microorganisms that might be transferred from the dispenser or bottle to hands are immediately reduced significantly by application of the hand rub. To maximize the use of ABHRs, wall-mounted dispensers should be placed in hallways near the doors of patient rooms in addition to having dispensers at bedsides or within a few feet of patient beds. Several studies have shown that HCP use dispensers located in hallways more frequently than those in patient rooms.[36,37] However, some personnel may be more likely to access bedside dispensers during invasive procedures or patient care that may expose personnel to a patient's body fluids or excretions.[36] Dispensers should be placed in locations that are in the line-of-sight of personnel and are consistent with workflow patterns.[38] Dispensers also should be available in perioperative areas, because surgical hand antisepsis can be performed with either an antimicrobial soap and water or an alcohol-based hand rub.[2,3]

Non–Alcohol-based Hand Rubs

Although a number of non-ABHRs have been marketed, current guidelines do not recommend the use of nonalcohol hand rubs for routine hand hygiene in health care settings.[2,3,39] Additional studies of such products are needed to establish their antimicrobial efficacy, impact on transmission of pathogens, and ability to reduce HAIs.

Soap

Soaps can help remove dirt, proteinaceous material, and some microorganisms from hands via mechanical action. Plain soaps have little or no antimicrobial activity. Washing hands with plain soap and water is less effective than performing hand hygiene with an ABHR.[2,3] Early studies reported that washing hands with plain soap and water for 15 seconds reduced bacteria on the hands by 0.6 to 1.1 $\log_{10}$, and washing for 30 seconds reduced bacteria by 1.8 to 2.8 $\log_{10}$.[2] A recent study of washing nonwetted hands for 30 seconds with a novel non-antimicrobial soap compared with washing with the standard plain soap reported $\log_{10}$ reductions of 1.46 and 1.12, respectively.[40] Interestingly, if soap was applied after hands were wetted, lower $\log_{10}$ reductions of 1.07 and 0.97, respectively, were achieved. In real-life clinical situations, $\log_{10}$ reductions achieved may be lower than those observed in laboratory studies because most HCP wash their hands for less than 15 seconds.[2] Washing hands with an antimicrobial soap is generally more effective than washing with plain soap, but less effective than performing hand hygiene with an alcohol-based hand rub.[2,3] Washing hands with hot water should be avoided, as it has no significant effect on antimicrobial efficacy, and can increase the risk of hand dermatitis.

GLOVES

Gloves help reduce, but do not eliminate, contamination of the hands of HCP that can occur when touching patients or their environment. Gloves represent the primary form of hand hygiene when caring for patients with *Clostridioides difficile* infection because ABHRs are not effective in reducing spores from hands. In routine or endemic settings, hand hygiene after caring for patients with *C difficile* infection can be performed after removing gloves with either soap and water or an alcohol-based hand rub.[41] If *C difficile* infections are epidemic or hyperendemic, handwashing with soap and water is the preferred method. Hand hygiene is always recommended after removing gloves, because gloves do not protect completely against hand contamination.[2] Although HCP frequently perform hand hygiene before donning nonsterile gloves, the need for this is somewhat controversial. A randomized controlled trial found that hand hygiene before donning nonsterile gloves did not significantly reduce bacterial counts on gloves,[42] suggesting that this issue requires reconsideration. If glove changes are indicated during an episode of care on the same patient, hand hygiene should be performed after removing gloves and before donning a new pair of nonsterile gloves.

HAND HYGIENE TECHNIQUE

Following publication of the CDC and WHO guidelines, most efforts to promote improved hand hygiene have focused on increasing hand hygiene compliance, with little attention paid to how hand hygiene is performed (hand hygiene technique). As an example, several studies have reported that high adherence rates were accompanied by poor hand hygiene technique.[43,44] Because approximately 80% of hand hygiene events are performed using ABHR,[36,45,46] studies of hand hygiene technique have focused on the use of ABHRs.

Factors affecting the adequacy of hand hygiene technique include the extent to which personnel cover all surfaces of their hands and fingers with ABHR, the volume of product applied, the duration of hand rubbing (dry-time), and hand size. Personnel often do not adequately apply hand rub to their fingertips and thumbs.[47] The WHO 6-

step hand hygiene protocol was designed to ensure coverage of all surfaces of hands, but compliance with the protocol is often suboptimal.[48] As a result, modifications of the WHO protocol have recently been described.[49] A greatly simplified procedure was developed that includes the following 3 steps: (1) cover all surfaces of the hand, (2) rotational rubbing of fingertips in the palm of the alternate hand, and (3) rotational rubbing of both thumbs (**Fig. 1**).[49] A cluster randomized trial comparing the simplified 3-step protocol with the 6-step WHO protocol revealed that the simplified method resulted in increased compliance, and was not microbiologically inferior to the WHO 6-step protocol.[44]

Inadequate coverage also may occur when personnel apply a small volume of ABHR to their hands to achieve short dry-times, which are often <15 seconds.[17,43,50] However, current studies suggest that dry-times of 15 seconds or longer should be applied to achieve desired reductions of pathogens.[51–53] Because applying volumes of less than 1 mL often results in dry-times of less than 15 seconds,[25,30,54] facilities should consider adjusting ABHR dispensers to deliver a minimum of 1 mL of product with one accession. Educating personnel about the importance of applying an amount of ABHR that yields adequate dry-times should be part of hand hygiene promotion programs.

Not surprisingly, hand size can also affect how well surfaces are covered and dry-times achieved with ABHRs.[28] When a given dose is applied to large hands, dry-times are shorter than when applied to small hands.[28] As a result, it has been suggested that dosing should be individualized to achieve adequate dry-times.[28] However, when nurses are given the opportunity to choose the dose they receive, those with large

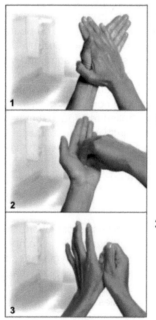

1. Cover all surfaces of the hands

2. Rotational rubbing of fingertips in the palm of the alternate hand

3. Rotational rubbing of both thumbs

Fig. 1. Simplified 3-step hand hygiene technique. (*From* Tschudin-Sutter S, Rotter ML, Frei R, Nogarth D, Hausermann P, Stranden A, Pittet D, Widmer AF. Simplifying the WHO 'how to hand rub' technique: three steps are as effective as sixdresults from an experimental randomized crossover trial. Clin Microbiol Infect 2017;23:409.e1- 409.e4; with permission.)

hands may not select larger doses than those with small hands.[55] Individualizing doses might be facilitated in the future if dispensers could deliver variable amounts based on an individual's hand size.

CDC guideline recommends that when washing hands with soap and water, personnel should first wet hands with water, apply an amount of soap recommended by the manufacturer, and rub hands together vigorously for at least 15 seconds, covering all surfaces of the hands and fingers.[2] Hands should then be rinsed with water and dried thoroughly with a disposable towel. The WHO guideline recommends wetting hands before applying an amount of soap necessary to cover all surfaces followed by rinsing hands with water and drying thoroughly with a single-use towel.[3] The duration of the entire process should be 40 to 60 seconds. Although some investigators have recommended against the use of jet-air electric dryers in hospitals,[56] further research is needed to establish with certainty the safest method for drying hands in health care settings.[57]

HAND HYGIENE ADHERENCE

Before publication of the CDC and WHO guidelines, HCP hand hygiene adherence rates averaged approximately 40%.[2,3] Hand hygiene adherence rates have improved in the ensuing years, although achieving and sustaining high rates of adherence remain challenges in many facilities. Reported adherence rates have varied tremendously, from less than 25% to more than 90%, depending on the country, health care setting (hospital vs long-term care facility), hospital bed size, type of nursing unit, HCP job category, indication for hand hygiene, promotional interventions, and methods used to estimate adherence rates (direct observation methods vs automated monitoring systems).[17,44–46,48,50,58–74] Due to the large number of factors affecting adherence rates, a comprehensive analysis of the topic is beyond the scope of this review. Accordingly, only a few factors are mentioned here.

Lambe and colleagues[61] found that adherence rates in ICUs were lower in low-income countries than in high-income countries. A study involving 5 acute-care hospitals revealed that adherence rates decreased as hospital bed size increased.[66] Several studies documented very low adherence rates in nursing homes.[62,63] In 1 of the 2 studies that was conducted in the United States, HCP performed hand hygiene more frequently with soap and water than with ABHR,[62] an issue that likely persists in some other nursing homes. Within a given facility, there is substantial individual variability in adherence rates,[37,75,76] with adherence by physicians often (but not always) lower than among nurses.[50,58,61,64,67] Adherence rates continue to vary depending on the type of patient care being provided, with personnel performing hand hygiene more frequently after patient contact (to protect themselves) than before contact (to protect patients).[37,62–64] In the context of the M5M; adherence to Moments 1 and 2 is sometimes lower than it is to Moments 3, 4, and 5.[50,61,77] As a result, ongoing efforts to improve adherence need to focus on reminding personnel of the importance of performing hand hygiene before touching patients and before performing aseptic procedures.

MONITORING HAND HYGIENE ADHERENCE
Direct Observation Method

Monitoring adherence to hand hygiene recommendations by HCP and providing them with feedback regarding their performance are essential elements of an effective multimodal strategy for improving hand hygiene.[2,3] Unfortunately, monitoring hand hygiene adherence has proven to be more complex than anticipated, and remains a challenge in many health care facilities. Direct observation of personnel by trained observers is by far the most common method for estimating adherence rates, and continues to be considered the "gold standard" method.

Advantages and disadvantages of the direct observation method are summarized in **Box 2**. Unlike other methods, direct observations can be used to monitor all M5M, although this may prove difficult in some settings.[64] Hand hygiene technique can be evaluated, although this is seldom recorded and analyzed. Unlike currently available automated monitoring systems, direct observations are feasible in virtually all types of health care facilities, including those with few resources.

The accuracy of hand hygiene adherence rates generated by direct observations is affected by multiple factors.[78,79] Despite some guidance provided by the WHO guidelines, there is a lack of standardization of the following factors: the type and time spent training of observers, the frequency of validating interobserver reliability, the type of personnel performing observations, the criteria for hand hygiene adherence (hand hygiene on room entry and exit, the M5M, 4 Moments for Hand Hygiene [eg, Canada]), and the duration of the observation sessions (range, 10 minutes to >1 hour).[70,73,80,81] Many hospitals in the United States observe hand hygiene adherence of personnel on room entry and room exit, whereas others monitor adherence to the M5M.[80] Monitoring personnel at room entry and exit is popular because it is easier to perform than attempting to observe all M5M. Covertly observing M5M, especially Moments 2 and 3, can be difficult due to privacy curtains being drawn or to architectural aspects of the nursing unit.[64] One comparative study found that adherence rates generated by the 2 methods were similar, whereas another study found that monitoring M5M resulted in significantly higher adherence rates than observing room entries and exits.[64,82] A review of 28 studies found that adherence rates for Moments 1, 4, and 5 combined were similar to rates for all M5M.[78]

Many hospitals perform observations only during day shifts during weekdays, and may observe as few as 10 to 30 hand hygiene opportunities/nursing unit/month.[80,81,83] However, the number of hand hygiene opportunities often varies from 10,000 to greater than 100,000/unit/month on medical and surgical wards, and from 20,000 to 150,000/unit/month in ICUs.[50,81,84–87] As a result, in many hospitals, direct observations often capture as few as $\leq$0.1% of all hand hygiene opportunities,[73,81,83,88] which is too small a sample to yield valid results. The WHO Hand Hygiene Implementation

---

Box 2
Advantages and disadvantages of monitoring hand hygiene using the direct observation method

Advantages
- Ability to estimate adherence with all "My 5 Moments for Hand Hygiene"
- Identify barriers to hand hygiene
- Evaluation of hand hygiene technique
- Most widely used method for monitoring adherence
- Applicable in virtually all facilities, regardless of the level of resources

Disadvantages
- Lack of standardized methods for training observers and conducting auditing sessions
- Periodic validation of observer accuracy is often not performed
- Inadequate sampling of hand hygiene opportunities
- Hawthorne effect results in exaggerated adherence rates
- Observing all indications for hand hygiene is difficult in some settings
- Conducting observations is time consuming
- Observers and frontline staff may have concerns regarding the accuracy of results

Guide and an analysis by Yin and colleagues[89] recommend that hospitals observe 150 to 200 hand hygiene opportunities/nursing unit/time period to obtain reasonable estimates of adherence rates.[90]

The Hawthorne effect is common with direct observation method, and varies with the type of observer, the presence of nearby HCP not involved in performing observations, and the duration of the observation sessions.[86,89,91–94] Adherence rates are higher when generated by unit-based observers than by non–unit-based observers, and when other HCP are nearby.[86,91] The Hawthorne effect increases significantly when observation periods are more than 15 minutes in duration.[89,92,94] As a result of the preceding issues, adherence rates generated by direct observations are 1.5-fold to 3-fold higher than those generated by automated monitoring systems.[60,77,95] Although some infection preventionists assume that the Hawthorne effect has a positive, long-term effect on adherence rates, 2 studies have found that increased adherence rates associated with the Hawthorne decrease by 50% to 100% within 1 hour after the observer has left the unit.[96,97] Overall, the lack of standardized methods for conducting direct observations precludes comparing rates between institutions.

Tips on how to optimize direct observations include the following:

- Provide observers with standardized training, including videos if possible
- Periodically validate observer accuracy
- Reduce impact of Hawthorne effect:
  ○ Use covert "secret shopper" observers
  ○ Avoid observers performing audits on their own units
  ○ Avoid having observers who collect adherence data provide immediate feedback
  ○ Have champions limit activities to coaching and promotional efforts
- If possible, observe ~150 to 200 opportunities/unit/time period, unless unit is small
- Consider using a digital app for recording observations, to facilitate processing data
- Monitor hand hygiene technique
  ○ Observe if ABHR is applied to all surfaces of hands (including thumbs and fingertips)
  ○ Monitor duration of hand rubs (should be ≥ 15 seconds of rubbing)

Automated Hand Hygiene Monitoring

Electronic counting devices installed in dispensers can record many more hand hygiene events (HHEs) than direct observations, and can be used to monitor trends in hand hygiene frequency, but do not provide adherence data.[78,98]

Group monitoring systems

Several group monitoring systems are available that estimate unit-level HCP adherence rates. One system uses dispensers equipped with sensors that record each accession (HHEs) and send data to a central server. Hand hygiene opportunities (HHOs) are estimated using a software algorithm based on initial observations of the distribution of M5M (or M4M) on different units, patient census, patient-to-nurse ratios, and adjustments.[69,99–101] Estimated adherence rates are calculated by dividing the number of HHEs by the estimated number of HHOs. Studies have validated the approach to estimating HHOs in several settings.[36,85,100,102] However, some facilities may encounter challenges in obtaining accurate census and staffing data.[103] Advantages of the system include its estimates of adherence with all M5M (or M4M), and a lack of need for sensors at patient doorways or specialized personnel badges. A recent 2-year stepped-wedge cluster randomized study conducted in 5 hospitals documented a significant overall improvement in hand hygiene adherence, from a baseline level of 29% to 53% after 10 months, and a trend toward reduced transmission of MRSA.[69] Importantly, system implementation was accompanied by multiple complementary measures, including several methods of providing HCP with feedback and encouraging accountability.

Other group "activity" monitoring systems use sensors in dispensers and at doorways to patient rooms to monitor each room entry and exit, which are considered HHOs.[83,87,104] Some systems can provide audible reminders on room entry and exit.[87] Compared with direct observations, advantages include the following:

- Capture 100 to greater than 10,000 times as many HHOs on a 24/7 basis compared to the number of direct observations performed per time period in many facilities
- Provide large amounts of data on estimated adherence rates
- Not affected by observer bias and Hawthorne effect
- Provide near real-time feedback on unit-level adherence rates
- Require much less personnel time than direct observation
- Perceived as less intrusive than badge-based systems
- Less expensive than badge-based systems

One group activity monitoring system also documented changes in room entry/exit frequency and adherence rates related to the COVID-19 pandemic.[105] One system reported to have a sensitivity of 92.7% and positive predictive value of 84.4% has been associated with significantly increased hand hygiene adherence in 2 studies (Abstract: Landon E et al. Open Forum Infect Dis 2017;4 (Suppl 1):S408).[83,104] In one study, implementing the system was associated with a trend toward fewer non–C difficile HAIs.[83]

Limitations of activity monitoring systems include their inability to differentiate visitors from HCP entering and exiting rooms, lack of individual-specific adherence rates, and limited published evidence regarding their ability to sustain improved hand hygiene performance and to reduce health care–associated infections.[78] Data on the relative frequency of room entries and exits by HCP and visitors are available,[106] and can be used to adjust estimated adherence rates.

Badge-based systems

Badge-based automated systems include sensors located in dispensers, patient rooms, and specialized electronic personnel badges.[78] These systems can detect entry of individual HCP into patient rooms, whether or not hand hygiene was performed just before or after entering the room, and provide individual feedback in a variety of forms.[71,72,74,81,88,107] Of the badge-based systems whose accuracy has been formally validated, one had an accuracy of 99%, and another correctly identified ~85% of HHOs.[73,107] Adherence rates have ranged from approximately 63% to 85% to 95%, with the highest rates more common in those with immediate reminder functions.[46,71,72,74,75,81,88] Additional advantages include the ability to identify significant variability in individual performance, the impact of duration of room visit on adherence rates, identify consecutive missed opportunities, and analyze the frequency of room visits by individuals, which may aid in outbreak investigations and contact tracing.[75,107] Limitations include the installation and maintenance costs of such systems, limited evidence on their cost-effectiveness, ability to yield long-term improvements in adherence rates, and HAI rates, accuracy and badge-related issues with some systems, and level of acceptance by HCP.[71,72,108,109]

Systems based on video cameras or other technologies
Few studies have evaluated the use of video cameras to evaluate hand hygiene adherence.[17,93,110–112] Implementation of a video camera system in a single institution achieved sustained adherence rates of ~80% in a medical ICU and surgical ICU.[111,112] Further research of video-based systems is needed to address concerns regarding personnel and patient privacy, cost-effectiveness, and impact on HAIs. Using machine learning and neural network techniques to combine computer vision with data from depth and thermal sensors shows promise for providing new approaches to automated hand hygiene monitoring.[113]

Importance of complementary strategies
A point that cannot be overemphasized is the need for automated hand hygiene monitoring systems to be incorporated into a multimodal promotion program.[69,71,73,76,83,114] Implementation plans should include validation of the system by hospital personnel using a 2-phase protocol.[104,108,115] Installing an automated system without implementing complementary strategies is very likely to lead to little or no improvement in adherence rates (Abstract: Edmonds-Wilson S et al. Am J Infect Control 2016;44(6):S6-7).[83] Hospitals that have successfully implemented automated monitoring systems have used a variety of complementary strategies, examples of which are available as abstracts (Abstract: Landon E et al. Open Forum Infect Dis 2017;4 (Suppl 1):S408; Abstract: Arbogast J et al. Infect Control Hosp Epidemiol 2020;41 (Suppl 1):S451-2), and others in full-length articles.[69,71,73,81,83,110,116]

- Engagement of hospital leadership
- Input of frontline staff before implementation regarding workflow patterns and concerns
- Interacting with system vendor during and after installation
- Weekly adherence reports e-mailed to department and unit managers
- Weekly feedback via emails or text messages to individuals when using badge-based system, which may include anonymized rates of other individuals in similar job positions
- Unit managers and champions attend weekly "accountability" meetings/calls to share adherence rates, challenges, and successful local initiatives
- Posting weekly unit-based adherence rates in areas visible to personnel and patients
- Recognition of top performers, and prize for top performer
- Periodic educational rounds or in-house webinars

Personnel attitudes toward automated monitoring
Before and during early phases of implementation, HCP may harbor concerns regarding the accuracy of automated systems, and have fears of potential punitive consequences.[117] It is essential to (1) explain to personnel in advance about how the systems work and their limitations, (2) alert personnel to expect lower adherence rates than those based on direct observations, and (3) be transparent about how adherence data will be used.[69,73,83,103,117,118]

Combining automated monitoring with direct observation
As additional information regarding the accuracy and effectiveness of automated systems becomes available, hospitals may want to consider combining automated monitoring with direction observations.[78] For example:

- Use automated systems as the primary source of quantitative data on adherence rates and feedback mechanisms

- Use direct observations for scenarios in which it has unique advantages
  - Monitor adherence to Moments 2 and 3
  - Evaluate adherence with performing hand hygiene between multiple tasks during an episode of care with the same patient
  - Monitor hand hygiene technique
    - Is ABHR applied to all surfaces of the hands (especially fingertips and thumbs)?
    - Are hands rubbed together for at least 15 seconds?

IMPACT OF HAND HYGIENE ON HEALTH CARE–ASSOCIATED INFECTIONS

Multiple studies have shown that improving hand hygiene can reduce HAIs.[3,9,70,119] A smaller number of studies have reported that automated monitoring systems have been associated with reductions in HAIs.[69,73,81,83,114,116] Additional studies are needed to determine the ability of different forms of automated monitoring to reduce HAIs.

ISSUES REQUIRING ADDITIONAL RESEARCH

Important aspects of hand hygiene not included in the present review include the role of patient hand hygiene in reducing HAIs, and improving adherence rates in long-term care facilities, outpatient hemodialysis centers, clinics, and dental facilities. Other issues that require additional research include (but are not limited to) the level of hand contamination needed to prevent pathogen transmission, optimum hand hygiene technique, and the most effective methods for providing personnel with feedback regarding their performance.

CLINICS CARE POINTS

- Perform hand hygiene before touching patients or performing aseptic procedures to reduce the chances of transmitting health care–associated pathogens to your patients.
- If an adequate amount of ABHR was applied to your hands, it should require rubbing your hands together for 15 seconds or longer before they feel dry.
- During a work shift, do not switch frequently between an ABHR and washing with soap and water, as this increases the risk of hand irritation. Wash only when indicated.
- Routinely wear gloves when caring for patients with C difficile infection.
- Always perform hand hygiene after removing gloves.

DISCLOSURE

J.M. Boyce is a consultant to, has received travel support from, and has presented at conference symposia sponsored by Diversey and by GOJO Industries, and is a consultant to Sodexo Healthcare.

REFERENCES

1. Vermeil T, Peters A, Kilpatrick C, et al. Hand hygiene in hospitals: anatomy of a revolution. J Hosp Infect 2019;101(4):383–92.
2. Boyce JM, Pittet D. Guideline for hand hygiene in health-care settings: recommendations of the healthcare infection control practices advisory committee and the HICPAC/SHEA/APIC/IDSA hand hygiene task force. Infect Control Hosp Epidemiol 2002;23(12 Suppl):S3–40.

3. World Health O. WHO guidelines for hand hygiene in health care. Geneva: World Health Organization; 2009.
4. Mortimer EA Jr, Lipsitz PJ, Wolinsky E, et al. Transmission of staphylococci between newborns. Am J Dis Child 1962;104:289–95.
5. Ayliffe GA, Babb JR, Quoraishi AH. A test for 'hygienic' hand disinfection. J Clin Pathol 1978;31(10):923–8.
6. Widmer AF. Replace hand washing with use of a waterless alcohol hand rub? Clin Infect Dis 2000;31:136–43.
7. Rotter M. Arguments for the alcoholic hand disinfection. J Hosp Infect 2001; 28(Suppl A):S4–8.
8. Voss A, Widmer AF. No time for handwashing!? Handwashing versus alcoholic rub: can we afford 100% compliance? Infect Control Hosp Epidemiol 1997;18: 205–8.
9. Pittet D, Hugonnet S, Harbarth S, et al. Effectiveness of a hospital-wide programme to improve compliance with hand hygiene. Lancet 2000;356:1307–12.
10. Ellingson K, Haas JP, Aiello AE, et al. Strategies to prevent healthcare-associated infections through hand hygiene. Infect Control Hosp Epidemiol 2014;35(Suppl 2):S155–78.
11. Hand hygiene: a handbook for medical professionals. Hoboken, NJ: Wiley-Blackwell; 2017.
12. Zapka C, Leff J, Henley J, et al. Comparison of standard culture-based method to culture-independent method for evaluation of hygiene effects on the hand microbiome. mBio 2017;8(2):e00093.
13. Edmonds-Wilson SL, Nurinova NI, Zapka CA, et al. Review of human hand microbiome research. J Dermatol Sci 2015;80(1):3–12.
14. Mukherjee PK, Chandra J, Retuerto M, et al. Effect of alcohol-based hand rub on hand microbiome and hand skin health in hospitalized adult stem cell transplant patients: A pilot study. J Am Acad Dermatol 2018;78(6):1218–21.e5.
15. Mody L, Washer LL, Kaye KS, et al. Multidrug-resistant organisms in hospitals: what is on patient hands and in their rooms? Clin Infect Dis 2019;69(11): 1837–44.
16. Shams AM, Rose LJ, Edwards JR, et al. Assessment of the overall and multidrug-resistant organism bioburden on environmental surfaces in healthcare facilities. Infect Control Hosp Epidemiol 2016;37(12):1426–32.
17. Clack L, Scotoni M, Wolfensberger A, et al. "First-person view" of pathogen transmission and hand hygiene - use of a new head-mounted video capture and coding tool. Antimicrob Resist Infect Control 2017;6:108.
18. Hajar Z, Mana TSC, Cadnum JL, et al. Dispersal of gram-negative bacilli from contaminated sink drains to cover gowns and hands during hand washing. Infect Control Hosp Epidemiol 2019;40(4):460–2.
19. Montoya A, Schildhouse R, Goyal A, et al. How often are health care personnel hands colonized with multidrug- resistant organisms? A systematic review and meta-analysis. Am J Infect Control 2019;47(6):693–703.
20. Chowdhury D, Tahir S, Legge M, et al. Transfer of dry surface biofilm in the healthcare environment: the role of healthcare workers' hands as vehicles. J Hosp Infect 2018;100(3):e85–90.
21. Bellissimo-Rodrigues F, Pires D, Soule H, et al. Assessing the likelihood of hand-to-hand cross-transmission of bacteria: an experimental study. Infect Control Hosp Epidemiol 2017;38(5):553–8.

22. Thakur M, Alhmidi H, Cadnum JL, et al. Use of viral DNA surrogate markers to study routes of transmission of healthcare-associated pathogens. Infect Control Hosp Epidemiol 2020;1–6.

23. Scotoni M, Koch J, Julian TR, et al. Silica nanoparticles with encapsulated DNA (SPED) - a novel surrogate tracer for microbial transmission in healthcare. Antimicrob Resist Infect Control 2020;9(1):152.

24. Wilkinson MAC, Ormandy K, Bradley CR, et al. Comparison of the efficacy and drying times of liquid, gel and foam formats of alcohol-based hand rubs. J Hosp Infect 2018;98(4):359–64.

25. Macinga DR, Shumaker DJ, Werner HP, et al. The relative influences of product volume, delivery format and alcohol concentration on dry-time and efficacy of alcohol-based hand rubs. BMC Infect Dis 2014;14:511.

26. Ory J, Zingg W, de Kraker MEA, et al. Wiping is inferior to rubbing: a note of caution for hand hygiene with alcohol-based solutions. Infect Control Hosp Epidemiol 2018;39(3):332–5.

27. Edmonds SL, Macinga DR, Mays-Suko P, et al. Comparative efficacy of commercially available alcohol-based hand rubs and World Health Organization-recommended hand rubs: formulation matters. Am J Infect Control 2012;40(6):521–5.

28. Suchomel M, Leslie RA, Parker AE, et al. How long is enough? Identification of product dry-time as a primary driver of alcohol-based hand rub efficacy. Antimicrob Resist Infect Control 2018;7:65.

29. Macinga DR, Edmonds SL, Campbell E, et al. Efficacy of novel alcohol-based hand rub products at typical in-use volumes. Infect Control Hosp Epidemiol 2013;34(3):299–301.

30. World Health Organization. Global guidelines on the prevention of surgical site infections. Geneva (Switzerland): WHO Press, World Health Organization; 2016.

31. World Health O. Global guidelines on the prevention of surgical site infection 2017.

32. Kratzel A, Todt D, V'Kovski P, et al. Inactivation of severe acute respiratory syndrome coronavirus 2 by WHO-recommended hand rub formulations and alcohols. Emerg Infect Dis 2020;26(7):1592–5.

33. Leslie RA, Zhou SS, Macinga DR. Inactivation of SARS-CoV-2 by commercially available alcohol-based hand sanitizers. Am J Infect Control 2012;49:401–2.

34. Boyce JM, Polgreen PM, Monsalve M, et al. Frequency of use of alcohol-based hand rubs by nurses: a systematic review. Infect Control Hosp Epidemiol 2017; 38(2):189–95.

35. Dear K, Grayson L, Nixon R. Potential methanol toxicity and the importance of using a standardised alcohol-based hand rub formulation in the era of COVID-19. Antimicrob Resist Infect Control 2020;9(1):129.

36. Conway L, Moore C, Coleman BL, et al. Frequency of hand hygiene opportunities in patients on a general surgery service. Am J Infect Control 2020; 48(5):490–5.

37. Iversen AM, Kavalaris CP, Hansen R, et al. Clinical experiences with a new system for automated hand hygiene monitoring: a prospective observational study. Am J Infect Control 2020;48(5):527–33.

38. Pennathur PR, Herwaldt LA. Role of human factors engineering in infection prevention: gaps and opportunities. Curr Treat Options Infect Dis 2017;9(2):230–49.

39. la Fleur P, Jones S. Non-alcohol based hand rubs: a review of clinical effectiveness and guidelines [Internet] 2017. Available at: https://ncbi.nlm.nih.gov/books/NBK470501. Accessed January 14, 2021.

40. Bingham J, Cartner TJ, Mays Suko PA, et al. Multifactor assessment of non-antimicrobial soap performance. Open Forum Infect Dis 2019;6(5):ofz151.

41. McDonald LC, Gerding DN, Johnson S, et al. Clinical practice guidelines for clostridium difficile infection in adults and children: 2017 update by the Infectious Diseases Society of America (IDSA) and Society for Healthcare Epidemiology of America (SHEA). Clin Infect Dis 2018;66(7):987–94.

42. Rock C, Harris AD, Reich NG, et al. Is hand hygiene before putting on nonsterile gloves in the intensive care unit a waste of health care worker time?–a randomized controlled trial. Am J Infect Control 2013;41(11):994–6.

43. Helder OK, Brug J, Looman CW, et al. The impact of an education program on hand hygiene compliance and nosocomial infection incidence in an urban neonatal intensive care unit: an intervention study with before and after comparison. Int J Nurs Stud 2010;47(10):1245–52.

44. Tschudin-Sutter S, Sepulcri D, Dangel M, et al. Simplifying the WHO protocol: Three steps versus six steps for performance of hand hygiene - a cluster-randomized trial. Clin Infect Dis 2019;69:614–20.

45. Stewardson AJ, Sax H, Gayet-Ageron A, et al. Enhanced performance feedback and patient participation to improve hand hygiene compliance of health-care workers in the setting of established multimodal promotion: a single-centre, cluster randomised controlled trial. Lancet Infect Dis 2016;16(12):1345–55.

46. Albright J, White B, Pedersen D, et al. Use patterns and frequency of hand hygiene in healthcare facilities: analysis of electronic surveillance data. Am J Infect Control 2018;46:1104–9.

47. Widmer AF, Dangel M. Alcohol-based handrub: evaluation of technique and microbiological efficacy with international infection control professionals. Infect Control Hosp Epidemiol 2004;25(3):207–9.

48. Tschudin-Sutter S, Sepulcri D, Dangel M, et al. Compliance with the World Health Organization hand hygiene technique: a prospective observational study. Infect Control Hosp Epidemiol 2015;36(4):482–3.

49. Tschudin-Sutter S, Rotter ML, Frei R, et al. Simplifying the WHO 'how to hand rub' technique: three steps are as effective as six-results from an experimental randomized crossover trial. Clin Microbiol Infect 2017;23(6):409.

50. Stahmeyer JT, Lutze B, von LT, et al. Hand hygiene in intensive care units: a matter of time? J Hosp Infect 2017;95(4):338–43.

51. Pires D, Soule H, Bellissimo-Rodrigues F, et al. Hand hygiene with alcohol-based hand rub: how long is long enough? Infect Control Hosp Epidemiol 2017;38(5):547–52.

52. Pires D, Soule H, Bellissimo-Rodrigues F, et al. Antibacterial efficacy of handrubbing for 15 versus 30 seconds: EN 1500-based randomized experimental study with different loads of Staphylococcus aureus and Escherichia coli. Clin Microbiol Infect 2019;25(7):851–6.

53. Harnoss JC, Dancer SJ, Kaden CF, et al. Hand antisepsis without decreasing efficacy by shortening the rub-in time of alcohol-based handrubs to 15 seconds. J Hosp Infect 2020;104(4):419–24.

54. Kenters N, Eikelenboom-Boskamp A, Hines J, et al. Product dose considerations for real-world hand sanitiser efficacy. Am J Infect Control 2020;48(5):503–6.

55. Martinello RA, Arbogast JW, Guercia K, et al. Nursing preference for alcohol-based hand rub volume. Infect Control Hosp Epidemiol 2019;40(11):1248–52.

56. Best E, Parnell P, Couturier J, et al. Environmental contamination by bacteria in hospital washrooms according to hand-drying method: a multi-centre study. J Hosp Infect 2018;100(4):469–75.

57. Reynolds KA, Sexton JD, Norman A, et al. Comparison of electric hand dryers and paper towels for hand hygiene: a critical review of the literature. J Appl Microbiol 2021;130(1):25–39.

58. Baek E-H, Kim S-E, Kim D-H, et al. The difference in hand hygiene compliance rate between unit-based observers and trained observers for World Health Oganization checklist and optimal hand hygiene. Int J Infect Dis 2020;90:197–200.

59. Kovacs-Litman A, Muller MP, Powis JE, et al. Association between hospital outbreaks and hand hygiene: Insights from electronic monitoring. Clin Infect Dis 2020. [Epub ahead of print].

60. McLaws ML, Kwok YLA. Hand hygiene compliance rates: fact or fiction? Am J Infect Control 2018;46(8):876–80.

61. Lambe KA, Lydon S, Madden C, et al. Hand hygiene compliance in the ICU: a systematic review. Crit Care Med 2019;47(9):1251–7.

62. Mills JP, Zhu Z, Mantey J, et al. The devil is in the details: factors influencing hand hygiene adherence and contamination with antibiotic-resistant organisms among healthcare providers in nursing facilities. Infect Control Hosp Epidemiol 2019;40(12):1394–9.

63. Teesing GR, Erasmus V, Nieboer D, et al. Increased hand hygiene compliance in nursing homes after a multimodal intervention: a cluster randomized controlled trial (HANDSOME). Infect Control Hosp Epidemiol 2020;41(10):1169–77.

64. Chang NC, Reisinger HS, Jesson AR, et al. Feasibility of monitoring compliance to the My 5 Moments and Entry/Exit hand hygiene methods in US hospitals. Am J Infect Control 2016;44(8):938–40.

65. Cure L, Van Enk R. Effect of hand sanitizer location on hand hygiene compliance. Am J Infect Control 2015;43(9):917–21.

66. Scherer AM, Reisinger HS, Goto M, et al. Testing a novel audit and feedback method for hand hygiene compliance: a multicenter quality improvement study. Infect Control Hosp Epidemiol 2019;40(1):89–94.

67. Le CD, Lehman EB, Nguyen TH, et al. Hand hygiene compliance study at a large central hospital in Vietnam. Int J Environ Res Public Health 2019;16(4):607.

68. Kingston L, O'Connell NH, Dunne CP. Hand hygiene-related clinical trials reported since 2010: a systematic review. J Hosp Infect 2016;92(4):309–20.

69. Leis JA, Powis JE, McGeer A, et al. Introduction of group electronic monitoring of hand hygiene on inpatient units: a multicenter cluster randomized quality improvement study. Clin Infect Dis 2020;71:e680–5.

70. Sickbert-Bennett EE, DiBiase LM, Willis TM, et al. Reduction of healthcare-associated infections by exceeding high compliance with hand hygiene practices. Emerg Infect Dis 2016;22(9):1628–30.

71. Edmisten C, Hall C, Kernizan L, et al. Implementing an electronic hand hygiene monitoring system: lessons learned from community hospitals. Am J Infect Control 2017;45(8):860–5.

72. Doll ME, Masroor N, Cooper K, et al. A comparison of the accuracy of two electronic hand hygiene monitoring systems. Infect Control Hosp Epidemiol 2019; 40(10):1194–7.

73. Knepper BC, Miller AM, Young HL. Impact of an automated hand hygiene monitoring system combined with a performance improvement intervention on hospital-acquired infections. Infect Control Hosp Epidemiol 2020;41(8):931–7.

74. Pong S, Holliday P, Fernie G. Effect of electronic real-time prompting on hand hygiene behaviors in health care workers. Am J Infect Control 2018;46(7): 768–74.

75. Pong S, Holliday P, Fernie G. Secondary measures of hand hygiene performance in health care available with continuous electronic monitoring of individuals. Am J Infect Control 2019;47(1):38–44.

76. Kerbaj J, Toure Y, Soto AA, et al. Smartphone text message service to foster hand hygiene compliance in health care workers. Am J Infect Control 2017; 45(3):234–9.

77. Hagel S, Trodvjlr J, Kesselmeier M, et al. Quantifying the Hawthorne effect in hand hygiene compliance through comparing direct observation with automated hand hygiene monitoring. Infect Control Hosp Epidemiol 2015;36: 957–62.

78. Boyce JM. Electronic monitoring in combination with direct observation as a means to significantly improve hand hygiene compliance. Am J Infect Control 2017;45:528–35.

79. Jeanes A, Coen PG, Gould DJ, et al. Validity of hand hygiene compliance measurement by observation: a systematic review. Am J Infect Control 2019;47(3): 313–22.

80. Reisinger HS, Yin J, Radonovich L, et al. Comprehensive survey of hand hygiene measurement and improvement practices in the Veterans Health Administration. Am J Infect Control 2013;41(11):989–93.

81. McCalla S, Reilly M, Thomas R, et al. An automated hand hygiene compliance system is associated with improved monitoring of hand hygiene. Am J Infect Control 2017;45(5):492–7.

82. Sunkesula VC, Meranda D, Kundrapu S, et al. Comparison of hand hygiene monitoring using the 5 moments for hand hygiene method versus a wash in-wash out method. Am J Infect Control 2015;43(1):16–9.

83. Boyce JM, Laughman JA, Ader MH, et al. Impact of an automated hand hygiene monitoring system and additional promotional activities on hand hygiene performance rates and healthcare-associated infections. Infect Control Hosp Epidemiol 2019;40(7):741–7.

84. Fisher DA, Seetoh T, Oh May-Lin H, et al. Automated measures of hand hygiene compliance among healthcare workers using ultrasound: validation and a randomized controlled trial. Infect Control Hosp Epidemiol 2013;34(9):919–28.

85. Nayyar D, Moore C, McCreight L, et al. Hand hygiene opportunities on Canadian acute-care inpatient units: a multicenter observational study. Infect Control Hosp Epidemiol 2018;39(11):1378–80.

86. Monsalve MN, Pemmaraju SV, Thomas GW, et al. Do peer effects improve hand hygiene adherence among healthcare workers? Infect Control Hosp Epidemiol 2014;35(10):1277–85.

87. Ellison RT III, Barysauskas CM, Rundensteiner EA, et al. A prospective controlled trial of an electronic hand hygiene reminder system. Open Forum Infect Dis 2015;2:ofv121.

88. Michael H, Einloth C, Fatica C, et al. Durable improvement in hand hygiene compliance following implementation of an automated observation system with visual feedback. Am J Infect Control 2017;45(3):311–3.

89. Yin J, Schacht Reisinger H, Vander Weg M, et al. Establishing evidence-based criteria for directly observed hand hygiene compliance monitoring programs: a prospective, multicenter cohort study. Infect Control Hosp Epidemiol 2014;35: 1163–8.

90. World Health OWPS. A guide to the implementation of the WHO multimodal hand hygiene improvement strategy. World Health Organization; 2009. Available at: https://apps.who.int/iris/handle/10665/70030. Accessed January 14, 2021.

91. Dhar S, Tansek R, Toftey EA, et al. Observer bias in hand hygiene compliance reporting. Infect Control Hosp Epidemiol 2010;31(8):869–70.

92. Chen LF, Carriker C, Staheli R, et al. Observing and improving hand hygiene compliance: implementation and refinement of an electronic-assisted direct-observer hand hygiene audit program. Infect Control Hosp Epidemiol 2013; 34(2):207–10.

93. Brotfain E, Livshiz-Riven I, Gushansky A, et al. Monitoring the hand hygiene compliance of health care workers in a general intensive care unit: use of continuous closed circle television versus overt observation. Am J Infect Control 2017; 45(8):849–54.

94. Werzen A, Thom KA, Robinson GL, et al. Comparing brief, covert, directly observed hand hygiene compliance monitoring to standard methods: a multi-center cohort study. Am J Infect Control 2019;47(3):346–8.

95. Srigley JA, Furness CD, Baker GR, et al. Quantification of the Hawthorne effect in hand hygiene compliance monitoring using an electronic monitoring system: a retrospective cohort study. BMJ Qual Saf 2014;23:974–80.

96. Filho MA, Marra AR, Magnus TP, et al. Comparison of human and electronic observation for the measurement of compliance with hand hygiene. Am J Infect Control 2014;42(11):1188–92.

97. Vaisman A, Bannerman G, Matelski J, et al. Out of sight, out of mind: a prospective observational study to estimate the duration of the Hawthorne effect on hand hygiene events. BMJ Qual Saf 2020;29(11):932–8.

98. Scheithauer S, Bickenbach J, Heisel H, et al. Do WiFi-based hand hygiene dispenser systems increase hand hygiene compliance? Am J Infect Control 2018;46(10):1192–4.

99. Steed C, Kelly JW, Blackhurst D, et al. Hospital hand hygiene opportunities: where and when (HOW2)? The HOW2 Benchmark Study. Am J Infect Control 2011;39(1):19–26.

100. Azim S, Juergens C, Hines J, et al. Introducing automated hand hygiene surveillance to an Australian hospital: Mirroring the HOW2 Benchmark Study. Am J Infect Control 2016;44(7):772–6.

101. Kwok YL, Juergens CP, McLaws ML. Automated hand hygiene auditing with and without an intervention. Am J Infect Control 2016;44(12):1475–80.

102. Diller T, Kelly JW, Blackhurst D, et al. Estimation of hand hygiene opportunities on an adult medical ward using 24-hour camera surveillance: validation of the HOW2 Benchmark Study. Am J Infect Control 2014;42(6):602–7.

103. Conway LJ, Riley L, Saiman L, et al. Implementation and impact of an automated group monitoring and feedback system to promote hand hygiene among health care personnel. Jt Comm J Qual Patient Saf 2014;40(9):408–17.

104. Limper HM, Slawsky L, Garcia-Houchins S, et al. Assessment of an aggregate-level hand hygiene monitoring technology for measuring hand hygiene performance among healthcare personnel. Infect Control Hosp Epidemiol 2017; 38(3):348–52.

105. Moore LD, Robbins G, Quinn J, et al. The impact of COVID-19 pandemic on hand hygiene performance in hospitals. Am J Infect Control 2021;49(1):30–3.

106. Arbogast JW, Moore L, Clark T, et al. Who goes in and out of patient rooms? An observational study of room entries and exits in the acute care setting. Am J Infect Control 2019;47(5):585–7.

107. Brouqui P, Boudjema S, Soto Aladro A, et al. New approaches to prevent healthcare-associated infection. Clin Infect Dis 2017;65(suppl_1):S50–4.
108. Pineles LL, Morgan DJ, Limper HM, et al. Accuracy of a radiofrequency identification (RFID) badge system to monitor hand hygiene behavior during routine clinical activities. Am J Infect Control 2014;42(2):144–7.
109. Boyce JM, Cooper T, Yin J, et al. Challenges encountered and lessons learned during a trial of an electronic hand hygiene monitoring system. Am J Infect Control 2019;47(12):1443–8.
110. Boudjema S, Tarantini C, Peretti-Watel P, et al. Merging video coaching and an anthropologic approach to understand health care provider behavior toward hand hygiene protocols. Am J Infect Control 2017;45(5):487–91.
111. Armellino D, Hussain E, Schilling ME, et al. Using high-technology to enforce low-technology safety measures: the use of third-party remote video auditing and real-time feedback in healthcare. Clin Infect Dis 2012;54(1):1–7.
112. Armellino D, Trivedi M, Law I, et al. Replicating changes in hand hygiene in a surgical intensive care unit with remote video auditing and feedback. Am J Infect Control 2013;41(10):925–7.
113. Yeung S, Downing NL, Fei-Fei L, et al. Bedside computer vision - moving artificial intelligence from driver assistance to patient safety. N Engl J Med 2018; 378(14):1271–3.
114. Larson EL, Murray MT, Cohen B, et al. Behavioral interventions to reduce infections in pediatric long-term care facilities: the keep it clean for kids trial. Behav Med 2018;44(2):141–50.
115. Limper HM, Garcia-Houchins S, Slawsky L, et al. A validation protocol: assessing the accuracy of hand hygiene monitoring technology. Infect Control Hosp Epidemiol 2016;37(8):1002–4.
116. McCalla S, Reilly M, Thomas R, et al. An automated hand hygiene compliance system is associated with decreased rates of healthcare-associated infections. Am J Infect Control 2018;46(12):1381–6.
117. Tarantini C, Brouqui P, Wilson R, et al. Healthcare workers' attitudes towards hand-hygiene monitoring technology. J Hosp Infect 2019;102(4):413–8.
118. Meng M, Sorber M, Herzog A, et al. Technological innovations in infection control: a rapid review of the acceptance of behavior monitoring systems and their contribution to the improvement of hand hygiene. Am J Infect Control 2019; 47(4):439–47.
119. Allegranzi B, Harbarth S, Pittet D. Effect of hand hygiene on infection rates. In: Pittet D, Boyce JM, Allegranzi B, editors. Hand hygiene: a handbook for medical professionals. Hoboken, NJ: Wiley-Blackwell; 2017. p. 299–316.

Disinfection and Sterilization in Health Care Facilities: An Overview and Current Issues

William A. Rutala, PhD, MPH[a],*, David J. Weber, MD, MPH[a,b]

KEYWORDS

- Disinfection • Sterilization • High-level disinfection • Disinfectants
- Room decontamination

KEY POINTS

- The level of disinfection or sterilization is dependent on the intended use of the object: critical (items that contact sterile tissue, such as surgical instrument); semicritical (items that contact mucous membranes, such as endoscopes), and noncritical (items that contact only intact skin, such as stethoscopes) require sterilization, high-level disinfection, or low-level disinfection, respectively.
- Current disinfection and sterilization guidelines must be strictly followed.
- Staff should receive training on reprocessing of medical and surgical equipment and be competency tested.
- Failure to properly disinfect semicritical devices used in health care (eg, endoscopes) has led to many outbreaks.
- New disinfection and sterilization technologies and practices could reduce the risk of infection associated with devices and surfaces.

INTRODUCTION

Each year in the United States, there are approximately 53,000,000 outpatient surgical procedures and 46,000,000 inpatient surgical procedures.[1] For example, there are at least 18 million gastrointestinal (GI) endoscopies per year.[2] Each of these procedures involves contact by a medical device or surgical instrument with a patient's sterile tissue and/or mucous membranes. A major risk of all such procedures is the introduction of infection. Failure to properly disinfect or sterilize medical devices and surgical instruments may lead to transmission via these devices (eg, endoscopes contaminated with carbapenem-resistant *Enterobacterales* [CRE]).[3]

[a] Division of Infectious Diseases, University of North Carolina School of Medicine, Chapel Hill, NC 27599-7030, USA; [b] Hospital Epidemiology, University of North Carolina Health, Chapel Hill, NC 27514, USA
* Corresponding author. Division of Infectious Diseases, Bioinformatics, UNC at Chapel Hill, 130 Mason Farm Road, Chapel Hill, NC 27599-7030.
E-mail address: brutala@med.unc.edu

Infect Dis Clin N Am 35 (2021) 575–607
https://doi.org/10.1016/j.idc.2021.04.004
0891-5520/21/© 2021 Elsevier Inc. All rights reserved.
id.theclinics.com

Achieving disinfection and sterilization through the use of disinfectants and sterilization practices is essential for ensuring that medical and surgical instruments do not transmit infectious pathogens to patients. Because it is unnecessary to sterilize all patient care items, health care policies must identify whether cleaning, disinfection, high-level disinfection (HLD), or sterilization is indicated based primarily on the items' intended use.

Multiple studies in many countries have documented lack of compliance with established guidelines for disinfection and sterilization.[4–6] Failure to comply with scientifically based guidelines has led to numerous outbreaks.[7] In this article, which is an update of previous publications,[8–17] a pragmatic approach to the judicious selection and proper use of disinfection and sterilization processes is presented, based on well-designed studies assessing the efficacy (via laboratory investigations) and effectiveness (via clinical studies) of disinfection and sterilization procedures.

RATIONAL APPROACH TO DISINFECTION AND STERILIZATION

More than 50 years ago, Earle H. Spaulding[18] devised a rational approach to disinfection and sterilization of patient care items or equipment. This classification scheme is so clear and logical that it has been retained, refined, and used successfully by infection control professionals and others when planning methods for disinfection or sterilization.[8–14,17–20] Spaulding believed that the nature of disinfection could be understood more readily if instruments and items for patient care were divided into 3 categories based on the degree of risk of infection involved in the use of the items. Although the scheme remains valid, there are some examples of disinfection studies with viruses, mycobacteria, and protozoa as well as disinfectants that challenge the current definitions and expectations of high-level and low-level disinfection.[21] The 3 categories Spaulding described were critical, semicritical, and noncritical.

Critical Items

Critical items are so called because of the high risk of infection if such an item is contaminated with any microorganism, including bacterial spores. Thus, it is critical that objects that enter sterile tissue or the vascular system be sterile because any microbial contamination could result in disease transmission. This category includes surgical instruments, cardiac and urinary catheters, implants, arthroscopes, laparoscopes, and ultrasound probes used in sterile body cavities. Most of the items in this category should be purchased as sterile or be sterilized by steam sterilization if possible. If heat-sensitive, the object may be treated with ethylene oxide (ETO), hydrogen peroxide gas plasma (HPGP), vaporized hydrogen peroxide (VHP), hydrogen peroxide vapor plus ozone, or liquid chemical sterilants if other methods are unsuitable. **Tables 1–3** summarize sterilization processes and liquid chemical sterilants and the advantages and disadvantages of each. Sterilization technologies can be relied on to produce sterility only if cleaning, to reduce or eliminate the organic and inorganic material as well as microbial load, precedes treatment.[22–24] Other issues that sterile reprocessing and operating room professionals must deal with when reprocessing instruments include weight limits for instrument trays, wet packs, packaging, loaned instruments, cleaning monitoring, and water quality.[25,26]

Semicritical Items

Semicritical items are those that come in contact with intact mucous membranes or nonintact skin. Respiratory therapy and anesthesia equipment, some endoscopes, laryngoscope blades and handles,[27–29] esophageal manometry probes, endocavitary

Table 1
Methods for high-level disinfection and sterilization of medical and surgical instruments

Process	Level of Microbial Inactivation	Method	Examples (with Processing Times)	Health Care Application (Examples)
Sterilization[a]	Destroys all microorganisms, including bacterial spores	High temperature	Steam (~40 min), dry heat (1–6 h depending on temperature)	Heat-tolerant critical (surgical instruments) and semicritical patient care items
		Low temperature	ETO gas (~15 h), HPGP (28–38 min, NX), hydrogen peroxide and ozone (46–60 min, VP4), hydrogen peroxide vapor (28–55 min, V-Pro MAX)	Heat-sensitive critical and semicritical patient care items
		Liquid immersion	Chemical sterilants[b]: >2% glut (10 h at 20°C –25°C); 1.12% glut with 1.93% phenol (12 h at 25°C); 7.35% HP with 0.23% PA (3 h at 20°C); 7.5% HP (6 h at 20°C); 1.0% HP with 0.08% PA (8 h at 20°C); ~0.2% PA (6 min at 46–55°C)	Heat-sensitive critical and semicritical patient care items that can be immersed
HLD	Destroys all microorganisms except some bacterial spores	Heat-automated	Pasteurization (65°C–77°C, 30 min)	Heat-sensitive semicritical items (eg, respiratory therapy equipment)
		Liquid immersion	Chemical sterilants/HLDs[b]: >2% glut (20–90 min at 20°C–25°C); 2.5% glut (5 min at 35°C); 0.55% OPA (12 min at 20°C); 1.12% glut with 1.93% phenol (20 min at 25°C); 7.35% HP with 0.23% PA (15 min at 20°C); 7.5% HP (30 min at 20°C); 1.0% HP with 0.08% PA (25 min at 20°C); 400–450 free chlorine (10 min at 30°C); 2.0% HP (8 min at 20°C); 3.4% glut with 20.1% isopropanol (5 min at 25°C)	Heat-sensitive semicritical items (eg, GI endoscopes, bronchoscopes, and endocavitary probes)

Abbreviations: glut, glutaraldehyde; HP, hydrogen peroxide; OPA, ortho-phthalaldehyde; PA, peracetic acid.
 [a] Prions (such as CJD) exhibit an unusual resistance to conventional chemical and physical decontamination methods and are not readily inactivated by conventional sterilization procedures.
 [b] Consult the FDA-cleared package insert for information about the cleared contact time and temperature, and see reference[32] for discussion why greater than 2% glut products are used at a reduced exposure time (2% glut at 20 min, 20°C). Increasing the temperature using an automated endoscope reprocess reduces the contact time (eg, OPA 12 min at 20°C but 5 min at 25°C in automated endoscope reprocess). Exposure temperatures for some HLDs varies from 20°C to 25°C; check FDA-cleared temperature conditions.[32] Tubing must be completely filled for HLD and liquid chemical sterilization. Material compatibility should be investigated when appropriate (for example, HP and HP with PA may cause functional damage to endoscopes).
Data from Refs.[8–17,169]

Table 2
Summary of advantages and disadvantages of commonly used sterilization technologies

Sterilization Method	Advantages	Disadvantages
Steam	• Nontoxic to patient, staff, environment • Cycle easy to control and monitor • Rapidly microbicidal • Least affected by organic/inorganic soils among sterilization processes listed • Rapid cycle time • Penetrates medical packing, device lumens	• Deleterious for heat-sensitive instruments • Microsurgical instruments damaged by repeated exposure • May leave instruments wet, causing them to rust • Potential for burns
HPGP	• Safe for the environment and HCP • Leaves no toxic residuals • Cycle time is 28–38 min and no aeration necessary • Used for heat-sensitive and moisture-sensitive items because process temperature <50°C • Simple to operate, install (208-V outlet), and monitor • Compatible with most medical devices • Requires only electrical outlet • Microbicidal efficacy data	• Cellulose (paper), linens, and liquids cannot be processed • Endoscope or medical device restrictions based on lumen internal diameter and length (see manufacturer's recommendations) (eg, single-channel and dual-channel device with stainless steel lumen that is ≥1.0 mm internal diameter and ≤150 mm in length) • Requires synthetic packaging (polypropylene wraps and polyolefin pouches) and special container tray • Hydrogen peroxide may be toxic at levels >1 ppm TWA • Organic matter reduces microbicidal activity
100% ETO (gas blends phased out in 2015)	• Penetrates packaging materials, device lumens • Single-dose cartridge and negative-pressure chamber minimizes the potential for gas leak and ETO exposure • Simple to operate and monitor • Compatible with most medical materials	• Requires aeration time to remove ETO residue • ETO is toxic, a probable carcinogen, and flammable • ETO emission regulated by states/countries. Catalytic converters and acid water scrubbers reduce ETO emissions. • ETO cartridges should be stored in flammable liquid storage cabinet • Lengthy cycle/aeration time • Organic matter reduces microbicidal activity

VHP	• Safe for the environment and HCP • It leaves no toxic residue; no aeration necessary • Cycle time, 28–55 min • Used for heat-sensitive and moisture-sensitive items (metal and nonmetal devices)	• Medical devices restrictions based on lumen internal diameter and length—see manufacturer's recommendations, (eg, single-channel device with stainless steel lumen that is ≥0.7 mm internal diameter and ≤500 mm in length) • Not used for liquid, linens, powders, or any cellulose materials • Requires synthetic packaging (polypropylene) • Limited materials compatibility data • Limited clinical use data • Limited comparative microbicidal efficacy data • Organic matter reduces microbicidal activity
Hydrogen peroxide and ozone	• Safe for the environment and HCP • Uses dual sterilants, hydrogen peroxide, and ozone • No aeration needed due to no toxic byproducts • Compatible with common medical devices • Cycle time, 46–70 min • FDA cleared for general instruments and multichannel flexible endoscopes (see manufacturer's instructions)	• Endoscope or medical device restrictions based on lumen internal diameter and length (see manufacturer's recommendations) (eg, single-channel and dual-channel device with stainless steel lumen that is ≥0.7 mm internal diameter and ≤500 mm in length) • Limited clinical use data • Limited materials compatibility data • Limited microbicidal efficacy data • Requires synthetic packaging (polypropylene wraps, polyolefin pouches) and special container tray • Organic matter reduces microbicidal activity

Abbreviation: TWA, time-weighted average.
Data from Refs.[8–17]

Table 3
Summary of advantages and disadvantages of chemical agents used as chemical sterilants or as high-level disinfectants

Sterilization Method	Advantages	Disadvantages
Peracetic acid/ hydrogen peroxide	• No activation required	• Material compatibility concerns (lead, brass, copper, and zinc) both cosmetic and functional • Limited clinical experience • Mucous membrane and respiratory health effects • Potential for eye and skin damage
Glutaraldehyde	• Numerous use studies published • Relatively inexpensive • Excellent material compatibility	• Respiratory irritation from glutaraldehyde vapor • Pungent and irritating odor • Relatively slow mycobactericidal activity (unless other disinfectants added, such as phenolic, alcohol) • Coagulates blood and fixes tissue to surfaces • Allergic contact dermatitis • ACGIH recommends limiting employee exposure to ceiling concentration of 0.05 ppm
Hydrogen peroxide (standard)	• No activation required • May enhance removal of organic matter and organisms • No disposal issues • No odor or irritation issues • Does not coagulate blood or fix tissues to surfaces • Inactivates *Cryptosporidium* at 6%–7.5% • Use studies published	• Material compatibility concerns (brass, zinc, copper, and nickel/ silver plating) both cosmetic and functional • Serious eye damage with contact
OPA	• Fast-acting HLDs • No activation required • Odor not significant • Excellent materials compatibility claimed • Does not coagulate blood or fix tissues to surfaces claimed • Relatively rapid mycobactericidal activity	• Stains protein gray (eg, skin, mucous membranes, clothing, and environmental surfaces) • More expensive than glutaraldehyde • Eye irritation with contact • Slow sporicidal activity • Anaphylactic reactions to OPA in bladder cancer patients with repeated exposure to OPA through cystoscopy

Peracetic acid	• Standardized cycle (eg, liquid chemical sterilant processing system using peracetic acid, rinsed with extensively treated potable water) • Low temperature (50°C–55°C) liquid immersion sterilization • Environmentally friendly by-products (acetic acid, O_2, H_2O) • Fully automated • Single-use system eliminates need for concentration testing • May enhance removal of organic material and endotoxin • No adverse health effects to operators under normal operating conditions • Compatible with many materials and instruments • Does not coagulate blood or fix tissues to surfaces • Sterilant flows through scope facilitating salt, protein, and microbe removal • Rapidly sporicidal • Provides procedure standardization (constant dilution, perfusion of channel, temperatures, exposure)	• Potential material incompatibility (eg, aluminum anodized coating becomes dull) • Used for immersible instruments only • Biological indicator may not be suitable for routine monitoring • One scope or a small number of instruments can be processed in a cycle • More expensive (endoscope repairs, operating costs, purchase costs) than HLD • Serious eye and skin damage (concentrated solution) with contact • Point-of-use system, no sterile storage • An automated endoscope reprocessor using 0.2% peracetic acid not FDA-cleared as sterilization process but HLD
Improved hydrogen peroxide (2.0%); HLDs	• No activation required • No odor • Nonstaining • No special venting requirements • Manual or automated applications • 12-mo shelf life, 14-d reuse • 8 min at 20°C HLDs claim	• Material compatibility concerns due to limited clinical experience • Organic material resistance concerns due to limited data

All products effective in presence of organic soil, relatively easy to use, and have a broad spectrum of antimicrobial activity (bacteria, fungi, viruses, bacterial spores, and mycobacteria). These characteristics are documented in the literature; contact the manufacturer of the instrument and HLDs/chemical sterilant for additional information. All products listed above are FDA-cleared as chemical sterilants except OPA and 2% accelerated hydrogen peroxide, which are FDA-cleared, HLD.

Abbreviation: ACGIH, American Conference of Governmental Industrial Hygienists.

Data from Refs.[8–17]

probes, nasopharyngoscopes, prostate biopsy probes,[30] infrared coagulation device,[31] anorectal manometry catheters, cystoscopes, and diaphragm fitting rings are included in this category.[27,28] These medical devices should be free of all microorganisms, although small numbers of bacterial spores may be present. The US Food and Drug Administration (FDA) definition of HLD is a sterilant used for a shorter contact time to achieve at least a 6-$\log_{10}$ kill of an appropriate *Mycobacterium* species. Cleaning followed by HLD should eliminate all pathogens capable of causing infection. Intact mucous membranes, such as those of the lungs or the GI tract, generally are resistant to infection by common bacterial spores but susceptible to other organisms, such as bacteria, mycobacteria, and viruses. Semicritical items minimally require HLD using chemical disinfectants. Glutaraldehyde, hydrogen peroxide, OPA, peracetic acid, hypochlorite (via superoxidized water), and peracetic acid with hydrogen peroxide are cleared by the FDA[32] and are dependable HLDs provided the factors influencing germicidal procedures are met (see **Tables 1** and **3**). When a disinfectant is selected for use with certain patient care items, the chemical compatibility after extended use with the items to be disinfected also must be considered.

Noncritical Items

Noncritical items are those that come in contact with intact skin but not mucous membranes. Intact skin acts as an effective barrier to most microorganisms; therefore, the sterility of items coming in contact with intact skin is "not critical." Examples of noncritical items are bedpans, blood pressure cuffs, crutches, bed rails, bedside tables, patient furniture, toys,[33] portable equipment (eg, wheel chairs, infusion pumps, pulse oximeters, and medication carts),[34,35] and floors.[36,37] The 5 noncritical items touched most commonly in the patient environment have been quantitatively shown to be bed rails, bed surface, supply cart, overbed table, and intravenous (IV) pump.[38] In contrast to critical and some semicritical items, most noncritical reusable items may be decontaminated where they are used and do not need to be transported to a central processing area. Noncritical items can be involved in indirect transmission. There is virtually no documented risk of transmitting infectious agents to patients via noncritical items[39] when they are used as noncritical items and do not contact nonintact skin and/or mucous membranes. These items (eg, ophthalmic equipment, bedside tables, and bed rails), however, potentially could contribute to secondary or indirect transmission by contaminating hands of health care personnel (HCP) or by contact with medical equipment that subsequently comes in contact with patients.[40] For example, an adenovirus outbreak occurred when provider-owned, contaminated handheld ophthalmologic equipment (ie, lenses or indirect ophthaloscope) was used in a neonatal intensive care unit for ophthalmic examinations. The variability in disinfecting the ophthalmic equipment and infection prevention practices (eg, glove use and inadequate hand hygiene) contributed to infants developing adenovirus infection. The implicated equipment was held or touched by providers' hands but did not contact patients directly.[41] **Table 4** lists several low-level disinfectants that may be used for noncritical items. Some Environmental Protection Agency (EPA)-registered liquid disinfectants have a 10-minute label claim. Multiple investigators have demonstrated, however, the effectiveness of these disinfectants against vegetative bacteria, yeasts, mycobacteria, and viruses at exposure times of 30 seconds to 60 seconds.[9,42–47] Thus, it is acceptable to disinfect noncritical medical equipment (eg, blood pressure cuff) and noncritical surfaces (eg, bedside table) with an EPA-registered disinfectant or disinfectant/detergent at the proper use dilution and a contact time of approximately 1 minute.[9,48,49] Because the typical drying time for a liquid disinfectant on a surface is 1 minute to 2 minutes (unless the product contains alcohol [eg, a 60%–

Table 4
Summary of advantages and disadvantages of disinfectants used as low-level disinfectants

Disinfectant Active	Advantages	Disadvantages
Alcohol	• Bactericidal, tuberculocidal, fungicidal, virucidal • Fast acting • Noncorrosive • Nonstaining • Easy to use • Used to disinfect small surfaces, such as rubber stoppers on medication vials[170] • No toxic residue	• Not sporicidal • Affected by organic matter • Slow acting against nonenveloped viruses (eg, norovirus) • No detergent or cleaning properties • Not EPA registered • Damage some instruments (eg, harden rubber, deteriorate glue) • Flammable (large amounts require special storage) • Evaporates rapidly making contact time compliance difficult • Not recommended for use on large surfaces • Outbreaks ascribed to contaminated alcohol[171]
Sodium hypochlorite	• Bactericidal, tuberculocidal, fungicidal, virucidal • Sporicidal • Fast acting • Inexpensive (in dilutable form) • Not flammable • Unaffected by water hardness • Reduces biofilms on surfaces • Relatively stable (eg, 50% reduction in chlorine concentration in 30 d)[172] • Used as the disinfectant in water treatment • EPA registered	• Reaction hazard with acids and ammonias • Leaves salt residue • Corrosive to metals (some ready-to-use products may be formulated with corrosion inhibitors) • Unstable active (some ready-to-use products may be formulated with stabilizers to achieve longer shelf life) • Affected by organic matter • Discolors/stains fabrics • Potential hazard is production of trihalomethane • Odor (some ready-to-use products may be formulated with odor inhibitors). Irritating at high concentrations

(continued on next page)

Table 4
(continued)

Disinfectant Active	Advantages	Disadvantages
Improved hydrogen peroxide	• Bactericidal, tuberculocidal, fungicidal, virucidal • Fast efficacy • Easy compliance with wet-contact times • Safe for workers (lowest EPA toxicity category, IV) • Benign for the environment • Surface compatible • Nonstaining • EPA registered • Not flammable	• More expensive that most other low-level disinfecting actives • Not sporicidal at low concentrations
Iodophors	• Bactericidal, tuberculocidal, virucidal • Not flammable • Used for disinfecting blood culture bottles	• Not sporicidal • Shown to degrade silicone catheters • Requires prolonged contact to kill fungi • Stains surfaces • Used mainly as an antiseptic rather than disinfectant
Phenolics	• Bactericidal, tuberculocidal, fungicidal, virucidal • Inexpensive (in dilutable form) • Nonstaining • Not flammable • EPA registered	• Not sporicidal • Absorbed by porous materials and irritate tissue • Depigmentation of skin caused by certain phenolics • Hyperbilirubinemia in infants when phenolic not prepared as recommended
Quaternary ammonium compounds (eg, didecyldimethylammonium bromide, dioctyldimethylammonium bromide)	• Bactericidal, fungicidal, virucidal against enveloped viruses (eg, HIV) • Good cleaning agents • EPA registered • Surface compatible • Persistent antimicrobial activity when undisturbed • Inexpensive (in dilutable form)	• Not sporicidal • In general, not tuberculocidal and virucidal against nonenveloped viruses • High water hardness and cotton/gauze can make less microbicidal • A few reports documented asthma as result of exposure to benzalkonium chloride. • Affected by organic matter • Absorption by cotton, some wipes • Multiple outbreaks ascribed to contaminated benzalkonium chloride[171]

| Peracetic acid/ hydrogen peroxide | • Bactericidal, fungicidal, virucidal and sporicidal (eg, C difficile)
• Active in the presence of organic material
• Environmentally friendly by-products (acetic acid, O_2, H_2O)
• EPA registered
• Surface compatible | • Lack of stability
• Potential for material incompatibility (eg, brass, copper)
• More expensive than most other disinfecting actives
• Odor may be irritating
• Can cause mucous membrane and respiratory health effects |

If low-level disinfectant is prepared on-site (not ready-to-use), document correct concentration at a routine frequency.
Data from Refs.[8–17]

70% alcohol dries in approximately 30 seconds]), 1 application of the germicide on all hand contact or touchable surfaces to be disinfected is recommended.

Hospital cleanliness continues to attract patient attention, and, in the United States, it still is assessed primarily via visual appearance, which is not a reliable indicator of surface cleanliness.[50] Three other methods have been offered for monitoring patient room hygiene and they include adenosine triphosphate (ATP) bioluminescence,[51,52] fluorescent markers,[53-55] and microbiologic sampling. Studies have demonstrated suboptimal cleaning by aerobic colony counts as well as the use of the ATP biolumi-nescence and fluorescent markers.[51,55] ATP bioluminescence and fluorescent markers are preferred to aerobic plate counts because they provide an immediate assessment of cleaning effectiveness. When the 4 major hospital cleaning validation methods (ie, visual, microbiological, ATP, and fluorescence) were compared, the fluo-rescent marker was the most useful tool in determining how thoroughly a surface was cleaned and mimics the microbiological data better than ATP (<500 relative light units). There was no statistical correlation between ATP levels and standard aerobic plate counts.[56,57]

STERILIZATION OF CRITICAL ITEMS

Most medical and surgical devices used in health care facilities are made of materials that are heat stable and thus are sterilized by heat, primarily steam sterilization. Since 1950, however, there has been an increase in medical devices and instruments made of materials (eg, plastics) that require low-temperature sterilization. ETO gas has been used since the 1950s for heat-sensitive and moisture-sensitive medical devices. Within the past 25 years, several new, low-temperature sterilization systems (eg, HPGP, VHP, and hydrogen peroxide plus ozone) have been developed and are used to sterilize medical devices.[9] A summary of the advantages and disadvantages for commonly used sterilization technologies is presented in **Table 2**.

Sterilization destroys all microorganisms on the surface of an article or in a fluid to prevent disease transmission associated with the use of that item. Although the use of inadequately sterilized critical items represents a high risk of transmitting pathogens, documented transmission of pathogens associated with an inadequately sterilized critical item is exceedingly rare.[58-61] This likely is due to the extraordinary margin of safety associated with the sterilization processes used in health care facilities (eg, $17\text{-}\log_{10}$ margin of safety for surgical instruments).[62] The concept of what constitutes "sterile" is measured as a probability of sterility for each item to be sterilized (ie, sterility assurance level of 10^{-6}).[63,64]

Health care facilities must ensure there is a quality process in place to ensure the adequacy of HCP training, competency testing (at employment and at least annually), compliance with evidence-based guidelines and/or manufacturer's instructions for use (IFU), and appropriate and adequate space and equipment as well as appropriate process monitoring (eg, cleaning monitors) with documentation.[25,65] All areas that reprocess semicritical or critical patient care equipment should be audited to ensure they comply with evidence-based guidelines and/or manufacturer's IFU, and, if defi-ciencies are identified, they should be corrected.[66] If noncompliance of evidence-based guidelines occurs during reprocessing of critical and semicritical equipment, a patient risk assessment using a 15-step protocol can guide an institution in deter-mining if and how patients should be notified of the potential adverse event.[67,68]

CURRENT ISSUES IN STERILIZATION
Inactivation of Creutzfeldt-Jakob Disease Agent

Creutzfeldt-Jakob disease (CJD) is a degenerative neurologic disorder of humans with an incidence in the United States of approximately 1 case/million population/year.[69,70] CJD is thought to be caused by a proteinaceous infectious agent or prion. Prions are relatively resistant to conventional disinfection and sterilization procedures, and, because of the invariably fatal outcome of CJD, the procedures for disinfection and sterilization of the CJD prion have been both conservative and controversial for many years.[69,71–75]

The current prion recommendations consider inactivation data but also use epidemiologic studies of prion transmission, infectivity of human tissues, and efficacy of removing proteins by cleaning.[69,71,72,75,76] On the basis of scientific data, only critical (eg, surgical instruments) and semicritical devices contaminated with high-risk tissue (ie, brain, spinal cord, and eye tissue) from high-risk patients (eg, known or suspected infection with CJD or other prion disease) require special prion reprocessing. A moist environment post-contamination reduces the attachment of both protein and prion amyloid to the stainless steel surface so as to maintain moist conditions.[77] After a device is clean, it should be sterilized by either autoclaving (ie, steam sterilization) or using a combination of sodium hydroxide and autoclaving using one of these options: option 1—autoclave at 134°C for 18 minutes in a prevacuum sterilizer; option 2—autoclave at 132°C for 1 hour in a gravity displacement sterilizer; option 3—immerse in 1N NaOH for 1 hour, remove and rinse in water, and then transfer to an open pan and autoclave (121°C gravity displacement or 134°C porous or prevacuum sterilizer) for 1 hour; or option 4—immerse in 1N NaOH for 1 hour, heat in a gravity displacement at 121°C for 30 minutes, and then clean and subject to routine sterilization.[69,71–75] Prion-contaminated medical devices that are impossible or difficult to clean should be discarded. To minimize environmental contamination, noncritical environmental surfaces should be covered with plastic-backed paper, and, when contaminated with high-risk tissues, the paper should be discarded properly. Noncritical environmental surfaces (eg, laboratory surfaces) contaminated with high-risk tissues should be cleaned and then spot decontaminated with a 1:10 dilution of hypochlorite solutions.[69,75]

Robustness of Sterilization Technologies

Despite careful surgical instrument reprocessing, surgeons and other HCP describe cases in which surgical instruments have been contaminated with organic material (eg, blood). Alfred and coworkers[78] found decontamination problems in approximately 1% of surgical cases and approximately 50% of the contamination type reported by operating room staff was bioburden related (M Alfred, written communication, 2020). Although most of these cases of instrument contamination are observed before the instrument reaches the patient, in some cases the contaminated instrument contaminates the sterile field or, rarely, the patient. Studies have evaluated the robustness of sterilization technologies when spores and bacteria mixed with blood and placed on dirty (noncleaned) instruments or the impact of protein, salt, or lubricating oils were placed on the instrument.[22,24,79]

In 1 experiment, test carriers were inoculated with *Pseudomonas aeruginosa*, *Escherichia coli*, *Staphylococcus aureus*, vancomycin-resistant *Enterococcus* (VRE), *M terrae*, *Bacillus atrophaeus* spores, *Geobacillus stearothermophilus* spores, or *Clostridioides difficile* spores in the presence of salt and serum and then subjected to sterilization technologies (ie, steam, ETO, VHP, and HPGP). Steam, ETO, and the

HPGP sterilizers were capable of inactivating the test organisms on stainless steel carriers with a failure rate of 0% (0/220), 1.9% (6/310), and 1.9% (5/270), respectively. The failure rate for VHP was 76.3% (206/270).[24] One possible reason for this difference in failure rate is the theoretic concentration of hydrogen peroxide for HPGP is higher than VHP (ie, 25.6 mg/L vs 9.1 mg/L hydrogen peroxide for the HPGP and VHP, respectively).[80] Steam sterilization is the most effective and had the largest margin of safety, followed by ETO and HPGP and, lastly, VHP.[24] The data demonstrate how important cleaning is prior to sterilization because salt and organic matter left on instruments can interfere with low-temperature sterilization.[80] The issue of "how clean is clean enough" remains unresolved but various cleaning markers (eg, protein ≤ 6.4 μg/cm^2) on when to consider a device clean can be used by manufacturers when preparing reprocessing IFU.[81,82]

Effects of Sterilization on 3-Dimensional Printed Models/Instruments

Three-dimensional (3-D) imaging technologies are used in medicine and dentistry to guide surgeons preoperatively, and 3-D printed models have been used to plan surgeries in several fields, including dental implant surgery, cardiothoracic surgery, orthopedic surgery, neurologic surgery, and plastic surgery. Like other instruments used in surgery, these items must be sterile to avoid infection. At present, the data show that both plasma sterilization and steam sterilization at 121°C are suitable for sterilizing tested 3-D printed guides.[83,84]

Recent Developments with the Use of Ethylene Oxide for Sterilization of Medical Devices

There are more than 20 billion medical devices and health care products sold every year in the United States that are sterilized by ETO. This accounts for approximately half of the medical devices that require sterilization (Medical Device Manufacturers Association, February 2020). For more than 50,000 medical devices and health care products, ETO is the only sterilization modality that has been validated through extensive testing. Many, if not all, of the devices cannot be sterilized by another sterilization method (eg, radiation) because of the heat sensitive nature of the device, composition (eg, plastic), or internal cavities or channels. In October 2019, the FDA warned that without the availability of ETO as a sterilization method, there would be a shortage of essential and life-saving critical devices, such as drug-eluting cardiac stents, feeding tubes, surgical kits, catheters, shunts, and other implantable devices.[85,86]

At present, there are no readily available processes that can serve as an alternative to ETO for sterilization of medical devices. Although there are no solutions, there are several initiatives to reduce the infection risk (eg, identifying alternatives to ETO and strategies to reduce ETO emissions).[85–87]

HIGH-LEVEL DISINFECTION OF SEMICRITICAL ITEMS

Semicritical items are those that come in contact with mucous membranes or nonintact skin. Semicritical items minimally require HLD using chemical disinfectants. Glutaraldehyde, hydrogen peroxide, OPA, peracetic acid, and peracetic acid with hydrogen peroxide, and a chlorine-based system are cleared by the FDA[32] and are dependable HLDs provided the factors influencing germicidal procedures are met. **Table 3** lists the FDA-cleared HLDs and chemical sterilants with the advantages and disadvantages of each. The exposure time for most HLDs varies from 8 minutes to 45 minutes at 20°C to 25°C (see **Table 1**).[32] As with all disinfectants, sterilizers, and devices, users must be familiar with the manufacturer's IFU. When a disinfectant is selected for use with certain patient care items, the chemical compatibility after extended use with the items to be disinfected also must be considered. Disinfection strategies for some semicritical items (eg, applanation tonometers and rectal/vaginal probes) are highly variable.[88]

Because semicritical equipment has been associated with reprocessing errors that result in patient lookback and patient notifications, it is essential that control measures be instituted to prevent patient exposures.[67,68] Before new equipment (especially semicritical equipment, because the margin of safety is significantly less than that for sterilization)[89] is used for patient care on more than 1 patient, reprocessing procedures for that equipment should be developed. The FDA requests that the device manufacturer include at least 1 validated cleaning and disinfection/sterilization protocol in the labeling for their device. HCP should receive training on the safe use and reprocessing of the equipment and be competency tested. Infection prevention rounds or audits should be conducted at least annually in all clinical areas that reprocess critical and semicritical devices to ensure adherence to the reprocessing guidelines, manufacturers' IFU, and/or institutional policies.[90] Results of infection prevention rounds should be provided to the unit managers and deficiencies in reprocessing should be corrected and the corrective measures documented to infection prevention.

Semicritical items that have contact with mucous membranes of the GI tract or upper respiratory tract should be rinsed with sterile water or filtered water or tap water followed by an alcohol rinse.[9,91] An alcohol rinse and forced-air drying markedly reduces the likelihood of contamination of the instrument (eg, endoscope), most likely by removing the wet environment favorable for bacterial growth.[92] After rinsing, items should be dried and stored (eg, packaged or hung) in a manner that protects them from damage or contamination. Drying also retards biofilm formation.[61,93] Using an automated drying and storage cabinet, a recent article demonstrated that internal channels were dry at 1 hour and external surfaces at 3 hours. With the standard storage cabinet, there was residual internal fluid at 24 hours, whereas external surfaces were dry at 24 hours.[94] There is no recommendation to use sterile or filtered water rather than tap water for rinsing semicritical equipment that will have contact with the mucous membranes of the rectum (eg, rectal probes and anoscope) or vagina (eg, vaginal probes).[9]

Semicritical items represent the greatest risk of disease transmission because far more health care–associated infections have been caused by reusable semicritical items than critical or noncritical items.[27,28] There is virtually no documented risk of transmitting infectious agents to patients via noncritical items[39] when they are used as noncritical items and do not contact nonintact skin and/or mucous membranes. Similarly, critical items are rarely[60,61] associated with disease transmission. In contrast, semicritical items (eg, GI endoscopes) have been associated with more than 150 outbreaks (**Table 5**).

CURRENT ISSUES FOR HIGH-LEVEL DISINFECTION
Endoscopes: A Challenge to Achieve High-Level Disinfection

Physicians use endoscopes to diagnose and treat numerous medical disorders. Although endoscopes represent a valuable diagnostic and therapeutic tool in modern medicine and the incidence of infection associated with use has been reported as low, more health care–associated outbreaks have been linked to contaminated endoscopes than to any other medical device. Over the past few years alone, there have been greater than 25 outbreaks of multidrug-resistant organisms, such as CRE, in major hospitals in the United States and the world that have killed dozens of patients and

Table 5
Infections/outbreaks associated with semicritical medical devices

Instruments[a]	Outbreaks/ Infections (No.)	Outbreaks/ Infections with Blood-borne Pathogens (No.)
Vaginal probes	0[b]	0
Nasal endoscopes	0	0
Hysteroscopes	0	0
Laryngoscopes	2[173–175]	0
Urologic instrumentation (eg, cystoscopes, ureteroscopes)	8[176–183]	0
Transrectal–ultrasound-guided prostate probes	1[184]	0
Transesophageal echocardiogram	5[181,185–188]	0
Applanation tonometers	2[189,190]	
GI endoscopes/bronchoscopes	>130[4,6]	1 HBV[191] 2 HCV[192,193]

[a] These infections/outbreaks were found in the peer-reviewed literature through PubMed and Google.
[b] Does not include outbreaks associated with contaminated ultrasound gel used with vaginal probes or transmission via HCP.
Modified from Rutala WA, Weber DJ. Reprocessing semicritical items: Outbreaks and current issues. Am J Infect Control. 2019 Jun;47S:A79-A89; with permission.

caused morbidity in hundreds more.[6] These outbreaks have been linked primarily to contaminated duodenoscopes that are used to diagnose and treat disease of the liver, bile ducts, and pancreas. Nine of these outbreaks occurred despite appropriate cleaning and HLD.[28] Other GI endoscopes (eg, colonoscopes and gastroscopes) and bronchoscopes, however, have been associated with about 100 more outbreaks causing additional death and illness.[4] The key concern raised by these outbreaks is whether current endoscope reprocessing guidelines are adequate to ensure a patient-safe endoscope (ie, one devoid of potential pathogens) or if endoscopes with their long, narrow channels, right-angle turns, difficult to clean and disinfect components, heavy microbial and soil contamination, and possibly biofilm development (and removal)[95] make them impossible to achieve HLD.[28,96] Because GI endoscopes and bronchoscopes contact intact mucous membranes but frequently have contact with nonintact mucous membranes and sterile tissue, there is a risk of patient-to-patient transmission of potential pathogens with a subsequent risk of infection.

Efforts to reduce the risk associated with reprocessing of endoscopes (eg, double HLD) have not been successful.[97,98] The transition from HLD to sterilization would provide a safety margin of 10^6 for endoscope reprocessing because HLD results in a 6-$\log_{10}$ reduction and sterilization results in a 12-$\log_{10}$ reduction of spores. It also would allow compliance with the Spaulding scheme because although these instruments enter a mucous membrane they indirectly contact normally sterile tissue and should be classified as critical (eg, cystoscope [bladder], bronchoscope [lung], and duodenoscope [duodenum and bile ducts]).[62] The critical need and rationale for this transition from disinfection to sterilization for endoscopes have been discussed in various peer-reviewed publications, including *JAMA*, *American Journal of Infection Control*, and *Infection Control and Hospital Epidemiology*.[3,62,89,99] Recommendations for the cleaning and disinfection of endoscopic equipment have been published and should be followed strictly.[9,91]

Ultrasound Transducer Disinfection for Assessment and Insert of Peripheral and Central Catheters

At present, there are no reported infections associated with the practice of cleaning/disinfecting ultrasound probes used for the assessment and insertion of peripheral and central venous catheters. As a result, an intersocietal position paper has agreed that cleaning and low-level disinfection are required for such probes.[100] The American Institute for Ultrasound in Medicine and the Association of Vascular Access guidelines recommend that all transducers used for peripheral or central venous access device insertion should undergo, at a minimum, low-level disinfection (ie, step 1—clean, and step 2—low-level disinfection) and be used in conjunction with a single-use sterile probe cover.[101,102] Should such a probe on occasion become contaminated with blood or other potentially infectious material, appropriate cleaning and low-level disinfection (with EPA-registered tuberculocidal claim or EPA-registered disinfectants that are labeled as effective against both human immunodeficiency virus [HIV] and hepatitis B virus [HBV])[103] would eliminate the key blood-borne pathogens (ie, HIV, HBV, and hepatitis C virus [HCV]).

Hydrogen Peroxide Mist System for Probes

An alternative procedure for disinfecting the endocavitary and surface probes is a hydrogen peroxide mist system, which uses 35% hydrogen peroxide at 56°C with the probe reaching no more than 40°C (ie, Trophon [Nanosonics, Indianapolis, IN, USA]).[104] The Trophon system processes the portion of the probe that has not only mucous membrane contact but also the handle of an endocavitary probe, which may be contaminated, and it is an alternative to high-level chemical disinfection for ultrasound probes.

Inactivation of Human Papillomavirus

Human papillomavirus (HPV) is an extremely common sexually acquired infection and is the most frequent cause of cervical cancer. An article in 2014 reported that the FDA-cleared high disinfectants (ie, glutaraldehyde and OPA) tested did not inactivate the HPV, a nonenveloped virus.[105] These findings are inconsistent with many articles in the peer-reviewed literature, which demonstrates that HLDs, such as OPA and glutaraldehyde, inactivate nonenveloped viruses, such as hepatitis A virus, polio, adenovirus, norovirus, and so forth.[9] In recent studies, Ozbun and coworkers[106] have demonstrated, using tissue-derived and recombinant HPV preparations, that both OPA and hypochlorite are effective disinfectants. Data suggest that viral RNA contamination led to the inaccurate results by Meyers and colleagues [105] Based on the findings of Ozbun and colleagues,[106] the authors believe that OPA is effective against HPV and can be used for reprocessing semicritical items.

A Look-Back or Exposure Investigation of Patients Potentially Exposed to Blood-Borne Pathogens via Failure to Follow Reprocessing Guidelines for Medical Instruments

When there is a failure to follow reprocessing guidelines for semicritical items, health care facilities should assess the risk of exposed patients to blood-borne pathogens using a 15-step protocol (**Box 1**).[67,68]

Box 1
Protocol for exposure investigation after a failure of disinfection and sterilization processes

- Confirm disinfection or sterilization reprocessing failure.
- Immediately embargo any possibly improperly disinfected/sterilized items.
- Do not use the questionable disinfection/sterilization unit (eg, sterilizer or automated endoscope reprocessor) until proper functioning has been assured.
- Inform key stakeholders.
- Conduct a complete and thorough evaluation of the cause of the disinfection/sterilization failure.
- Prepare a line listing of potentially exposed patients.
- Assess whether the disinfection/sterilization failure increases a patient's risk for infection.
- Inform expanded list of stakeholders of the reprocessing issue.
- Develop a hypothesis for the disinfection/sterilization failure and initiate corrective action.
- Develop a method to assess potential adverse patient events.
- Consider notification of appropriate state and federal authorities (eg, state health department and FDA).
- Consider patient notification.
- If patients are notified, consider whether such patients require medical evaluation for possible postexposure therapy with appropriate anti-infectives. In addition, appropriate follow-up to detect infection (eg, HIV, HBV, and HCV) should be offered, if warranted.
- Develop a detailed plan to prevent similar failures in the future.
- Perform after-action report.

Data from Refs.[67,68]

LOW-LEVEL DISINFECTION ON NONCRITICAL ENVIRONMENTAL SURFACES AND MEDICAL DEVICES

Over the past decade, there is excellent evidence in the scientific literature that contaminated environmental surfaces and noncritical patient care items play an important role in the transmission of several key health care–associated pathogens including methicillin-resistant *S aureus* (MRSA), VRE, *Acinetobacter*, norovirus, and *C difficile*.[40,107–115] All these pathogens have been demonstrated to persist in the environment for days (in some cases, months),[111,115–117] frequently contaminate the environmental surfaces in rooms of colonized or infected patients,[118] transiently colonize the hands of HCP,[119,120] be transmitted by HCP, and cause outbreaks in which environmental transmission was deemed to play a role. A study by Stiefel and colleagues[119] demonstrated that contact with the environment was just as likely to contaminate the hands of HCP as was direct contact with the patient. Furthermore, admission to a room in which the previous patient had been colonized or infected with MRSA, VRE, *Acinetobacter*, or *C difficile* has been shown to be a risk factor for the newly admitted patient to develop colonization or infection.[54,121] Thus, surface disinfection of noncritical environmental surfaces and medical devices (defined as those that contact intact skin) is one of the important infection prevention strategies to prevent pathogen transmission.

This infection risk from environmental surfaces is not surprising because multiple studies have demonstrated that environmental surfaces and objects in rooms frequently are not cleaned properly, and these surfaces may be important in transmission of health care–associated pathogens.[110] Furthermore, although interventions aimed at improving cleaning thoroughness have demonstrated the effectiveness of surface disinfection in reducing microbial contamination and/or health care–associated infections,[112,114,122–127] many surfaces remain inadequately cleaned and, therefore, potentially contaminated. Now investigators are using 16S rRNA amplicon sequencing and quantitative polymerase chain reaction to investigate the microbial diversity of the hospital environment.[128]

CURRENT ISSUES FOR LOW-LEVEL DISINFECTION
Role of the Health Care Surface Environment in Severe Acute Respiratory Syndrome Coronavirus 2 Transmission and Potential Control Measures

In recent years, there has been an emergence of several new infectious diseases, many of which were major public health threats that were met with important infection prevention strategies. Now, an outbreak of novel coronavirus (severe acute respiratory syndrome coronavirus 2 [SARS-CoV-2]), which causes the coronavirus disease 2019 (COVID-19) has spread rapidly, with greater than 20 million cases in the United States in January 2021 and cases confirmed in approximately 220 countries.

The health care environment serves as one of the possible routes of transmission of epidemiologically important pathogens, but the role of the contaminated environment on SARS-CoV-2 transmission remains unknown. Recent reviews evaluated the survival, contamination, and transmission of SARS-CoV-2 via environmental surfaces and shared medical devices as well as environmental disinfection of COVID-19 in health care settings.[129] Coronaviruses, including SARS-CoV-2, have been demonstrated to survive for hours to days on environmental surfaces, depending on experimental conditions. The health care environment frequently is contaminated with SARS-CoV-2 RNA in most studies but without evidence of viable virus. Direct exposure to respiratory aerosols is the main transmission route of SARS-CoV-2. The contaminated health care environment potentially can result in transmission of SARS-CoV-2 by touching a contaminated surface or object and then touching their own mouth, nose, or eyes, but this is not thought to be the main way the virus spreads. It is important to improve thoroughness of cleaning/disinfection practice in health care facilities and select adequate disinfectants to decontaminate inanimate surfaces and shared patient care items.[130,131]

As of July 15, 2020, the Centers for Disease Control and Prevention (CDC) recommendation on disinfectant products for COVID-19 is to use an EPA-registered disinfectant on List N on the EPA Web site,[132] which identifies which registered products are qualified under the EPA emerging viral pathogens program for use against SARS-CoV-2. The CDC guideline recommends routine cleaning and disinfection of a List N disinfectant to frequently touched surfaces or objects for appropriate contact times as indicated on the products label.[131]

Electrostatic Spraying

Most cleaning and disinfection in health care facilities are done using a moistened, disposable wipe or via the application of a disinfectant with a cloth (eg, cotton or microfiber). One strategy that may improve application is the use of a disinfectant as a spray with minimal precleaning to remove visible soil. Cadnum and colleagues[133] evaluated an electrostatic sprayer device, which delivers electrostatically charged droplets, with an average size of 40 μ to 80 μ, that are attracted to the surface to improve thoroughness of surface coverage. The disinfectant used contained 0.25%

sodium hypochlorite. This concentration of chlorine reduced *C difficile* spores by greater than or equal to 6-$\log_{10}$ colony-forming units with a 5-minute contact time and bacteriophage MS2 by greater than or equal to 6-$\log_{10}$ PFU with a 2-minute contact time. The use of the sprayer provided a rapid and effective means to reduce microbial contamination on wheelchairs, portable equipment, and waiting room chairs.[133]

Decontamination of Sink Drains

Sink drains have been recognized as an important reservoir and source of CRE. Based on the high prevalence of CRE-positive sinks, investigators have attempted to identify a practical approach for routine disinfection. They found that a hydrogen peroxide–based foaming disinfectant was more effective at decreasing bacterial counts after 24 hours than bleach or no-treatment controls. The effect of the hydrogen peroxide–based disinfectant disappeared completely after 7 days of initial application.[134] Jones and colleagues[135] found foaming application of a hydrogen peroxide and peracetic acid–based disinfectant suppressed sink drain colonization for at least 3 days. With repeated treatments every 3 days, a progressive decrease in the bacterial load recovered from sinks was achieved.[135]

Mops and Wipes

Reusable cleaning cloths (eg, cotton), disposable wipes, and sprays are used regularly to achieve low-level disinfection.[136–139] Disinfectant cleaning wipes and sprays (eg, quaternary ammonium compounds and alcohol and chlorine) and disinfectant impregnated wipes have been found highly effective (>4-$\log_{10}$ reduction) in removing/inactivating epidemiologically important pathogens.[57,138–142] Disinfectant impregnated wipes (towelettes) remove by mechanical action and release the disinfectant on the surface, which is responsible for the microbicidal activity.[138,139,142]

Mops (especially cotton string mops) are used for floor decontamination and commonly are not kept adequately cleaned and disinfected. If the water-disinfectant mixture is not changed regularly (eg, after every 3 to 4 rooms, no longer than 60-min intervals), the mopping procedure actually may spread heavy microbial contamination throughout the health care facility.[143] The frequent laundering of cotton string mops (eg, daily) is recommended. Microfiber mops have demonstrated superior microbial removal compared with cotton string mops when used with detergent cleaner (ie, 95% vs 68%, respectively). Use of a disinfectant did significantly improve microbial removal when a cotton string mop was used compared with the detergent cleaner (ie, 95% vs 68%, respectively).[137]

Quaternary Ammonium Compounds Absorption to Wipes

Several studies have demonstrated the decreased activity of quaternary ammonium compounds via binding when exposed to cotton wipes, microfiber, and 1 of 2 disposable wipes.[144,145] These evaluations demonstrated a significant reduction (>50%) of quaternary ammonium compounds concentrations after exposure to the wipes/towels.[144–146] Manufacturers of disposable wipes believe they have addressed this issue because any absorption of the quaternary ammonium compounds that may occur has been taken into account because the wipes are tested via EPA registration tests for active ingredient content from the expressed liquid.

Floors

Studies have evaluated hospital floors as a potential source of pathogen dissemination. Deshpande and colleagues[36] found floors in patient rooms frequently were contaminated with health care pathogens (eg, *C difficile*, MRSA, and VRE [contamination range was 35%–53% during the patient stay]) and high-touch objects (eg, blood pressure cuffs and call buttons) often (41%) were in contact with the floor. Contact with objects on the floors resulted in transfer of pathogens to hands or gloves at varying frequencies (eg, *C difficile*—3%, VRE—6%, and MRSA—18%).[36] Another study found that a nonpathogenic virus inoculated onto floors in hospital rooms disseminated rapidly to the footwear and hands of patients and to high-touch surfaces in the rooms. The virus was frequently found on high-touch surfaces in adjacent rooms and nursing stations. This suggest that HCP contributed to dissemination after acquiring the virus during contact with surfaces or patients.[37] Although further studies are needed to determine if floors contribute to pathogen transfer, these data support the disinfection of floors.

Biofilms

Biofilms traditionally are associated with wet environments, such as indwelling medical devices. In 2019, Alfa[61] described 3 types of biofilms: traditional hydrated biofilm (water content 90%); build-up biofilm—occurs in endoscope channels; and dry surface biofilm—heterogenous accumulation of organisms and other material in a dry matrix (water content 61%).[61,147,148]

Biofilms are less susceptible to disinfectants but oxidizing agents (eg, chlorine) are more effective.[149,150] Many investigators have studied the efficacy of disinfection technologies. For example, Almatroudi and colleagues[149] tested the efficacy of sodium hypochlorite solution against *S aureus* dry surface biofilms. They found that treatment of dry surface biofilms with chlorine from 1000 ppm to 20,000 ppm resulted in a greater than 7-$\log_{10}$ reduction in *S aureus*. Even when treated with 20,000 ppm of chlorine, however, the biofilm recovered with prolonged incubation, releasing planktonic *S aureus*.[149] This raises questions about the inactivation of microbes with a dry surface biofilm by currently used cleaning/disinfecting methods.

A Bundle Approach to Disinfection of Noncritical Surfaces and Equipment

A bundle is a set of evidence-based practices, generally 3 to 5, that, when performed collectively and reliably, have proved to improve patient outcomes. The power of a bundle comes from a body of science that supports it and execution of the components of the bundle with complete consistency.[148]

The bundle, identified by Havill for surface disinfection, has 5 components.[107,151] They are creating policies and procedures; appropriate selection of cleaning/disinfecting products; educating staff to include environmental services, patient equipment, and nursing; monitoring compliance (eg, thoroughness of cleaning, product use) with feedback; and implementing a no-touch room decontamination technology and ensuring compliance for patients on contact and enteric precautions.

No-touch (or Mechanical) Methods for Room Decontamination

As discussed previously, multiple studies have demonstrated that environmental surfaces and objects in rooms frequently are not cleaned properly and these surfaces may be important in transmission of health care–associated pathogens. Furthermore, interventions aimed at improving cleaning/disinfection thoroughness (eg, disinfectant product substitution and no-touch room decontamination) have demonstrated effectiveness in reducing microbial contamination on surfaces and/or health care–associated infections.[112,114,122–127,151,152] Nonetheless, many surfaces remain inadequately cleaned/disinfected and therefore potentially contaminated, and that puts the next patient at risk for the previous patient's pathogen. For this reason, several manufacturers have developed room disinfection units that can effectively decontaminate environmental surfaces and objects and/or inoculated test surfaces. The 2 systems that have been studied most comprehensively are UV light and hydrogen peroxide systems.[152] Boyce and Donskey[153] recently summarized the UV-C doses needed to yield a 3-$\log_{10}$ reduction of health care–associated pathogens and factors affecting UV-C efficacy. Heilingloh and coworkers demonstrated that SARS-CoV-2 is highly susceptible to UV-C.[154] These technologies supplement, but do not replace, standard cleaning and disinfection because surfaces must be physically cleaned of dirt and debris.

Continuous Room Decontamination

Even after cleaning and disinfection, surfaces rapidly can become recontaminated. Thus, hands of HCP can become colonized by touching contaminated environmental surfaces and patient care equipment[33] and then, via inadequate hand hygiene or inappropriate glove use, can transfer health care pathogens from health care provider-to-patient. Because routine cleaning of room surfaces by environmental services frequently is inadequate, continuous room decontamination methods are being evaluated. The intent of this technology is to make surfaces hygienically clean (not sterile), that is, free of pathogens in sufficient numbers to prevent human disease. These methods include visible light disinfection (high-intensity narrow-spectrum light),[155,156] dry hydrogen peroxide,[157] far-UVC light (222 nm),[158] continuously active disinfectants,[155,159–164] multijet cold air plasma,[165] and self-disinfection surfaces (eg, copper).[166–168] Several of these technologies are under active investigation and some have demonstrated their ability to reduce microbial contamination and infections[161,167] and present an opportunity for controlling transmission from inanimate objects.

SUMMARY

When properly used, disinfection and sterilization can ensure the safe use of invasive and noninvasive medical devices. Strict adherence to current disinfection and sterilization guidelines is essential to prevent patient infections and exposures to infectious agents.

- Cleaning always must precede HLD and sterilization.
- Sterilization
  - Steam sterilization is the most robust method of sterilization.
  - Sterilization should be validated with the use of physical indicators (eg, temperature and duration), chemical indicators, and biological indicators.
- High-level disinfection
  - Endoscopes are devices most commonly linked to outbreaks.
  - Follow professional organization and/or manufacturer recommendations for HLD.
  - Train staff performing HLD at initiation of employment and at least yearly.
- Low-level disinfection of health care room surfaces
  - Standardize cleaning/disinfection of patient rooms and shared equipment/devices throughout the hospital.
  - Develop checklists for who is responsible for cleaning/disinfection of room surfaces and devices (ie, environmental services or nursing).
  - All touchable room surfaces should be disinfected daily, when spills occur, and when the surfaces are visibly soiled.
  - All noncritical medical devices should be disinfected daily and when soiled.

  ○ Monitor cleaning effectiveness (eg, fluorescent dye) with immediate feedback.
  ○ Use room disinfection devices (eg, UV-C/VHP) for contact precaution patient rooms.

ACKNOWLEDGMENTS

The authors thank Amy W. Powell for recovering articles on disinfection and sterilization in the peer-reviewed literature from 2012 to 2020.

DISCLOSURE

Drs W.A. Rutala and D.J. Weber are consultants for Professional Disposables International (PDI) and Dr W.J. Weber is a consultant for Germitec.

REFERENCES

1. Martin R. U.S. outpatient surgery passes inpatient, to 53 million a year. Tampa Bay Times; 2010.
2. Peery AF, Dellon ES, Lund J, et al. Burden of gastrointestinal disease in the United States: 2012 update. Gastroenterol 2012;143:1179–87.
3. Rutala WA, Weber DJ. Outbreaks of carbapenem-resistant *Enterobacteriaceae* infections associated with duodenoscopes: What can we do to prevent infections? Am J Infect Control 2016;44:e47–51.
4. Kovaleva J, Peters FT, van der Mei HC, et al. Transmission of infection by flexible gastrointestinal endoscopy and bronchoscopy. Clin Microbiol Rev 2013;26:231–54.
5. Ofstead CL, Wetzler HP, Snyder AK, et al. Endoscope reprocessing methods: a prospective study on the impact of human factors and automation. Gastroenterol Nurs 2010;33:304–11.
6. Murray P. Preventable tragedies: Superbugs and how ineffective monitoring of medical device safety fails patients. 2016. Available at: https://www.help.senate.gov/imo/media/doc/Duodenoscope%20Investigation%20FINAL%20Report.pdf. Accessed July 4, 2021. United States Senate Minority Report.
7. Kovalena J. Endoscope drying and its pitfalls. J Hosp Infect 2017;97:319–28.
8. Rutala WA, Weber DJ. Cleaning, disinfection and sterilization. In: Grota P, editor. APIC text of infection control and epidemiology. 4 ed. Washington, DC: Association for Professionals in Infection Control and Epidemiology, Inc.; 2014. 31.1-.15.
9. Rutala WA, Weber DJ, Healthcare Infection Control Practices Advisory Committee. Guideline for disinfection and sterilization in healthcare facilities, 2008. Centers for Disease Control and Prevention. 2008. Available at: https://www.cdc.gov/infectioncontrol/guidelines/disinfection/. Accessed December 2020.
10. Rutala WA, Weber DJ. Disinfection, sterilization, and antisepsis: An overview. Am J Infect Control 2016;44:e1–6.
11. Rutala WA, Weber DJ. Disinfection and sterilization in health care facilities: An overview and current issues. Infect Dis Clin North Am 2016;30:609–37.
12. Rutala WA, Weber DJ. Disinfection and sterilization in healthcare facilities. In: Lautenbach E, Preeti MN, Woeltje KF, et al, editors. Practical healthcare epidemiology. 4th edition. Cambridge University Press; 2018.
13. Rutala WA, Weber DJ. High-level disinfection and sterilization. In: Talbot T, Weber DJ, eds. Hospital epidemiology and infection control. New York: Lippincott Williams & Wilkins; In press.

14. Rutala WA, Weber DJ. Disinfection and sterilization in healthcare facilities. In: Jarvis WR, ed. Hospital infections. Philadelphia: Lippincott Wiliams & Wilkins; In press.

15. Rutala WA, Weber DJ. Disinfection, sterilization, and antispesis: An overview. Am J Infect Control 2019;47:A3–9.

16. Rutala WA, Weber DJ. Disinfection and sterilization: an overview. Am J Infect Control 2013;41:S2–5.

17. Rutala WA, Weber DJ. Disinfection, sterilization and control of hospital waste. In: Bennett JE, Dolan R, Blaser MJ, editors. Mandell, Douglas, and Bennett's Principles and practices of infectious diseases. Philadephia, PA: Elsevier; 2020. p. 3543–59.

18. Spaulding EH. Chemical disinfection of medical and surgical materials. In: Lawrence C, Block SS, editors. Disinfection, sterilization, and preservation. Philadelphia, PA: Lea & Febiger; 1968. p. 517–31.

19. Favero MS, Bond WW. Chemical disinfection of medical and surgical materials. In: Block SS, editor. Disinfection, sterilization, and preservation. Philadelphia, PA: Lea & Febiger; 2001. p. 881–917.

20. Simmons BP. CDC guidelines for the prevention and control of nosocomial infections. Guideline for hospital environmental control. Am J Infect Control 1983;11: 97–120.

21. McDonnell G, Burke P. Disinfection: Is it time to reconsider Spaulding? J Hosp Infect 2011;78:163–70.

22. Alfa MJ, DeGagne P, Olson N, et al. Comparison of ion plasma, vaporized hydrogen peroxide, and 100% ethylene oxide sterilizers to the 12/88 ethylene oxide gas sterilizer. Infect Control Hosp Epidemiol 1996;17:92–100.

23. Alfa MJ. Monitoring and improving the effectiveness of cleaning medical and surgical devices. Am J Infect Control 2013;41:S56–9.

24. Rutala WA, Gergen MF, Sickbert-Bennett EE, et al. Comparative evaluation of the microbicidal activity of low-temperature sterilization technologies to steam sterilization. Infect Control Hosp Epidemiol 2020;41:391–5.

25. Alfa MJ. Medical instrument reprocessing: Current issues with cleaning and cleaning monitoring. Am J Infect Control 2019;47:A10–6.

26. Seavey R. High-level disinfection, sterilization, and antisepsis: Current issues in reprocessing medical and surgical instruments. Am J Infect Control 2013;41:S111–7.

27. Rutala WA, Weber DJ. Reprocessing semicritical items: Current issues and new technologies. Am J Infect Control 2016;44:e53–62.

28. Rutala WA, Weber DJ. Reprocessing semicritical items: Outbreaks and current issues. Am J Infect Control 2019;47S:A79–89.

29. Rutala WA, Weber DJ. New developments in reprocessing semicritical items. Am J Infect Control 2013;41:S60–6.

30. Rutala WA, Gergen MF, Weber DJ. Disinfection of a probe used in ultrasound-guided prostate biopsy. Infect Control Hosp Epidemiol 2007;28:916–9.

31. Rutala WA, Gergen MF, Weber DJ. Disinfection of an infrared coagulation device used to treat hemorrhoids. Am J Infect Control 2012;40:78–9.

32. Food and Drug Administration. FDA-cleared sterilants and high level disinfectants with general claims for processing reusable medical and dental devices. FDA-cleared sterilants and high level disinfectants with general claims for processing reusable medical and dental devices. 2019. Available at: https://www.fda.gov/medical-devices/reprocessing-reusable-medical-devices-information-manufacturers/fda-cleared-sterilants-and-high-level-disinfectants-general-claims-processing-reusable-medical-and. Accessed December 2020.

33. Kanamori H, Rutala WA, Weber DJ. The role of patient care items as a fomite in healthcare-associated outbreaks and infection prevention. Clin Infect Dis 2017; 65:1412–9.

34. John A, Alhmidi H, Cadnum JL, et al. Contaminated portable equipment is a potential vector for dissemination of pathogens in the intensive care unit. Infect Control Hosp Epidemiol 2017;38:1247–9.

35. Suwantarat N, Supple LA, Cadnum JL, et al. Quantitative assessment of interactions between hospitalized patients and portable medical equipment and other fomites. Am J Infect Control 2017;45:1276–8.

36. Deshpande A, Cadnum JL, Fertelli D, et al. Are hospital floors an underappreciated reservoir for transmission of health care-associated pathogens. Am J Infect Control 2017;45:336–8.

37. Koganti S, Alhmidi H, Tomas ME, et al. Evaluation of hospital floors as a potential source of pathogen dissemination using a nonpathogenic virus as a surrogate marker. Infect Control Hosp Epidemiol 2016;37:1374–7.

38. Huslage K, Rutala WA, Sickbert-Bennett E, et al. A quantitative approach to defining "high-touch" surfaces in hospitals. Infect Control Hosp Epidemiol 2010;31:850–3.

39. Weber DJ, Rutala WA. Environmental issues and nosocomial infections. In: Wenzel RP, editor. Prevention and control of nosocomial infections. 3rd ed. Baltimore, MD: Williams and Wilkins; 1997. p. 491–514.

40. Weber DJ, Rutala WA, Miller MB, et al. Role of hospital surfaces in the transmission of emerging health care-associated pathogens: norovirus, *Clostridium difficile*, and *Acinetobacter species*. Am J Infect Control 2010;38:S25–33.

41. Sammons JS, Graf EH, Townsend S, et al. Critical importance of equipment cleaning during inpatient ophthalmologic examination. Ophthalmology 2018; 126:137–43.

42. Best M, Kennedy ME, Coates F. Efficacy of a variety of disinfectants against *Listeria* spp. Appl Environ Microbiol 1990;56:377–80.

43. Best M, Sattar SA, Springthorpe VS, et al. Efficacies of selected disinfectants against *Mycobacterium tuberculosis*. J Clin Microbiol 1990;28:2234–9.

44. Best M, Springthorpe VS, Sattar SA. Feasibility of a combined carrier test for disinfectants: studies with a mixture of five types of microorganisms. Am J Infect Control 1994;22:152–62.

45. West AM, Teska PJ, Oliver HF. There is no additional bactericidal efficacy of Environmental Protection Agency-registered disinfectant towelettes after surface drying or beyond label contact time. Am J Infect Control 2019;47:27–32.

46. Rutala WA, Barbee SL, Aguiar NC, et al. Antimicrobial activity of home disinfectants and natural products against potential human pathogens. Infect Control Hosp Epidemiol 2000;21:33–8.

47. Rutala WA, Gergen MF, Weber DJ. Efficacy of improved hydrogen peroxide against important healthcare-associated pathogens. Infect Control Hosp Epidemiol 2012;33:1159–61.

48. Rutala WA, Weber DJ. Selection of the ideal disinfectant. Infect Control Hosp Epidemiol 2014;35:855–65.

49. Rutala WA, Weber DJ. Surface disinfection: Treatment time (wipes and sprays) versus contact time (liquids). Infect Control Hosp Epidemiol 2018;39:329–31.

50. Cooper RA, Griffith CJ, Malik RE, et al. Monitoring the effectiveness of cleaning in four British hospitals. Am J Infect Control 2007;35:338–41.

51. Boyce JM, Havill NL, Dumigan DG, et al. Monitoring the effectiveness of hospital cleaning practices by use of an adenosine triphosphate bioluminescence assay. Infect Control Hosp Epidemiol 2009;30:678–84.

52. Lewis T, Griffith C, Gallo M, et al. A modified ATP benchmark for evaluating the cleaning of some hospital environmental surfaces. J Hosp Infect 2008;69: 156–63.

53. Carling PC, Briggs JL, Perkins J, et al. Improved cleaning of patient rooms using a new targeting method. Clin Infect Dis 2006;42:385–8.

54. Carling PC, Huang SS. Improving healthcare environmental cleaning and disinfection: current and evolving issues. Infect Control Hosp Epidemiol 2013;34: 507–13.

55. Carling PC. Evaluating the thoroughness of environmental cleaning in hospitals. J Hosp Infect 2008;68:273–4.

56. Rutala WA, Kanamori H, Gergen MF, et al. Comparative analysis of four major hospital cleaning validation methods. Am J Infect Control 2017;45:S37.

57. Kenters N, Huijskens EGW, de Wit SCJ, et al. Effectiveness of cleaning-disinfection wipes and sprays against multidrug-resistant outbreak strains. Am J Infect Control 2017;45:e69–73.

58. Singh J, Bhatia R, Gandhi JC, et al. Outbreak of viral hepatitis B in a rural community in India linked to inadequately sterilized needles and syringes. Bull World Health Organ 1998;76:93–8.

59. Eickhoff TC. An outbreak of surgical wound infections due to Clostridium perfringens. Surg Gynecol Obstet 1962;114:102–8.

60. Tosh PK, Disbot M, Duffy JM, et al. Outbreak of Pseudomonas aeruginosa surgical site infections after arthroscopic procedures: Texas, 2009. Infect Control Hosp Epidemiol 2011;32:1179–86.

61. Alfa MJ. Biofilms on instruments and environmental surfaces: Do they interfere with instrument reprocessing and surface disinfection? Review of the literature. Am J Infect Control 2019;47:A39–45.

62. Rutala WA, Kanamori H, Sickbert-Bennett EE, et al. What's new in reprocessing endoscopes: Are we going to ensure "the needs of the patient come first" by shifting from disinfection to sterilization? Am J Infect Control 2019;47:A62–6.

63. Favero MS. Sterility assurance: concepts for patient safety. In: Rutala WA, editor. Disinfection, sterilization and antisepsis: principles and practices in healthcare facilities. Washington, DC: Association for Professional in Infection Control and Epidemiology; 2001. p. 110–9.

64. Oxborrow GS, Berube R. Sterility testing-validation of sterilization processes, and sporicide testing. In: Block SS, editor. Disinfection, sterilization, and preservation. Philadelphia, PA: Lea & Febiger; 1991. p. 1047–57.

65. Alfa MJ. Current issues result in a paradigm shift in reprocessing medical and surgical instruments. Am J Infect Control 2016;44:e41–5.

66. Centers for Disease Control and Prevention. Immediate need for healthcare facilities to review procedures for cleaning, disinfecting, and sterilizing reusable medical devices. 2015. Available at: http://emergency.cdc.gov/han/han00382.asp. Accessed December 2020.

67. Rutala WA, Weber DJ. How to assess risk of disease transmission to patients when there is a failure to follow recommended disinfection and sterilization guidelines. Infect Control Hosp Epidemiol 2007;28:146–55.

68. Weber DJ, Rutala WA. Assessing the risk of disease transmission to patients when there is a failure to follow recommended disinfection and sterilization guidelines. Am J Infect Control 2013;41:S67–71.

69. Rutala WA, Weber DJ. Guideline for disinfection and sterilization of prion-contaminated medical instruments. Infect Control Hosp Epidemiol 2010;31: 107–17.

70. Centers for Disease Control and Prevention. Surveillance for Creutzfeldt-Jakob disease–United States. MMWR Morb Mortal Wkly Rep 1996;45:665–8.

71. Rutala WA, Weber DJ. Disinfection and sterilization of prion-contaminated medical instruments, Reply to Belay. Infect Control Hosp Epidemiol 2010;31:1306–7.

72. Belay ED, Schonberger LB, Brown P, et al. Disinfection and sterilization of prion-contaminated medical instruments. Infect Control Hosp Epidemiol 2010;31: 1304–6, author reply 6-8.

73. Belay ED, Blase J, Sehulster LM, et al. Management of neurosurgical instruments and patients exposed to Creutzfeldt-Jakob disease. Infect Control Hosp Epidemiol 2013;34:1272–80.

74. WHO infection control guidelines for transmissible spongiform encephalopathies. 2003. Available at: http://www.who.int/csr/resources/publications/bse/whocdscsraph2003.pdf. Accessed December 2020.

75. Rutala WA, Weber DJ. Creutzfeldt-Jakob disease: recommendations for disinfection and sterilization. Clin Infect Dis 2001;32:1348–56.

76. Kampf G, Jung M, Suchomel M, et al. Prion disease and recommended procedures for flexible endoscope reprocessing- a review of policies worldwide and proposal for a simplified approach. J Hosp Infect 2020;104:92–110.

77. Secker TJ, Herve R, Keevil CW. Adsorption of prion and tissue proteins to surgical stainless steel surfaces and the efficacy of decontamination following dry and wet storage conditions. J Hosp Infect 2011;78:251–5.

78. Alfred M, Catchpole K, Huffer E, et al. Work systems analysis of sterile processing: decontamination. BMJ Qual Saf 2020;29:320–8.

79. Rutala WA, Gergen MF, Weber DJ. Impact of an oil-based lubricant on the effectiveness of the sterilization processes. Infect Control Hosp Epidemiol 2008;29: 69–72.

80. Rutala WA, Gergen MF, Sickbert-Bennett EE, et al. Reply to Randal W. Eveland regarding comparative evaluation of the microbicidal activity of low-temperature sterilization technologies to steam sterilization. Infect Control Hosp Epidemiol 2020;41:1000–1.

81. Food and Drug Administration. Reprocessing Medical Devices in Health Care Settings: Validation Methods and Labeling. Guidance for Industry and Food and Drug Administration. Available at: https://www.fda.gov/regulatory-information/search-fda-guidance-documents/reprocessing-medical-devices-health-care-settings-validation-methods-and-labeling https://www.fda.gov/media/80265/download. Accessed December 2020.

82. Richter SG. Reusable medical device disinfection and cleaning validation requirements. Infection Control Today. 2011. Available at: https://www.infectioncontroltoday.com/view/reusable-medical-device-disinfection-and-cleaning-validation-requirements. Accessed December 2020.

83. Torok G, Gombocz P, Bognar E, et al. Effects of disinfection and sterilization on the dimensional changes and mechanical properties of 3D printed surgical guides for implant therapy - pilot study. BMC Oral Health 2020;20:19.

84. Chen JV, Tanaka KS, Dang ABC, et al. Identifying a commercially-available 3D printing process that minimizes model distortion after annealing and autoclaving and the effect of steam sterilization on mechanical strength. 3D Print Med 2020; 6:9.

85. Food and Drug Administration. Reduction or elimination of ethylene oxide emissions for medical device sterilization. 2019. p. 1–221. GHPUDP-11.6.19-Transcript (fda.gov). Accessed July 4, 2021.

86. Food and Drug Administration. Reduction or elimination of ethylene oxide emissions for medical device sterilization. 2019. p. 222–427. GHPUDP-11.7.19-Transcript (fda.gov). Accessed July 4, 2021.

87. Food and Drug Administration. Ethylene oxide sterilization for medical devices. Available at: https://www.fda.gov/medical-devices/general-hospital-devices-and-supplies/ethylene-oxide-sterilization-medical-devices. Accessed July 4, 2021.

88. Ragan A, Cote SL, Huang JT. Applanation tonometer disinfection: a national benchmarking study. Can J Ophthalmol 2017;52:e46–9.

89. Rutala WA, Weber DJ. ERCP scopes: what can we do to prevent infections? Infect Control Hosp Epidemiol 2015;36:643–8.

90. Bringhurst J. Special problems associated with reprocessing instruments in outpatient care facilities. Am J Infect Control 2016;2016:e63–7.

91. Petersen B, Cohen J, Hambrick RD, et al. Multisociety guideline on reprocessing flexible gastrointestinal endoscopes, 2016. Gastrointest Endosc 2017;85:282–94.

92. Gerding DN, Peterson LR, Vennes JA. Cleaning and disinfection of fiberoptic endoscopes: evaluation of glutaraldehyde exposure time and forced-air drying. Gastroenterology 1982;83:613–8.

93. Kovaleva J, Degener JE, van der Mei HC. Mimicking disinfection and drying of biofilms in contaminated endoscopes. J Hosp Infect 2010;76:345–50.

94. Perumpail RB, Marya N, McGinty BL, et al. Endoscope reprocessing: Comparison of drying effectiveness and microbial levels with an automated drying and storage cabinet with forced filtered air and a standard storage cabinet. Am J Infect Control 2019;47:1083–9.

95. da Costa LC, Olson N, Tipple AE, et al. Evaluation of the ability of different detergents and disinfectants to remove and kill organisms in traditional biofilm. Am J Infect Control 2016;44:e243–9.

96. Ofstead CL, Hopkins KM, Buro BL, et al. Challenges in achieving effective high-level disinfection in endoscope reprocessing. Am J Infect Control 2020;48:309–15.

97. Synder GM, Wright SB, Smithey A, et al. Randomized comparison of 3 high-level disinfection and sterilization procedures for duodenoscopes. Gastroenterol 2017;153:1018–25.

98. Bartles RL, Leggett JE, Hove S, et al. A randomized trial of single versus double high-level disinfection of duodenoscopes and linear echoendoscopes using standard automated reprocessing. Gastrointest Endosc 2018;88:306–13.e2.

99. Rutala WA, Weber DJ. Gastrointestinal endoscopes: a need to shift from disinfection to sterilization? JAMA 2014;312:1405–6.

100. American Institute of ultrasound in Medicine. Intersocietal Position Paper. Disinfection of ultrasound transducers used for percutaneous procedures. J Ultrasound Med 2021;9999:1–3.

101. Thompson J, Garrett JH Jr. Guidance document: transducer disinfection for assessment and insertion of peripheral and central catheters. Association for Vascular Access; 2018. p. 1–13.

102. American Institute of Ultrasound in Medicine. Guidelines for cleaning and preparing external and internal ultrasound probes between patients, safe handling,

and use of ultrasound coupling gel. 2018. Available at: https://www.aium.org/officialStatements/57. Accessed July 4, 2021.

103. Occupational Safety and Health Administration. Most frequently asked questions concerning the bloodborne pathogen standard. Available at: https://www.osha.gov/laws-regs/standardinterpretations/1993-02-01-0. Accessed July 4, 2021.

104. Rutala WA, Gergen MF, Sickbert-Bennett EE. Effectiveness of a hydrogen peroxide mist (Trophon®) system in inactivating healthcare pathogens on surface and endocavitary probes. Infect Control Hosp Epidemiol 2016;37:613–4.

105. Meyers J, Ryndock E, Conway MJ, et al. Susceptibility of high-risk human papillomavirus type 16 to clinical disinfectants. J Antimicrob Chemother 2014;69(6):1546–50.

106. Ozbun MA, Bondu V, Patterson NA, et al. Infectious titers of human papillomavirus (HPVs) in patient lesions, methodological considerations in evaluaring HPV infectivity and implications for the efficacy of high-level disinfectants. E Bio Med 2021;63:103165.

107. Rutala WA, Weber DJ. Best practices for disinfection of noncritical environmental surfaces and equipment in health care facilities: A bundle approach. Am J Infect Control 2019;47S:A96–105.

108. Otter JA, Yezli S, Salkeld JA, et al. Evidence that contaminated surfaces contribute to the transmission of hospital pathogens and an overview of strategies to address contaminated surfaces in hospital settings. Am J Infect Control 2013;41:S6–11.

109. Boyce JM. Environmental contamination makes an important contribution to hospital infection. J Hosp Infect 2007;65(Suppl 2):50–4.

110. Han JH, Sullivan N, Leas BF, et al. Cleaning hospital room surfaces to prevent health care-associated infections. Ann Intern Med 2015;163(8):598–607.

111. Hota B. Contamination, disinfection, and cross-colonization: are hospital surfaces reservoirs for nosocomial infection? Clin Infect Dis 2004;39:1182–9.

112. Donskey CJ. Does improving surface cleaning and disinfection reduce health care-associated infections? Am J Infect Control 2013;41:S12–9.

113. Doll M, Stevens M, Bearman G. Environmental cleaning and disinfection of patient areas. Int J Infect Dis 2018;67:52–7.

114. Datta R, Platt R, Yokoe DS, et al. Environmental cleaning intervention and risk of acquiring multidrug-resistant organisms from prior room occupants. Arch Intern Med 2011;171:491–4.

115. Piedrahita CT, Cadnum JC, Jencson AL, et al. Environmental surfaces in healthcare facilities are a potential source for transmission of *Candida auris* and other *Candida* species. Infect Control Hosp Epidemiol 2017;38:1107–9.

116. Kramer A, Schwebke I, Kampf G. How long do nosocomial pathogens persist on inanimate surfaces? A systematic review. BMC Infect Dis 2006;6:130.

117. Suleyman G, Alangaden G, Bardossy AC. The role of environmental contamination in the transmission of nosocomial pathogens and healthcare-associated infections. Curr Infect Dis Rep 2018;20:12.

118. Shams AM, Rose LJ, Edwards JR, et al. Assessment of the overall and multidrug-resistant organism bioburden on environmental surfaces in healthcare facilities. Infect Control Hosp Epidemiol 2016;37:1426–32.

119. Stiefel U, Cadnum JL, Eckstein BC, et al. Contamination of hands with methicillin-resistant *Staphylococcus aureus* after contact with environmental surfaces and after contact with the skin of colonized patients. Infect Control Hosp Epidemiol 2011;32:185–7.

120. Siani H, Maillard JY. Best practice in healthcare environment decontamination. Eur J Clin Microbiol Infect Dis 2015;34:1–11.
121. Shaughnessy MK, Micielli RL, DePestel DD, et al. Evaluation of hospital room assignment and acquisition of Clostridium difficile infection. Infect Control Hosp Epidemiol 2011;32:201–6.
122. Hayden MK, Bonten MJ, Blom DW, et al. Reduction in acquisition of vancomycin-resistant enterococcus after enforcement of routine environmental cleaning measures. Clin Infect Dis 2006;42:1552–60.
123. Falk PS, Winnike J, Woodmansee C, et al. Outbreak of vancomycin-resistant enterococci in a burn unit. Infect Control Hosp Epidemiol 2000;21:575–82.
124. Denton M, Wilcox MH, Parnell P, et al. Role of environmental cleaning in controlling an outbreak of *Acinetobacter baumannii* on a neurosurgical intensive care unit. J Hosp Infect 2004;56:106–10.
125. Grabsch EA, Mahony AA, Cameron DR, et al. Significant reduction in vancomycin-resistant enterococcus colonization and bacteraemia after introduction of a bleach-based cleaning-disinfection programme. J Hosp Infect 2012;82:234–42.
126. Wilson AP, Smyth D, Moore G, et al. The impact of enhanced cleaning within the intensive care unit on contamination of the near-patient environment with hospital pathogens: A randomized crossover study in critical care units in two hospitals. Crit Care Med 2011;39:651–8.
127. Eckstein BC, Adams DA, Eckstein EC, et al. Reduction of *Clostridium difficile* and vancomycin-resistant *Enterococcus* contamination of environmental surfaces after an intervention to improve cleaning methods. BMC Infect Dis 2007;7:61.
128. Chen CH, Tu CC, Kuo HY, et al. Dynamic change of surface microbiota with different environmental cleaning methods between two wards in a hospital. Appl Microbiol Biotechnol 2017;101:771–81.
129. Kampf G, Bruggemann Y, Kaba HEJ, et al. Potential sources, modes of transmission and effectiveness of prevention measures against SARS-CoV-2. J Hosp Infect 2020;106:678–97.
130. Kanamori H, Weber DJ, Rutala WA. The role of the healthcare surface environment in SARS-CoV-2 transmission and potential control measures. Clin Infect Dis 2020. https://doi.org/10.1093/cid/ciaa1467.
131. Interim infection prevention and control recommendation for healthcare personnel during the coronavirus disease (COVID-19) pandemic. Available at: https://www.cdc.gov/coronavirus/2019-ncov/hcp/infection-control-recommendations.html. Accessed July 15, 2020.
132. List N. Disinfectants for Use Against SARS-CoV-2 (COVID-19). Available at: https://www.epa.gov/pesticide-registration/list-n-disinfectants-use-against-sars-cov-2-covid-19. Accessed August 20, 2020.
133. Cadnum JL, Jencson AL, Livingston SH, et al. Evaluation of an electrostatic spray disinfectant technology for rapid decontamination of portable equipment and large open areas in the era of SARS-CoV-2. Am J Infect Control 2020;48:951–4.
134. Buchan BW, Arvan JA, Graham MB, et al. Effectiveness of a hydrogen peroxide foam against bleach for the disinfection of sink drains. Infect Control Hosp Epidemiol 2019;40:724–6.
135. Jones LD, Mana TSC, Cadnum JL, et al. Effectiveness of foam disinfectants in reducing sink-drain gram-negative bacterial colonization. Infect Control Hosp Epidemiol 2020;41:280–5.

136. Rutala WA, Weber DJ. Monitoring and improving the effectiveness of surface cleaning and disinfection. Am J Infect Control 2016;44:e69–76.

137. Rutala WA, Gergen MF, Weber DJ. Microbiologic evaluation of microfiber mops for surface disinfection. Am J Infect Control 2007;35:569–73.

138. Song X, Vossebein L, Zille A. Efficacy of disinfectant-impregnated wipes used for surface disinfection in hospitals: a review. Antimicrob Resist Infect Control 2019;8:139.

139. Boyce JM. A review of wipes used to disinfect hard surfaces in health care facilities. Am J Infect Control 2020;49(1):104–14.

140. Rutala WA, Gergen MF, Weber DJ. Efficacy of different cleaning and disinfection methods against *Clostridium difficile* spores: importance of physical removal versus sporicidal inactivation. Infect Control Hosp Epidemiol 2012;33:1255–8.

141. Gonzalez EA, Nandy P, Lucas AD, et al. Ability of cleaning-disinfecting wipes to remove bacteria from medical device surfaces. Am J Infect Control 2015;43:1331–5.

142. West AM, Nkemngong CA, Voorn MG, et al. Surface area wiped, product type, and target strain impact bactericidal efficacy of ready-to-use disinfectant Towelettes. Antimicrob Resist Infect Control 2018;7:122.

143. Westwood JC, Mitchell MA, Legace S. Hospital sanitation: the massive bacterial contamination of the wet mop. Appl Microbiol 1971;21:693–7.

144. Engelbrecht K, Ambrose D, Sifuentes L, et al. Decreased activity of commercially available disinfectants containing quaternary ammonium compounds when exposed to cotton towels. Am J Infect Control 2013;41:908–11.

145. MacDougall KD, Morris C. Optimizing disinfectant application in healthcare facilities. Infect Control Today 2006;62–7.

146. Boyce JM. Quaternary ammonium disinfectant issues encountered in an environmental services department. Infect Control Hosp Epidemiol 2016;37:340–2.

147. Vickery K, Deva A, Jacombs A, et al. Presence of biofilm containing viable multiresistant organisms despite terminal cleaning on clinical surfaces in an intensive care unit. J Hosp Infect 2012;80:52–5.

148. Otter JA, Vickery K, Walker JT, et al. Surface-attached cells, biofilms and biocide susceptibility: implications for hospital cleaning and disinfection. J Hosp Infect 2015;89:16–27.

149. Almatroudi A, Gosbell IB, Hu H, et al. *Staphylococcus aureus* dry-surface biofilms are not killed by sodium hypochlorite: Implications for infection control. J Hosp Infect 2016;93:263–70.

150. Song L, Wu J, Xi C. Biofilms on environmental surfaces: Evaluation of the disinfection efficacy of a novel steam vapor system. Am J Infect Control 2012;40:926–30.

151. Havill NL. Best practices in disinfection of noncritical surfaces in the health care setting: creating a bundle for success. Am J Infect Control 2013;41:S26–30.

152. Weber DJ, Rutala WA, Anderson DJ, et al. Effectiveness of ultraviolet devices and hydrogen peroxide systems for terminal room decontamination: Focus on clinical trials. Am J Infect Control 2016;44:e77–84.

153. Boyce JM, Donskey CJ. Understanding ultraviolet light surface decontamination in hospital rooms: A primer. Infect Control Hosp Epidemiol 2019;40:1030–5.

154. Heilingloh CS, Aufderhorst UW, Schipper L, et al. Susceptibility of SARS-CoV-2 to UV irradiation. Am J Infect Control 2020;48:1273–5.

155. Rutala WA, Kanamori H, Gergen MF, et al. Antimicrobial activity of a continuous visible light disinfection system. Infect Control Hosp Epidemiol 2018;39:1250–3.

156. Bache SE, MacClean M, Gettinby G, et al. Universal decontamination of hospital surfaces in an occupied inpatient room with a continuous 405 nm light source. J Hosp Infect 2018;98:67–73.

157. Rutala WA, Kanamori H, Gergen MF, et al, CDC Prevention Epicenters Program. Evaluation of dilute hydrogen peroxide technology for continuous room decontamination of multidrug-resistant organisms. Infect Control Hosp Epidemiol 2019;40:1438–9.

158. Buonanno M, Welch D, Shuryak I, et al. Far-UVC light (222nm) efficiently and safely inactivates airborne human coronaviruses. Sci Rep 2020;10(1):10285.

159. Tamimi AH, Carlino S, Gerba CP. Long-term efficacy of a self-disinfecting coating in an intensive care unit. Am J Infect Control 2014;42:1178–81.

160. Ikner LA, Torrey JR, Gundy PM, et al. A continuously active antimicrobial coating effective against human coronavirus 229E 2020. https://doi.org/10.1101/2020.05.10.20097329.

161. Ellingson KD, Pogreba-Brown K, Gerba CP, et al. Impact of a novel antimicrobial surface coating on health care–associated infections and environmental bioburden at 2 urban hospitals. Clin Infect Dis 2020;71:1807–13.

162. Rutala WA, Weber DJ. New disinfection and sterilization methods. Emerg Infect Dis 2001;7:348–53.

163. Rutala WA, White MS, Gergen MF, et al. Bacterial contamination of keyboards: efficacy and functional impact of disinfectants. Infect Control Hosp Epidemiol 2006;27:372–7.

164. Fitton K, Barber K, Karamon A, et al. Long acting water-stable organosilane and its sustained effect on reducing microbial load in the intensive care unit. Am J Infect Control 2017;45:S23.

165. Cahill OJ, Claro T, Cafolla AA, et al. Decontamination of hospital surfaces with multijet cold plasma: A method to enhance infection prevention and control? Infect Control Hosp Epidemiol 2017;38:1182–7.

166. Weber DJ, Rutala WA. Self-disinfecting surfaces: review of current methodologies and future prospects. Am J Infect Control 2013;41:S31–5.

167. Salgado CD, Sepkowitz KA, John JF, et al. Copper surfaces reduce the rate of healthcare-acquired infections in the intensive care unit. Infect Control Hosp Epidemiol 2013;34:479–86.

168. Schmidt MG, von Dessauer B, Benavente C, et al. Copper surfaces are associated with significantly lower concentrations of bacteria on selected surfaces within a pediatric intensive care unit. Am J Infect Control 2016;44:203–9.

169. Kohn WG, Collins AS, Cleveland JL, et al. Guidelines for infection control in dental health-care settings–2003. MMWR Recomm Rep 2003;52:1–61.

170. Boyce JM. Alcohols as surface disinfectants in healthcare settings. Infect Control Hosp Epidemiol 2018;39:323–8.

171. Weber DJ, Rutala WA, Sickbert-Bennett EE. Outbreaks associated with contaminated antiseptics and disinfectants. Antimicrob Agents Chemother 2007;51:4217–24.

172. Rutala WA, Cole EC, Thomann CA, et al. Stability and bactericidal activity of chlorine solutions. Infect Control Hosp Epidemiol 1998;19:323–7.

173. Cullen MM, Trail A, Robinson M, et al. *Serratia marcescens* outbreak in a neonatal intensive care unit prompting review of decontamination of laryngoscopes. J Hosp Infect 2005;59:68–70.

174. Associated Press. L.A. hospital cited for deadly bacterial outbreak. Associated Press. 2007. Available at: https://www.nbcnews.com/health/health-news/l-

hospital-cited-deadly-bacterial-outbreak-flna1c9471261.   Accessed   July   4, 2021.

175. Muscarella LF. Reassessment of the risk of healthcare-acquired infection during rigid laryngoscopy. J Hosp Infect 2008;68:101–7.

176. Wendelboe AM, Baumbach J, Blossom DB, et al. Outbreak of cystoscopy related infections with *Pseudomonas aeurginosa*: New Mexico, 2007. J Urol 2008;180:588–92.

177. Koo VS, O'Neill P, Elves A. Multidrug-resistant NDM-1 *Klebsiella* outbreak and infection control in endoscopic urology. BJU Int 2012;110:E922–6.

178. Jimeno A, Alcalde MM, Ortiz M, et al. Outbreak of urinary tract infections by *Salmonella spp*. after cystoscopic manipulation. Actas Urol Esp 2016;40:646–9.

179. OYong K, Coelho L, Bancroft E, et al. Health care-associated infection outbreak Investigations in outpatient settings, Los Angeles County, California, USA, 2000-2012. Emerg Infect Dis 2015;21:1317–21.

180. Chang CL, Su LH, Lu CM, et al. Outbreak of ertapenem-resistant *Enterobacter cloacae* urinary tract infections due to a contaminated ureteroscope. J Hosp Infect 2013;85:118–24.

181. Strand CL, Bryant JK, Morgan JW, et al. Nosocomial *Pseudomanas aeruginosa* urinary tract infections. JAMA 1982;248:1615–8.

182. Echols RM, Palmer DL, King RM, et al. Multidrug-resistant *Serratia marcescens* bacteriuria related to urologic instrumentation. South Med J 1984;77:173–7.

183. Climo MW, Pastor A, Wong ES. An outbreak of *Pseudomonas aeruginosa* related to contaminated urodynamic equipment. Infect Control Hosp Epidemiol 1997;18:509–10.

184. Gillespie JL, Arnold KE, Noble-Wang J, et al. Outbreak of *Pseudomonas aeruginosa* infections after transrectal ultrasound-guided prostate biopsy. Urology 2007;69:912–4.

185. Seki M, Machida N, Yamagishi Y, et al. Nosocomial outbreak of multidrug-resistant *Pseudomonas aeurginosa* caused by damaged transesphageal echocardiogram probe used in cardiovascular surgical operations. J Infect Chemother 2013;19:677–81.

186. Bancroft EA, English L, Terashita D, et al. Outbreak of *Escherichia coli* infections associated with a contaminated transesophageal echocardiography probe. Infect Control Hosp Epidemiol 2013;34:1121–3.

187. Kanemitsu K, Endo S, Oda K, et al. An increased incidence of Enterobacter cloacae in a cardiovascular ward. J Hosp Infect 2007;66:130–4.

188. Levy PY, Teysseire N, Etienne J, et al. A nosocomial outbreak of *Legionella pneumophila* caused by contaminated transesophageal echocardiography probes. Infect Control Hosp Epidemiol 2003;24:619–22.

189. Viney KA, Kehoe Pj, Doyle B, et al. An outbreak of epidemic keratoconjunctivitis in a regional ophthalmology clinic in New South Wales. Epidemiol Infect 2007; 136:1197–206.

190. Montessori V, Scharf S, Holland S, et al. Epidemic keratoconjunctivitis outbreak at a tertiary referral eye care clinic. Am J Infect Control 1998;26:399–405.

191. Birnie GG, Quigley EM, Clements GB, et al. Endoscopic transmission of hepatitis B virus. Gut 1983;24:171–4.

192. Bronowicki JP, Venard V, Botte C, et al. Patient-to-patient transmission of hepatitis C virus during colonoscopy. N Engl J Med 1997;337:237–40.

193. Le Pogam S, Gondeau A, Bacq Y. Nosocomial transmission of hepatitis C virus. Ann Intern Med 1999;131:794.

Health Care Environmental Hygiene

New Insights and Centers for Disease Control and Prevention Guidance

Philip C. Carling, MD[a,b,*]

KEYWORDS

- Hygienic practice • Hand hygiene • Environmental hygiene
- Optimizing disinfection cleaning

KEY POINTS

- Optimizing patient-zone environmental hygiene plays a critical role in mitigating the transmission of health care-associated pathogens, particularly *Clostridioides difficile*.
- New research is clarifying the important role of asymptomatic carriers of *Clostridioides difficile* in transmission.
- The development of new hydrogen peroxide/peroxy acetic acid-based patient-zone surface disinfectants provides a potential for more effective approaches to patient-zone environmental hygiene.
- Although hand hygiene and environmental hygiene individually represent basic horizontal interventions to prevent transmission of health care-associated pathogens, there is a need for these 2 interventions to be recognized as interdependent.

INTRODUCTION

As a result of epidemiologic and microbiologic studies over the past decade, it has become increasingly evident that interventions to mitigate environmental surface pathogen contamination are an important component of health care-associated infection (HAI) prevention. During this time it has become widely appreciated that, "Cleaning of hard surfaces in hospital rooms is critical for reducing healthcare-associated infections."[1] Unfortunately, the complexity of the interrelated factors necessary to optimize the cleanliness of surfaces in the patient zone remains an evolving challenge. Despite such ongoing challenges, it is important to recognize that environmental hygiene represents a critical element of what Wenzel and Edmonds defined as

[a] Department of Infectious Diseases, Boston University School of Medicine, Boston, MA, USA;
[b] Carney Hospital, 2100 Dorchester Avenue, Boston, MA 02124, USA
* Carney Hospital, 2100 Dorchester Avenue, Boston, MA 02124.
E-mail address: Philip.Carling.MD@Steward.org

Infect Dis Clin N Am 35 (2021) 609–629
https://doi.org/10.1016/j.idc.2021.04.005   **id.theclinics.com**

"horizontal interventions" that are central to mitigating a wide range of HAIs.[2,3] These approaches aim to reduce the risk of infections caused by a broad range of pathogens by the implementation of standard practices that are effective regardless of patient-specific conditions.[4] In contrast to the horizontal interventions, "vertical interventions" are pathogen and/or condition specific. Vertical interventions include nasal decolonization specific to methicillin-resistant *Staphylococcus aureus* (MRSA) and transmission-based isolation precautions. These interventions are narrowly focused on preventing transmission of specific pathogens.

These interventions remain important in defined settings and become most cost effective when the indications for their use are most clearly defined. Although vertical and horizontal approaches are not mutually exclusive, there is evolving evidence that horizontal interventions in endemic situations may represent the best use of HAI prevention resources.[4]

To facilitate discussion of the many elements necessary to optimize health care hygienic cleaning, it is useful to put these interventions into a defined construct of HAI prevention activities. As noted in **Fig. 1**, hygienic cleaning and hand hygiene as well as interventions related to instrument reprocessing, air quality, water quality, and physical setting design are all horizontal interventions. All these horizontal interventions represent elements of *health care hygienic practice*. Although these elements have traditionally been discussed independently, their effectiveness in clinical settings is substantially interrelated, particularly environmental hygiene and hand hygiene, as will subsequently be discussed. The term "environmental hygiene" can be defined as "cleaning activities directed at removing and/or killing potentially harmful pathogens capable of being transmitted directly from surfaces or indirectly to susceptible individuals or other surfaces."[5] As noted, it consists of both the physical cleaning of surfaces and surface disinfection cleaning. Although liquid chemistries are well established as the most clinically useful approach to surface disinfection, innovative no-touch technologies that have the potential for complementing traditional liquid chemistry have been developed over the past several years. Each of these components of environmental hygiene will be discussed in detail in later sections, whereas the other components of health care hygienic practice noted in **Fig. 1** will be addressed in other reviews in this issue.

DISINFECTION CLEANING OF ENVIRONMENTAL SURFACES

Chemical Disinfectants: The use of Environmental Protection Association-registered hospital-grade disinfectants to clean and disinfect patient-zone surfaces has been

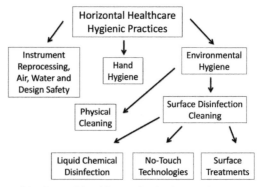

Fig. 1. The elements of horizontal health care hygienic practice.

considered the cornerstone of health care environmental cleaning for many years.[6] As recommended by the Centers for Disease Control and Prevention (CDC), disinfectants are used on all such surfaces in US hospitals.[7] Given the recent detailed review of disinfectant choice and use,[6] the following discussion will focus only on some important generalizations.

Over the past several years, the traditional use of disinfectants on noncritical patient-zone surfaces has been profoundly impacted by the development of broad-spectrum chemistries that are at least as effective as bleach, are not associated with significant damage to surfaces, and are not associated with potentially toxic residuals during either their use or disposal.[8] These chemistries are rapidly sporicidal and effective against *Candida auris* and all viral pathogens, including coronaviruses. Although studies to further quantify the relative clinical value of both hydrogen peroxide/peroxyacetic acid formulations and chlorinated hydrogen peroxide are warranted, these new chemistries have the potential for substantially improving the effectiveness and scope of use of patient-zone surface disinfection cleaning. In clinical studies a hydrogen peroxide/peroxyacetic acid formulation was found to be approximately twice as effective as a quaternary ammonium compound in surface bioburden reduction and as effective as bleach in clinical use.[4,9,10] Given the numerous traditional hospital-grade disinfectants currently marketed and the ongoing development of new chemistries it is critically important that all chemical disinfectants undergo rigorously designed comparative studies in actual clinical settings to quantify their clinical efficacy, similarities, differences, and potential limitations.[6,11,12]

Although premoistened disposable wipes are widely used to clean surfaces in health care settings, their clinical effectiveness has yet to be evaluated in comparative studies. The lack of such studies is particularly notable, given the evidence of the spread of health care-associated pathogens (HAPs) from contaminated to noncontaminated surfaces by wipes.[13–15] Given this important limitation, all premoistened disposable wipes should be tested to ensure that they do not transfer organisms between surfaces. The validity of this approach was confirmed by the recently approved American Society for Testing and Materials standard E2967-15 test. All the 5 wipes tested by the 3 independent testing sites confirmed a greater than 4 $\log_{10}$ reduction in *S aureus* and *Acinetobacter baumannii* on seeded surfaces, but only a wipe using 0.5% accelerated H_2O_2 prevented transfer of the test bacteria to another surface.[15]

Surface Disinfection Technologies

As previously noted, the past decade has seen the development of technological interventions designed to augment physical cleaning of patient-zone surfaces. These innovative technologies using hydrogen peroxide vapor or ultraviolet light systems have been advocated to augment traditional chemical-based disinfection cleaning at the time of discharge or patient transfer. Although these no-touch technologies have shown microbicidal efficacy in laboratory studies, clinical assessment of their effectiveness and potential for augmenting physical disinfection cleaning has been challenging. Ultimately, well-designed, independent, controlled, comparative studies are needed to objectively quantify the cost and potential added value of such technologies when routine cleaning and disinfection has been sustainably optimized.[16]

OPTIMIZING PATIENT-ZONE SURFACE SAFETY

Evaluating disinfection cleaning: The importance of physically removing visible dirt and soil from surfaces in hospitals has been recognized for more than 150 years.[17] Consequently, acute care hospitals have developed policies and procedures to define the role of environmental services (EVS) personnel for cleaning surfaces in all patient care areas. EVS managers and infection preventionists had implemented joint visual inspection of surfaces in patient care areas well before the CDC recommended that hospitals clean and disinfect "high-touch surfaces" in 2003.[7] EVS managers further recommended that hospitals "monitor, (i.e., supervise and inspect cleaning performance) to insure consistent cleaning and disinfection of surfaces in close proximity to the patient and likely to be touched by the patient and healthcare professionals" in 2006.[18] Such monitoring, referred to as "environmental rounds" in the United States and "visual audits" in Great Britain, is used primarily to identify cleaning deficiencies.[19] Unfortunately, the intrinsically subjective nature of such monitoring along with its episodic and deficiency-oriented features limit its ability to accurately assess the thoroughness of day-to-day cleaning activity. Preliminary studies documenting patient-zone surface contamination with HAPs raised concerns that cleaning practice should be improved.[20] It was not until actual cleaning practice was objectively monitored, initially using a covert visual monitoring program[21] and later with covertly applied fluorescent markers, that actual cleaning practice was objectively evaluated.[22,23] The identification of opportunities to improve the thoroughness of patient-zone surface cleaning as part of discharge cleaning in acute care hospitals spurred an evaluation of cleaning practice in other important venues within hospitals, including the operating rooms (both between-case and terminal cleaning), emergency departments, outpatient clinics, and chemotherapy administration suites.[24] Similar studies have been extended to long-term care facilities and dialysis units as well as dental clinics and EMS vehicles.[24] The evaluations were done in a standardized manner with a metered fluorescent marking system (DAZO, Ecolab Inc, St Paul, MN, USA). The outcome measured was the actual thoroughness of cleaning expressed as the "thoroughness of disinfection cleaning" or "TDC." The TDC score is an expression of the proportion of actual cleaning documented in comparison with the cleaning expected to be done according to the relevant cleaning policy.[25] As noted in **Fig. 2**, these studies consistently identified substantial opportunities for improving practice in all settings.[24] Visual monitoring as part of environmental rounds remains important for evaluating individual cleaning technique, whereas there are many advantages to the objective monitoring of disinfection cleaning practice.[26,27] Published reports have now confirmed the effectiveness of such programs in more than 120 hospitals in the United States, Canada,

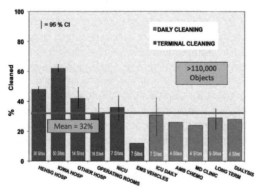

Fig. 2. Thoroughness of environmental cleaning in multiple health care settings. AMB, ambulatory; EMS, emergency medical services; HEHSG, Healthcare Environmental Hygiene Study Group; HOSP, hospitals.

and Australia.[24,28–31] In these hospitals, not only has the thoroughness of cleaning improved from TDC scores in the range of 40% to 60% to 80% to 90% or higher as a result of similar programmatic interventions but also the results have been sustained over at least 3 years where ongoing programs have been evaluated.[32] It has now been shown that improved environmental cleaning decreases HAP contamination of surfaces. In 4 comparable clinical studies objectively evaluating thoroughness of environmental cleaning over many months, contamination of patient-zone surfaces decreased an average of 64% as a result of an average 80% improvement in thoroughness of environmental disinfection cleaning with nonsporicidal disinfectants.[5] Environmental cleaning is not important unless it positively impacts patient outcomes. The complexity and cost of studies to evaluate the clinical impact of decreased patient-zone HAP contamination on patient acquisition has limited research in this area. Two landmark studies found similar statistically significant results. The 2006 study by Hayden confirmed a 66% ($P < .001$) reduction in vancomycin resistant enterococci (VRE) acquisition as a result of a 75% improvement in TDC.[21] A more recent study by Datta and colleagues[33] found a 50% ($P < .001$) reduction in MRSA acquisition and a 28% ($P < .001$) reduction in VRE acquisition as a result of an 80% improvement in environmental cleaning. This study also confirmed significantly decreased prior room occupant transmission for both pathogens during the intervention period. These studies clearly show that direct patient safety benefits can be realized by improving the thoroughness of patient-zone surface cleaning.

Evaluating environmental cleaning—the 2010 CDC guidance: As a result of published evidence supporting objective monitoring to evaluate surface cleaning processes and the subsequent improved patient outcomes, the CDC developed the guidance "Options for Evaluating Environmental Cleaning" in 2010.[25] This guidance recommends that all hospitals implement methods to objectively monitor environmental cleaning (**Box 1**). As noted in the guidance, 2 different testing systems can be used to evaluate the TDC, metered fluorescent markers and the adenosine triphosphate technology (ATP), as discussed later.

Fluorescent markers: As discussed earlier, studies in the United States and abroad during the past 10 years have used a specially developed fluorescent gel or "test soil" to covertly evaluate environmental cleaning in a wide range of health care settings.[22,28–31,34] These studies have used a standardized metered transparent gel specifically formulated for the covert evaluation of health care surface cleaning. While nonstandardized fluorescent powders and lotions have been used in a noncovert

---

Box 1
CDC environmental hygiene guidance recommendations 2010

Hospitals should implement programs to improve current environmental hygiene practice by adopting a 2-phase stepwise programmatic approach:

Level I program:
   Basic interventions to optimize disinfection cleaning policies, procedures, and ES staff education and practice. When completed move to Level II program.

Level II program:
   All elements of Level 1 program + objective monitoring

Data from Guh A, Carling P, and the environmental cleaning work group. Options for monitoring environmental cleaning. December 2010. Available at: http://www.cdc.gov/HAI/toolkits/Evaluating-Environmental-Cleaning.html. Accessed January 10, 2021.

manner for education,[35] studies by Munoz-Price[36,37] demonstrated that the visibility of these substances in ambient light limits their effective use in programs to objectively monitor cleaning practice as a result of their ability to induce a Hawthorne effect. In 2019 a study from Johns Hopkins compared the clinical use of the metered applicator to a cotton swab applicator of a nonstandardized fluorescent gel and found the metered applicator to provide a more accurate assessment of cleaning practice. The investigators concluded that, "Infection control programs implementing Evaluation of Environmental Cleaning programs should carefully consider the type and method of applying fluorescent gel marks to standardize and optimize the measurement of fluorescent gel removal."[38] As noted in an Agency for Healthcare Research and Quality[11(p14)] technical brief, "Metered fluorescent gel is the most commonly used formulation because it dries to a transparent finish on surfaces, it is abrasion-resistant, and unlike powder, is not easily disturbed. For these reasons, the fluorescent gel formulation has been the most well-studied method to assess surface disinfection and to quantify the impact of educational interventions." The report also notes that additional advantages of the made-for-purpose fluorescent surface markers include their "relatively low cost, ease of implementation and their use for direct feedback to the EVS staff."[11(p14)]

Adenosine triphosphate assays: ATP bioluminescence technology detects the presence of organic material, including viable and nonviable bioburden, on surfaces. Although ATP systems are easy to use, attempts to quantify health care surface bioburden have been challenging because of the presence of nonviable organic material and the systems' relative insensitivity to some HAPs.[39–41] As noted by Mulvey and colleagues[42(p29)] in a detailed evaluation of the ATP technology, "Sensitivity and specificity of 57% (with the ATP tool) means that the margin for error is too high to justify stringent monitoring of the hospital environment (with ATP technology) at present." Furthermore, significant intrinsic limitations of the technology that would impact its use in objectively monitoring cleaning practice have been recently identified by Whitley and colleagues[40,43] who noted both the poor sensitivity in measuring viable surface bioburden and the absence of standardization between luminometers by different manufacturers. Additional challenges to using an ATP tool to assess hospital cleaning were noted in a review by Nante and colleagues[44] in 2017, which pointed out the variation in sensitivity between systems made by different manufacturers as well as their lack of standardization. Although not yet investigated, it is plausible that the ATP assay could be used for prospective monitoring of cleaning practice over time if the type of prepost cleaning target evaluation system recommended in the 2010 guidance is followed.

Benefits and Challenges of Environmental Cleaning Monitoring

Although disinfection cleaning process improvement programs developed in accordance with the CDC 2010 guidance have been successful in improving patient zone cleaning as well as decreasing HAP surface contamination and transmission as discussed earlier, recent studies have begun to identify both the collateral benefits and the challenges of these programs.

As part of an HAI prevention initiative in Iowa, a diverse group of 56 hospitals implemented objective monitoring and standardized process improvement activities for discharge cleaning practice using the fluorescent marking system and programmatic interventions modeled after previously published reports.[28,32] Preintervention cleaning thoroughness averaged 60% and was similar in most hospitals (95% confidence interval [CI], 56.7–64.4). As noted in **Fig. 3**, following education and ongoing feedback of performance to the EVS staff, cleaning ultimately improved to 89% for the group (*P*

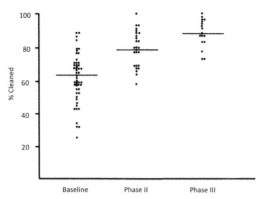

Fig. 3. Thoroughness of discharge cleaning (TDC) during the three phases of the Iowa disinfection cleaning project. Phase I is TDC after a single standardized educational intervention and Phase II is following 2 to 3 cycles of monitoring and feedback. (*Adapted from* Carling PC, Herwaldt LA, VonBeheren S. The Iowa Disinfection Cleaning Project: Opportunities, Successes and Challenges of a Structured Intervention Project in 56 Hospitals. *Infect Control Hosp Epidemiol.* 2017 Aug;38(8):960965; with permission.)

< .001).[32] A structured questionnaire by the hospitals completing the project found that the EVS staff at all hospitals appreciated and were enthusiastic about being evaluated, particularly because the program provided them with a new and unique opportunity to show other health care workers how well they were performing disinfection cleaning activities. Approximately half of the sites noted that the program led to new senior management recognition of the value of the patient safety-oriented work performed by EVS personnel, that the program redefined EVS' role in patient safety, and that the targeting system was valuable for one-on-one training. Twenty percent of the hospitals noted that the study led to identification of opportunities for improving EVS program issues related to manpower resources and communication. A similar number of sites commented on the favorable response the program received from the Board of Trustees. Three of 20 sites (15%) noted that the program initially met resistance from EVS management. Three other sites noted that the program resulted in some transient anxiety among the EVS personnel, which resolved once the value of the program and its nonpunitive orientation was understood. Although the study confirmed the value of an objective structured programmatic process to broadly improve cleaning practice, it also documented the challenges of implementing such activities. Owing primarily to resource limitations (infection preventionists' time constraints) and personnel turnover, more than one-third (23 of 56, 41%) of the sites that likely could have benefitted significantly from the program withdrew from the study before achieving cleaning scores of greater than 80% (see **Fig. 3**). In contrast, it is notable that 71% of the sites in which the initial assessment disclosed opportunities to improve disinfection cleaning were motivated enough to pursue the study and ultimately achieve cleaning scores of greater than 80%. Furthermore, 27% of the hospitals completing the study independently maintained cleaning thoroughness at greater than 90% for more than 3 years.[32] Similar sustainability of cleaning thoroughness (92%) was also found in a group of 14 hospitals in California using the same program for more than a year.[45]

An important component of these monitoring and process improvement programs relates to the importance of their having a validation component. As noted in the 2010

CDC guidance, "It is important that the monitoring be performed by hospital epidemiologists, infection preventionists or their designees who are not part of the actual EVS cleaning program. Such an approach assures the validity of the information collected".[25] [Appendix B, (p1)] The importance of this issue was confirmed in a study that found that when EVS managers monitored the discharge room cleaning, they documented an average TDC score of 82.5%, whereas a research team covertly evaluating the same 2 hospitals documented an average score of 52.4%.[46] Given that neither the Joint Commission nor the World Health Organization considers self-monitoring of hand hygiene practice to be acceptable, it seems reasonable that a similar expectation should be applied to monitoring disinfection cleaning activities.

Mitigating Clostridiodes difficile Spore Transfer from Environmental Surfaces

For more than 50 years, disinfection cleaning in hospitals has primarily used chemical disinfectants based on quaternary ammonium compounds because of their ease of use and good vegetative bacterial killing. Unfortunately, the evolution of *Clostridiodes difficile* (CD) as a major pathogen contaminating the environment in hospitals led to the recognition that these ammonium-based compounds were ineffective in killing CD spores. Research on this issue led to studies using chlorine-based disinfectants, particularly diluted commercial-grade bleach, confirming the clinical effectiveness of bleach-based disinfecting in reducing environmental contamination with CD spores[47] and reducing transmission of CD from surfaces to patients in several studies.[48,49] Unfortunately, the impact of bleach on patient-zone surfaces and the resulting physical damage to both hard and soft materials has precluded it from being widely used as a general disinfectant for daily patient-zone cleaning. Although many hospitals use bleach-based disinfectants for terminal cleaning of rooms vacated by patients with confirmed CD infection, its general use in discharge cleaning is currently recommended by the CDC only for outbreak settings.[50] In the context of these issues, the development of the previously sporicidal disinfectant chemistries raises the possibility that there may be clinical benefit of substituting these newer chemistries for quaternary ammonium disinfectants for daily cleaning of all patient-zone surfaces.

Evolving insights into environmental C difficile epidemiology: While it has long been recognized that spore-contaminated environments have a role in CD transmission, recent studies have clarified and quantified many aspects of the environmental epidemiology of CD in hospitals as outlined in **Table 1**. Several of these elements are of particular note. As noted in Elements 1 and 2, recent studies have shown that asymptomatic patients are CD colonized at the time of admission (average incidence density 10.6%, range 2.8%–21%)[48–60] or during their hospitalization (average prevalence density 12.5%, range 2.9%–21%).[48,61–66] As a result, approximately 11% of acute care hospitalized patients represent an ongoing risk of CD transmission to the environment and susceptible patients. Genomic epidemiology has now confirmed the environmental transmission of spores from these patients to other patients.[62,63,67–69] As noted in Element 3, patients recovering from acute CD infection are associated with significant transmission of spores to their environment.[70–72] This issue was carefully analyzed in a multisite study by Davies and colleagues[73] in 2020 that evaluated the impact of treatment of CD infection on patient-zone environmental contamination. Treatment of CD infection with metronidazole, vancomycin, or fidaxomicin similarly decreased a proportion of patients with positive stool cultures from 100% to 35% immediately after treatment. After treatment the rate rebounded to 80% to 90% by 2 to 4 weeks later. Although there was some decrease in the proportion of environmental sites contaminated with CD spores from 36% before treatment to 20% immediately following treatment, environmental contamination by these patients was still at

Table 1	
Elements of *Clostridioides difficile* environmental epidemiology	
1. At the time of hospitalization 10.6% of patients (range 2.8%–21%) are CD carriers	48–60
2. During hospitalization 12.5% of patients (range 2.9%–21%) are CD carriers	48,61–66
3. Transmission of CD spores to environmental surfaces is associated with: Patients with acute infection Patients recovering from acute infection Asymptomatic CD-colonized patients	70–72
4. Treatment does not decrease ongoing environmental spore contamination for more than a month	73
5. Widespread surface contamination far from known CD-infected patients	47,60
6. Increased cleaning and disinfection result in: Decreased surface and hand contamination Decreased CD acquisition	47,69,70,75
7. Genomic confirmation of the role of asymptomatic CD carriers in transmission	62,63,67–69
8. Acquisition of CD from a prior room occupant is significantly dependent on the prior room occupant receiving antibiotics	74

27% 4 weeks after completing treatment, confirming the significant ongoing risk of transmission of CD to other patients and health care workers by patients who had completed treatment of CD infection. The most striking new insight into the elemental epidemiology of CD was reported by Freedburg and colleagues[74] in 2016. As noted in **Table 1**, Element 8, a cohort of more than 100,000 patients who sequentially occupied a given hospital bed was evaluated to assess the factors relevant to CD spore transmission. The investigators found that administration of antibiotics to the prior bed occupant was the most significant risk factor associated with an increased risk of the subsequent bed occupant developing CD infection, independent of prior room occupants' CD infection status. This finding can only be explained by recipient acquisition of residual CD spores asymptomatically shed onto patient-zone surfaces by the preceding room occupant.

Assessment of the impact of daily sporicidal disinfection cleaning: Given the understanding that CD spore shedding is ongoing in both symptomatic and asymptomatic patients, the inability to clinically recognize CD-colonized patients, and the now feasible general use of sporicidal disinfectants on patient-zone surfaces, it has recently become feasible to consider the potential clinical value of moving to daily sporicidal disinfection cleaning of all high-touch objects. The feasibility of this structured intervention to objectively monitor and improve the thoroughness of daily sporicidal disinfection cleaning on health care-onset CD infection (HO-CDI) was first evaluated in a single-site quasi-experimental study in 2016.[75] As noted in **Fig. 4**, during the 33-month intervention period, TDC rapidly improved from 81% to 92% and remained greater than 88% during the remainder of the study ($P = . 01$). HO-CDI rates decreased significantly during the intervention period from an average of 8.9 to 3.2 per 10,000 patient-days ($P = .0001$, 95% CI 3.48–7.81). The potential value of such daily sporicidal cleaning was also evaluated in 2018 using an agent-based model of CD transmission in a 200-bed hospital, and it was found that daily cleaning with a

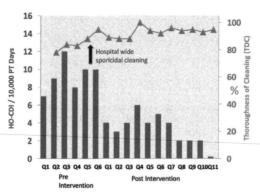

Fig. 4. The impact of optimizing environmental hygiene to decrease *Clostridoides difficile* transmission (*From* Carling P, Scott M. Optimizing envitonmental hygiene to successfully decrease Clostridiun difficile transmission. *Open Forum Infect Dis.* Volume 4, Issue suppl_1, 1 October 2017, Pages S404–S405, https://doi.org/10.1093/ofid/ofx163.1011 Accessed 10 January 2021; with permission.)

sporicidal disinfectant had the potential for reducing hospital-onset CD infections by 68.9%.[76]

The potential clinical usefulness of daily hospital-wide sporicidal disinfectant (Oxy-Cide, Ecolab Inc) for all patient-zone hygienic cleaning was recently evaluated using a quasi-experimental interrupted time series in a group of 8 acute care hospitals with stable endemic Standardized Infection Ratio (SIR) (mean 1.0 for the group) during an 18-month preintervention period.[77] Thoroughness of cleaning was programmatically monitored in accordance with the 2010 CDC guidance using a standardized metered fluorescent marking system (DAZO). As noted in **Fig. 5**, TDC following educational activities during the 3-month wash-in period improved rapidly from 52% to 88%. Ongoing monitoring and education resulted in a further sustained improvement to greater than 90% for all sites. During the initial quarter following the wash-in the SIRs for all hospitals dropped to 60% for the group, as noted in **Fig. 6**. During the final 9 months of the study the mean SIR for the group had decreased to 0.3, representing a greater than 60% improvement from the 18-month preintervention period ($P = .001$), a result highly consistent with the modeling study noted previously.[76] Seven potentially significant confounders were evaluated preintervention and postintervention and were found not to have had an impact on the results. Although a randomized controlled trial could further clarify and quantify the results of this intervention, such an undertaking would require considerable resources as well as the need for sites to defer implementing potentially effective design elements of the intervention. Given the challenges of a randomized trial, it should be noted that an agent-based modeling study by Barker and colleagues[78] (2020) evaluating the impact of multiple single and bundled interventions on HO-CDI prevention found that the single most clinically effective as well as cost-effective intervention was daily sporicidal cleaning of all patient-zone surfaces. Furthermore, quantitative input analysis of the model found only a limited additional incremental benefit from increasing modeling parameters of thoroughness of cleaning from an "enhanced level" (80% TDC) to an "ideal level" (94% TDC), suggesting that daily patient-zone sporicidal cleaning could have a substantial impact on CD transmission when TDC is lower than those achieved by the intervention group of hospitals discussed earlier.[78]

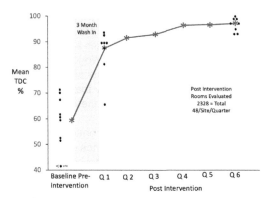

Fig. 5. Thoroughness of daily hospital-wide sporicidal cleaning of patient-zone surfaces. (*From* Carling P, O'Hara L, Harris A, Olmstead R. Mitigating hospital onset *C. difficile*: evaluation of a standardized environmental hygiene program in eight hospitals. The Sixth Decennial International Conference on Healthcare-Associated Infections Abstracts, March 2020. Infect Control Hosp Epidemiol 2020 October;41(S1):s43; with permission.)

ENVIRONMENTAL HYGIENE AND HAND HYGIENE: AN INTEGRATED APPROACH

Over the past several years it has become increasingly evident that infection prevention initiatives focused on optimizing hand hygiene have not realized their hoped-for impact on HAP transmission in well-resourced health care settings.[79–83] Accepting our inability to quantify the absolute risk of pathogen acquisition directly from health care workers' hands, there is good circumstantial evidence that such transmission accounts for a substantial proportion of HAP transmission. Indeed, it has become widely accepted that hand hygiene, as noted by Palamore and Henderson,[84(p8)] is "critically important for the prevention of HAIs". In response many health care organizations have undertaken extensive, resource-intensive efforts to improve hand hygiene compliance.[85] Despite extensive translational research and strong support from accrediting institutions, the enthusiasm for quickly reaping substantial benefits from optimizing hand hygiene practice has been tempered by the realization that

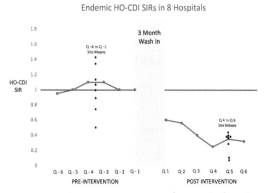

Fig. 6. Endemic HO-CDI SIRs in the study hospitals before and after the study intervention. (*From* Carling P, O'Hara L, Harris A, Olmstead R. Mitigating hospital onset *C. difficile*: evaluation of a standardized environmental hygiene program in eight hospitals. The Sixth Decennial International Conference on Healthcare-Associated Infections Abstracts, March 2020. Infect Control Hosp Epidemiol 2020 October;41(S1):s43; with permission.)

acceptance inertia, psychological barriers, suboptimal application technique, and most particularly, the pressures of providing direct patient care adversely impact the effectiveness of this intervention.[86] These issues along with the challenges of performing hand hygiene as recommended by the World Health Organization Five Moments construct while caring for acutely ill patients and the fact that 10% to 60% of patient-zone surfaces contain HAPs make it likely that pathogen-contaminated environmental surfaces will negate some of the benefits of optimized hand hygiene practice.[87]

Given the fact that patient-zone surfaces not contaminated by HAPs cannot be a source of pathogen transmission even in the absence of hand hygiene, further consideration must be given to viewing both environmental hygiene and hand hygiene as being interdependent interventions. As these 2 interventions are intrinsically relevant, together they represent what can be termed "hygienic practice." When viewed in this manner, it becomes evident that the mandates and challenges of these 2 interventions represent an inverse continuum as noted in **Fig. 7**. For example, in the intensive care unit (ICU) setting where hand hygiene often becomes logistically challenging and glove use without hand hygiene is frequent, there would be a particularly strong mandate to optimize hygienic cleaning. In contrast, in ambulatory and nonpatient care settings where there are few intrinsic barriers to hand hygiene, enhanced hygienic cleaning practices would not be as strongly mandated. In this context, the specific elements of hygienic practice can be characterized along a complexity gradient. By relating these constructs to the various settings noted in **Fig. 8**, interventions can be defined along the continuum outlined to provide a framework for analyzing and prioritizing the relative cost/benefit of different levels of complementary hygienic practices. By characterizing intrinsic patient/personnel risk and setting modifiers, a particular site can be moved up or down diagonally along the range of settings. For example, if an immunologically compromised person was in an ambulatory care setting, it would be reasonable to consider moving to a higher level of hygienic cleaning intervention than would otherwise be warranted. Similarly, if the patient population assisted living arrangements required only minimal assistance, it would be reasonable to move down the intervention continuum toward simpler interventions as noted in **Fig. 8**. Once the particular features of a setting are defined in this manner, programmatic interventions that maximize the components of health care hygienic practice for the best cost/benefit to improving patient/personnel safety can be identified and optimized.

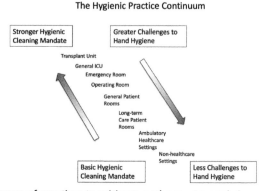

The Hygienic Practice Continuum

Stronger Hygienic Cleaning Mandate

Greater Challenges to Hand Hygiene

Transplant Unit
General ICU
Emergency Room
Operating Room
General Patient Rooms
Long-term Care Patient Rooms
Ambulatory Healthcare Settings
Non-healthcare Settings

Basic Hygienic Cleaning Mandate

Less Challenges to Hand Hygiene

Fig. 7. The Continuum of practices to mitigate pathogen transmission.

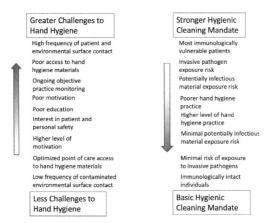

Fig. 8. Elements of hygienic practice.

IMPLEMENTING THE 2020 CDC GUIDANCE: CORE COMPONENTS OF ENVIRONMENTAL CLEANING AND DISINFECTION IN HOSPITALS

In October 2020 the CDC published a guidance document to provide hospitals with a detailed roadmap for the development of programs to optimize all aspects of patient-zone environmental hygiene because "maintaining a clean hospital environment and minimizing the presence of hospital pathogens is critical for keeping patients safe."[88(pe1)] The 6 individual "core components" (**Box 2**) and the specific recommendations within each of the strategies specify what "every healthcare facility should consider to ensure appropriate environmental cleaning and disinfection."[89(pe1)] The components described were developed primarily for acute care hospitals, but the document notes that "they can be applied to all healthcare facilities including long-term care facilities and outpatient settings, although special considerations may be needed for these other healthcare settings." Although not specifically discussed in the document, describing the EVS staff involved in patient-zone cleaning and disinfection as "healthcare personnel" represents a reflection of the relevance these activities have to safe patient care.

Box 2
Core components of environmental cleaning and disinfection in hospitals

1. Integrate environmental services into the hospital's safety culture

2. Educate and train all healthcare providers responsible for cleaning and disinfecting patient care areas

3. Select appropriate cleaning and disinfection technologies and products

4. Standardize setting-specific cleaning and disinfection protocols

5. Monitor effectiveness and adherence to cleaning and disinfection protocols

6. Provide feedback on adequacy and effectiveness of cleaning and disinfection to all responsible healthcare providers as well as relevant stakeholders (eg, infection control, hospital leadership)

Adapted from Reducing risk from surfaces: core components of environmental cleaning and disinfection in hospitals. Available at: https://www.cdc.gov/hai/prevent/environment/surfaces. html Accessed 10 January 2021.

Component 1: Integrate Environmental Services into the Hospital's Safety Culture

This component provides specific recommendations that define institutional responsibilities related to the development and ongoing maintenance of an integrated program to optimize infection prevention activities related to environmental hygiene. Recommendations related to specific pragmatic elements include leadership, multidepartmental involvement, and the need to define programmatic responsibilities including reporting and accountability. Also addressed are the development of both performance evaluation based on objective monitoring procedures (see Component 5) and career advancement opportunities for EVS personnel. .

Component 2: Educate and Train all Health Care Providers Responsible for Cleaning and Disinfecting Patient Care Areas

This component provides a detailed set of recommendations on critical elements of an optimized approach to the education and training of health care professionals involved in environmental hygiene activities along with the components of such training. Additional recommendations include documentation of such training, as well as the need for documentation of corrective actions disclosed as part of ongoing performance monitoring activities (see Component 5). It is also noted that training include information related to facility infection rates and prevention practices.

Component 3: Select Appropriate Cleaning and Disinfection Technologies and Products

This core component emphasizes the importance of validating the clinical and cost benefits of any product or technology being considered; it reflects the recognition that hospitals have adopted technologies and products whose clinical effectiveness and cost benefit value have been incompletely scientifically validated. In response to this issue, it is specifically recommended that hospitals use a prospective "systematic process" to evaluate all such technologies and products, which incorporates analysis by relevant leadership personnel to consider the clinical value, as well as direct and indirect costs, before implementing new programs and technologies.

Component 4: Standardize Setting-Specific Cleaning and Disinfection Protocols

This multifaceted component begins by noting the need for cleaning and disinfection procedures to account for differences in the specialized use of distinct patient care areas (ie, ICU, patient room, emergency department, etc.), taking into account the layout, equipment, and patient exposure with specific protocols in each setting. To ensure optimally effective cleaning disinfection practices, hospitals are also asked to develop specific "minimal cleaning times," which are to be monitored to ensure that they are being appropriately maintained. It is further recommended that the EVS staff be empowered to require adherence to these defined minimal cleaning times.

Component 5: Monitor Effectiveness and Adherence to Cleaning and Disinfection Protocols

This core component defines the need for institutions to develop a patient-zone cleaning disinfection monitoring strategy, as detailed in the 2010 CDC Guidance Options for Monitoring Environmental Cleaning.[25] In addition to implementing a level II program (see **Box 1**), the need to define who should do such monitoring and how data collected will be used is noted. Specific reference to the need for validation of the monitoring program by a person who is not directly responsible for cleaning practice was based on research that confirmed the need for such validation (see previous discussion).

Component 6: Provide Feedback on Adequacy and Effectiveness of Cleaning and Disinfection to all Responsible healthcare providers as well as Relevant Stakeholders (eg, Infection Control, Hospital Leadership)

The final core component addresses the need to have a structured ongoing system for process improvement using the objective monitoring results from the program developed in component 5 and the 2010 CDC guidance referenced earlier. In addition to using such a program for improving patient safety, it is further recommended that the audit data be presented to hospital leadership to "identify active issues and strategies to mitigate opportunities for improvement while validating the effectiveness of the overall cleaning strategy."

Taken together, these core components provide a detailed, clearly structured, and comprehensive template, based on implementation science studies over the past 20 years, to optimize all aspects of environmental hygiene practice for acute care hospitals, which can be adapted to a wide range of patient care settings.

RESEARCH OPPORTUNITIES AND CHALLENGES

Along with an evolving awareness of the need to optimize both the process and structural elements of hygienic cleaning as noted in **Fig. 1**, it has become increasingly evident that there is a need to develop quantifiable evidence to guide best practices.[11,90,91]

During the past 20 years many published reports have described improved outcomes as the result of modifications in basic hygienic cleaning. Unfortunately, causal analysis of almost all of these studies has been greatly hampered by the simultaneous implementation of multiple interventions in addition to "improved cleaning." This issue is particularly well illustrated by the reports of interventions to minimize health care-onset CD infection beginning in the mid-1980s. Although more than 20 quasi-experimental, often outbreak-associated, studies have supported the likely role of improved environmental hygiene on CD transmission, all these studies consist of several interventions implemented simultaneously. Because of confounding variables (some known, some unknown) in each study, it has been impossible to specifically quantify the impact of disinfection cleaning on CD transmission. Even when a single environmental intervention such as cleaning agent change or no-touch technology is being evaluated, published studies have not separated the thoroughness of cleaning from the specific intervention being tested.[92,93]

CLINICS CARE POINTS

- Implementing the CDCs 2020 guidance Core Components of Environmental Cleaning and Disinfection in Hospitals will provide hospitals with a detailed roadmap for the development of programs to optimize all aspects of patient zone environmental hygiene.

- "Hygienic practice" is optimized through coordinated, objectively monitored compliance practice of environmental hygiene and hand hygiene as integrated horizontal infection prevention interventions.

- Objectively validated, daily, hospital-wide patient-zone disinfection cleaning with advanced formula surface disinfectants has the potential for providing optimal mitigation of HAP transmission from environmental surfaces.

ACKNOWLEDGMENTS

This review is dedicated to the memory of Judene Bartley, MS, MPH, CIC, recipient of the prestigious Carol DeMille Achievement Award from the Association for Professionals in Infection Control, whose insight and leadership related to health care environmental hygiene science greatly influenced the development of the field. The author acknowledges editorial guidance and assistance from Hilary Humphreys, MD, and Linda Homan, RN, CIC.

DISCLOSURE

The author reports having served as a consultant to AORN and Ecolab and has licensed patents to Ecolab.

REFERENCES

1. Han JH, Sullivan N, Leas BF, et al. Cleaning hospital room surfaces to prevent healthcare-associated infections. Ann Intern Med 2015;163(8):598–607.
2. Wenzel RP, Edmond MB. Infection Control: The case for horizontal rather than vertical interventional programs. Int J Inf Dis 2010;(Suppl 4):S3–5.
3. Edmond MB, Wenzel RP. Screening inpatients for MRSA - Case Closed. N Engl J Med 2013;368(24):2314.
4. Septimus E, Weinstein A, Perl T, et al. Approaches for preventing healthcare-associated infections: Go long or go wide? Infect Control Hosp Epidemiol 2014;35(7):797–801.
5. Carling PC. Optimizing healthcare environmental hygiene. Infect Dis Clin North Am 2016;30:639–60.
6. Rutala WA, Weber DJ. Selection of the ideal disinfectant. Infect Control Hosp Epidemiol 2014;35(7):855–65.
7. Centers for disease control and prevention/Healthcare Infection Control Advisory Committee (HICPAC) Guidelines for environmental infection control in healthcare facilities. Atlanta, FA: Centers for Disease Control and Prevention; 2003. Available at: http://www.cdc.gov/hicpac/pdf/guidelines/eic_in_HCF_03.pdf. Accessed January 10, 2021.
8. Cadnum JL, Jencson A, Thriveen J, Mana SC, Donskey J. Evaluation of real-world materials compatibility of OxyCide daily disinfectant cleaner versus sodium hypochlorite. Abstract 7202. Presented at the Society for Healthcare Epidemiology Meeting, Orlando, FL, May 14, 2015.
9. Haider S, Moshos J, Burger T, et.al. Impact of QxyCide™ on environmental contamination and infection rates compared to standard cleaning practice. Abstract 1437, ID Week 2014, San Diego, CA October 2014.
10. Huang S, Datta R, Platt R. Risk of acquiring antibiotic-resistant bacteria from prior room occupants. Arch Intern Med 2006;166:1945–51.
11. Environmental cleaning for the prevention of healthcare-associated infections (HAI). Rockville (MD): Agency for Healthcare Research and Quality (US); 2015. Report No.: 15-EHC020-EF. Available at: https://effectivehealthcare.ahrq.gov/

sites/default/files/related_files/healthcare-infections_disposition-comments.pdf - 140k - 2020-12-27. Accessed January 10, 2021.

12. Carling PC, Perkins J, Ferguson J, et al. Evaluating a new paradigm for company surface disinfection in clinical practice. Infect Control Hosp Epidemiol 2014; 35(11):1349–55.

13. Ramm L, Siani S, Westgate R, et al. Pathogen transfer and high variability in pathogen removal by detergent wipes. Am J Infect Control 2015;43:724–8.

14. Sattar SA, Maillard J. The crucial role of wiping in decontamination of high-touch environmental surfaces: A review of current status and directions for the future. Am J Infect Control 2013;41:S97–104.

15. Sattar SA, Bradley C, Kibbee R, et al. Disinfectant wipes are appropriate to control microbial bioburden from surfaces: use of a new ASTM standard test protocol to demonstrate efficacy. J Hosp Infect 2015;91:319–25.

16. McDonald LC, Arduino M. Climbing the evidentiary hierarchy for environmental infection control. Clin Infect Dis 2013;56(1):36–9.

17. Smith P, Watkins K, Hewlett A. Infection control through the ages. Am J Infect Control 2012;40:35–42.

18. Siegel JD, Rhinehart E, Jackson M, et al. Healthcare infection control practices advisory committee. Management of multi-drug-resistant organisms in healthcare settings 2006. Available at: http://www.cdc.gov/hicpac/pdf/guidelines/eic_in_HCF_03.pdf. Accessed January 10, 2021.

19. Carling PC, Bartley JM. Evaluating hygienic cleaning in healthcare settings: what you do not know can harm your patients. Am J Infect Control 2010;38:S41–50.

20. Dancer SJ. How do we assess hospital cleaning? A proposal for microbiological standards for surface hygiene in hospitals. J Hosp Infect 2004;56:10–5.

21. Hayden MK, Bonten MJ, Blom DW, et al. Reduction in acquisition of vancomycin-resistant enterococcus after enforcement of routine environmental cleaning measures. Clin Infect Dis 2006;42(11):1552–60.

22. Carling PC, Brigs J, Hylander D, et al. Evaluation of patient area cleaning in 3 hospitals using a novel targeting methodology. AM J Infect Control 2006;34:513–9.

23. Carling PC, Parry MF, Von Beheren SM. Identifying Opportunities to enhance environmental cleaning in 23 acute care hospitals. Infect Control Hosp Epidemiol 2008;29(1):1–7.

24. Carling PC, Po JL, Bartley J, Herwaldt L; Healthcare environmental hygiene group Identifying opportunities to improve environmental hygiene in multiple healthcare settings. Abstract 908. Fifth Decennial International Conference on Healthcare-Associated Infections. Atlanta, GA, December 10, 2010.

25. Guh A, Carling P, the environmental cleaning work group. Options for monitoring environmental cleaning. Available at: http://www.cdc.gov/HAI/toolkits/Evaluating-Environmental-Cleaning.html. Accessed January 10 2021.

26. Association for the healthcare environment of the American Hospital Association. Curriculum for the Certified Healthcare Environmental Services Technician (TM). Available at: http://www.ahe.org/ahe/lead/CHEST/curriculum.shtml. Accessed January 10, 2021.

27. Carling P. Methods for assessing the adequacy of practice and improving room disinfection. Am J Infect Control 2013;14(5 Suppl):S20–5.

28. Carling PC, Parry MM, Rupp ME, et al. Improving cleaning of the environment surrounding patients in 36 acute care hospitals. Infect Control Hosp Epidemiol 2008; 29(11):1035–41.

29. Carling P, Briggs J, Perkins J, et al. Improving Cleaning of Patient Rooms Using a New Targeting Method. Clin Infect Dis 2006;42:385–8.

30. Carling PC, Eck EK. Achieving sustained improvement in environmental hygiene using coordinated benchmarking in 12 hospitals. Abstracts of the SHEA Fifth Decennial Meeting; Atlanta, GA; March 18-22, 2010.

31. Murphy CL, Macbeth DA, Derrington P, et al. An assessment of high touch object cleaning thoroughness using a fluorescent marker in two Australian hospitals. Healthc Infect 2012;16(4):156–63.

32. Carling PC, Herwaldt LA, VonBeheren S. The Iowa disinfection cleaning project: opportunities, successes and challenges of a structured intervention project in 56 hospitals. Infect Control Hosp Epidemiol 2017;38(8):960965.

33. Datta R, Platt R, Yokoe DS, et al. Environmental cleaning intervention and risk of acquiring multidrug-resistant organisms from prior room occupants. Arch Intern Med 2011;171(6):491–4.

34. Munoz-Price LS, Bimbach DJ, Lubarsky DA, et al. Decreasing operating room environmental pathogen contamination through improved cleaning practice. Infect Control Hosp Epidemiol 2012;33(9):897–904.

35. Gillespie E, Wright P, Snook K, et al. The role of ultraviolet marker assessments in demonstrating cleaning efficacy. Am J Infect Control 2015;43:1347–9.

36. Munoz-Price LS, Fajardo-Aquino Y, Arheart KL, et al. Ultraviolet powder versus ultraviolet gel for assessing environmental cleaning. Infect Control Hosp Epidemiol 2012;33(2):192–5.

37. Munoz-Price LS. Controlling multidrug-resistant gram-negative bacilli in your hospital: a transformational journey. J Hosp Infect 2015;89:254–8.

38. Rock C, Small BA, Hsu YJ, et al. Evaluating accuracy of sampling strategies for fluorescent gel monitoring of patient room cleaning. Infect Control Hosp Epidemiol 2019;40(7):794–7.

39. Boyce JM, Havill NL, Havill HL, et al. Comparison of fluorescent marker systems with 2 quantitative methods of assessing terminal cleaning practices. Infect Control Hosp Epidemiol 2011;32:1187–93.

40. Whiteley GS, Derry C, Glasbey T. A comparative performance of three brands of portable ATP – bioluminometers intended for use in hospital infection control. Healthc Infect 2012;73:4–9.

41. Malik DJ, Shama G. Estimating surface contamination by means of ATP determinations: 20 pence short of a pound. J Hosp Infect 2012;80(4):354–5.

42. Mulvey D, Redding P, Robertson C, et al. Finding a benchmark for monitoring hospital cleanliness. J Hosp Infect 2011;77(1):25–30.

43. Whiteley GS, Derry C, Glasbey T, et al. The perennial problem of variability in adenosine triphosphate (ATP) tests for hygiene monitoring within healthcare settings. Infect Control Hosp Epidemiol 2015;36(6):658–63.

44. Nante N, Ceriale E, Messina G, et al. Effectiveness of ATP bioluminesence to assess hospital cleaning: a review. J Prev Med Hyg 2017;58:E117–83.

45. Holmer L, Russell D, Steger P, Creed J, Speer R, Lakhanpal A. Sustainability of an environmental cleaning program in California small and critical access hospitals. Abstract presented at the Annual Meeting of the Association for Infection Control Professionals. San Diego, CA, May 2014.

46. Knelson LP, Ramadanovic G, Chen L, et al. Self-monitoring of hospital room cleaning by Environmenal Services (EVS) may not accurately measure cleanliness. Infect Control Hosp Epidemiol 2017;38(11):1371–3.

47. Kaatz GW, Gitlin SD, Schaberg DR. Acquisition of *Clostridium difficile* from the hospital environment. Am J Epidemiol 1988;127(6):1289–94.

48. Furuya-Kanamori L, Marquess J, Yakob L. Asymptomatic *Clostridium difficile* colonization: epidemiology and clinical implications. BMC Infect Dis 2015;15:516.

49. Weber DJ, Anderson DJ, Sexton DJ. Role of the environment in the transmission of *Clostridium difficile* in healthcare facilities. Am J Infect Control 2013;41(5 Supl): S105–10.

50. Recommendations of CDC and the healthcare infection control practices Advisor committee (HICPAC). Guidelines for environmental infection control in health-care facilities. Available at: https://www.cdc.gov/mmwr/preview/mmwrhtml/rr5210a1. htm. Accessed January 10, 2021.

51. Loo VG, Bourgault A, Poirier L. Host and pathogen for *Clostridium difficile* infection and colonization. N Engl J Med 2011;365:1693–703.

52. Hung Y, Tsai P, Hung K. Impact of *Clostridium difficile* colonization and infection among hospitalized adults at a district hospital in southern Taiwan. PLoS One 2012;7(8):1.

53. Eyre DW, Griffiths D, Vaughan A. Asymptomatic *Clostridium difficile* and Onward Transmission. PLoS One 2013;8(11):1.

54. Alasmari F, Seiler SM, Hink T. Prevalence and risk factors for asymptomatic *Clostridium difficile* carriage. Clin Infect Dis 2014;59(2):216–22.

55. Kong LY, Dendukuri N, Schiller I. Predictors of asymptomatic *Clostridium difficile* colonization on hospital admission. Am J Infect Control 2015;43:248–53.

56. Nissle K, Kopf D, Rosler A. Asymptomatic and yet *C. difficile*-toxin positive? Prevalence and risk factors of carriers of toxigenic *Clostridium difficile* among geriatric in-patients. BMC Geriatr 2016;16:185.

57. Longtin Y, Paquet-Bolduc B, Gilca R. Effect of detecting and isolating *Clostridium difficile* carriers at hospital admission on the incidence of *C. difficile* infections . A Quasi-experimental controlled study. JAMA Intern Med 2016;176(6):796–804.

58. Rea MC, O'Sullivan O, Shanahan F. *Clostridium difficile* carriage in elderly subjects and associated changes in the intestinal microbiota. J Clin Microbiol 2011;867–75.

59. Sheth PM, Douchant K, Uyanwune Y. Evidence of transmission of *Clostridium difficile* in asymptomatic patients following admission screening in a tertiary care hospital. PLoS One 2019;1–14.

60. Gonzalez-Orta M, Saldana C, Ng-Wong Y. Are many patients diagnosed with healthcare-associated *Clostridioides difficile* infections colonized with the infecting strain on admission? Clin Infect Dis 2019;69:1801–4.

61. Galdys AL, Nelson JS, Shutt KA. Prevalence and duration of asymptomatic *Clostridium difficile* carriage among healthy subjects in Pittsburgh, Pennsylvania. J Clin Microbiol 2014;52(7):2406–9.

62. Blixt T, Gradel KO, Homann C. Asymptomatic carriers contribute to nosocomial *Clostridium difficile* infection: A cohort study of 4508 patients. Gastroenterology 2017;152:1031–41.

63. Kong LY, Eyre DW, Corbeil J. *Clostridium difficile*: Investigating transmission patterns between infected and colonized patients using whole genome sequencing. Clin Infect Dis 2019;68(2):204–9.

64. Koo H, Van J, Zhao M. Real-time polymerase chain reaction detection of asymptomatic *Clostridium difficile* colonization and rising *C. difficile*-associated disease rates. Infect Control Hosp Epidemiol 2014;35(6):667–73.

65. Guerrero DM, Becker JC, Eckstein EC. Asymptomatic carriage of toxigenic *Clostridium difficile* by hospitalized patients. J Hosp Infect 2013;85:155–8.

66. Halstead FD, Ravi A, Thomson N. Whole genome sequencing of toxigenic *Clostridium difficile* in asymptomatic carriers: insights into possible role in transmission. Microb Genom 2019;(9):e000293.

67. Kumar N, Miyajima F, HE M. Genome-based infection tracking reveals dynamics of *Clostridium difficile* transmission and disease recurrence. Clin Infect Dis 2016; 62(6):746–52.

68. Endres BT, Dotson KM, Poblete K. Environmental transmission of *Clostridioides difficile* ribotype 027 at a long-term care facility; an outbreak investigation guided by whole genome sequencing. Infect Control Hosp Epidemiol 2018;39(11): 1322–9.

69. Chen LF, Knelson LP, Gergen MF. A prospective study of transmission of multidrug resistant organisms (MDROs) between environmental sites and hospitalized patients-the TransFER study. Infect Control Hosp Epidemiol 2019;40·47–52.

70. Jinno S, Kundrapu S, Gurrero DM, et al. Potential for transmission of *Clostridium difficile* by asymptomatic acute care patients and long-term care facility residents with prior *C. difficile* infection. Infect Control Hosp Epidemiol 2012;33(6):638–9.

71. Shrestha SK, Sunkesula CK, Kundrapu S. Acquisition of *Clostridium difficile* on hands of healthcare personnel caring for patients with resolved *C. difficile* infection. Infect Control Hosp Epidemiol 2016;37(4):45–7.

72. Reigadas E, Vazquez-Cuesta S, Villar-Gomara L. Role of *Clostridioides difficile* in hospital environment and healthcare workers. Anaerobe 2020;63:102204.

73. Davies K, Mawer D, Walker AS, et al. An analysis of Clostridium difficile environmental contamination During and after treatment for C difficile Infection. Available at: https://academic.oup.com/ofid/article/7/11/ofaa362/5893473. Accessed January 10, 2021.

74. Freedberg DE, Salmasian J, Cohen B. Receipt of antibiotics in hospitalized patients and risk for *Clostridium difficile* infection in subsequent patients who occupy the same bed. JAMA Intern Med 2016;176(12):1801–8.

75. Carling P, Scott M. Optimizing environmental hygiene to successfully decrease Clostridiun difficile transmission. Open Forum Infect Dis 2017;4(suppl_1): S404–5. Available at: https://doi.org/10.1093/ofid/ofx163.1011 Accessed January 10, 2021.

76. Barker AK, Alagoz O, Safdar N. Interventions to reduce the incidence of hospital-onset Clostridium difficile infection: An Agent-Based Modeling Approach to Evaluate Clinical Effectiveness in Acute Care Hospitals. Clin Infect Dis 2018;66(8): 1192–203.

77. Carling P, O'Hara L, Harris A, et al. Mitigating Hospital Onset *C. difficile*: Evaluation of a Standardized Environmental Hygiene Program in Eight Hospitals. The Sixth Decennial International Conference on Healthcare-Associated Infections Abstracts, March 2020. Infect Control Hosp Epidemiol 2020;41(S1):s43.

78. Barker A, Scaria E, Safdar N. Evaluation of the cost-effectiveness of infection control strategies to reduce hospital-onset *Clostridioides difficile* infection. JAMA Netw Open 2020;3(8):1–11.

79. Silvestri L, Petros AJ, Sarginson RE, et al. Hand washing in the intensive care unit: a big measure with modest effects. J Hosp Infect 2005;59:172–9.

80. Rupp M, Fitzgerald T, Puumala S, et al. Prospective, controlled, cross-over trial of alcohol-based hand gel in critical care units. Infect Control Hosp Epidemiol 2008; 29(1):8–15.

81. Sepkowitz KA. Why doesn't hand hygiene work better? Lancet Infect Dis 2012; 12:96–7.

82. Smiddy M, O'Connell R, Creedon S. Systematic qualitative literature review of health care worker's compliance with hand hygiene guidelines. Am J Infect Control 2015;43:269–74.

83. Graves N. It's not all about hand hygiene – other measures are at least that impor- tant. Controversies Infection Control and Prevention. Presented at the Inter- science Conference on Antimicrobial Agents and Chemotherapy 2015. San Diego, CA. September 17, 2015.

84. Palmore T, Henderson D. Big brother is washing . . . video surveillance for hand hygiene adherence, through the lenses of efficacy and privacy. Clin Infect Dis 2012;54(1):8–9.

85. Page K, Barnett A, Campbell M, et al. Costing the Australian national hand hy- giene initiative. J Hosp Infect 2014;88:141–8.

86. Conway L, Riley L, Saiman L, et al. Implementation and impact of an automated group monitoring and feedback system to promote hand hygiene among health care personnel. Jt Comm J Qual Patient Saf 2014;40(9):408–17.

87. Sax H, Allegranzi B, Uckay I, et al. "My five moments of hand hygiene": a user- centered design approach to understand, train, monitor and report hand hy- giene. J Hosp Infect 2007;67:9–21.

88. Reddy S. Core strategies of environmental cleaning and disinfection in hospitals. Minutes of the Healthcare Infection Control and Prevention Advisory Committee. page 74-81. November 14-15, 2019. Available at: https://www.cdc.gov/hicpac/ pdf/2019-Nov-HICPAC-Summary-508.pdf. Accessed October 6, 2020.

89. Reducing risk from surfaces: Core components of environmental cleaning and Disinfection in hospitals. Available at: https://www.cdc.gov/hai/prevent/ environment/surfaces.html. Accessed January 10, 2021.

90. Carling PC. Optimizing environmental hygiene: the Key to C. Difficile control 2012. Available at: http://www.webbertraining.com/files/library/docs/416.pdf. Ac- cessed January 30, 2021.

91. Safdar N, Anderson D, Braun B, et al. The evolving landscape of healthcare- associated infections: Recent advances in prevention and a road map for research. Infect Control Hosp Epidemiol 2014;35(5):480–93.

92. Carling PC. What is the role of mobile no-touch disinfection technology in opti- mizing healthcare environmental hygiene?. In: Berman R, Munoz-Price S, Morgan D, et al, editors. New perspectives and controversies in infection preven- tion. Springer; 2018.

93. Dancer SJ. How Much Impact Do Antimicrobial Surfaces Really Have on Health- care Acquired Infection? Clin Infect Dis 2020;71(8):1816.

Outbreaks in Health Care Settings

Geeta Sood, MD, MSc[a],*, Trish M. Perl, MD, MSc[b]

KEYWORDS

- Outbreaks • Clusters • Health care settings • Sources of outbreaks • Evaluation
- Review

KEY POINTS

- Outbreaks and pseudo-outbreaks occurring in health care settings should be approached systematically using advanced laboratory testing and epidemiologic tools to guide evaluation of events and to determine courses of action.
- Most often, no single source is identified and outbreaks arise because of failures in following processes, guidance, or policies; inadequate training or education; and inadequate resources. In cases where a single source is identified, health care personnel who are carriers or fail to follow appropriate practices, contaminated environment, supplies and equipment, potable water, and inadequate ventilation and construction or other processes have been associated with outbreaks.
- Multiple organisms including nontuberculous mycobacteria, antimicrobial-susceptible and resistant strains of *Acinetobacter*, *Pseudomonas*, *S aureus*, Enterobacteriales including carbapenem-resistant Enterobacteriaceae, influenza, coronaviruses, and fungal species cause outbreaks in health care settings.
- Health care settings can see dramatic spread because of the types of patient populations that are cared for in these settings and procedures these patients receive. Certain settings including intensive care units (ICUs), neonatal intensive care units, endoscopy units, oncology, and transplant units have at-risk populations and specific processes that impact the approach to investigation and control of outbreaks.
- Health care epidemiologists and infection preventionists have training in and are well equipped to lead and support outbreak investigations in health care settings.

OUTBREAKS

Health care settings generally provide a safe environment for patient care; however, these settings are complex and can facilitate the transmission of organisms and outbreaks. First, patients are vulnerable hosts because of immunosuppressive

[a] Division of Infectious Diseases, Johns Hopkins University School of Medicine, Johns Hopkins Bayview Medical Center, Mason F. Lord Building, Center Tower, 3rd Floor, 5200 Eastern Avenue, Baltimore, MD 21224, USA; [b] Division of Infectious Diseases and Geographic Medicine, UT Southwestern Medical Center, 5323 Harry Hines Boulevard, Y7;302, Dallas, TX 75390, USA
* Corresponding author.
E-mail address: gsood1@jhmi.edu

Infect Dis Clin N Am 35 (2021) 631–666
https://doi.org/10.1016/j.idc.2021.04.006
0891-5520/21/© 2021 Elsevier Inc. All rights reserved.

conditions, disruptions of their skin and mucous membranes, medications, and extremes of age. The facility design, the multitude of life-saving invasive procedures performed using complicated equipment, contamination of the hospital environment with organisms, including multidrug resistant organisms, the close proximity of patients that harbor transmissible organisms to one another, and frequent contact with health care personnel, who can themselves transmit organisms, can provide abundant opportunities for the propagation of an infectious agent.

As more health care delivery has shifted from acute care hospitals to outpatient settings, long-term or skilled nursing facilities and home settings, complexities have expanded into these nontraditional settings. These facilities are not designed for medical care and often have goals that require socialization of residents, which increases contact between patients. Staff may have less training in infection prevention practices yet the host risk factors that place these individuals at risk in acute care settings are still present. Hence, outbreaks are increasingly recognized in these types of alternative settings.

Outbreaks can lead to significant morbidity, mortality, costs, and stress among staff and patients. They are expensive, time-consuming, and can cause significant disruptions in health care operations.[1–3] A recent review found the costs for seven outbreaks ranged from €10,778 to €356,754 (~$12,934–$428,105).[4] The cost per day per patient involved in the outbreak was between €10 ($12) and €1369 ($1642) (95% confidence interval, €49–€1042). Almost 50% of the costs were associated with bed closure because of the outbreak.[4] Data show that 12% of published outbreaks led to closures of medical units, which is likely an underestimate of the true incidence.[5] The most common pathogens associated with unit closure were not highly resistant bacterial organisms but rather, viruses, such as influenza and norovirus.[5] Rotavirus and severe acute respiratory syndrome (SARS) were also associated with high closure rates.[5] These closures can also impact specialty units. In a review of outbreaks in burn units, 5 of 28 burn unit outbreaks required unit closure.[6]

The greatest challenges in outbreak management pertain to the delay in identification of an outbreak and the delay in determining the source of the outbreak. In 37% of published outbreaks, the source is not identified. When the source is identified, it can be traced back to patients (25.7%), medical equipment or devices (11.9%), the environment (11.6%), and the staff (10.9%).[7] The most common pathogens identified in outbreaks are *Staphylococcus aureus* (14.8%), *Pseudomonas* spp (8.9%), and *Klebsiella* spp (7.1%) and these organisms are rarely associated with unit closures.[7,8]

APPROACH TO AN OUTBREAK

An outbreak is defined as an increase in "events," such as infections or number of organisms, above the baseline rate for a geographic area during a specified period of time. Some experts use a statistical definition. This increase may be a single infection, as in the cases of anthrax, health care–associated Legionella, or group A Streptococcal infection, or it may be many infections. The increase may occur over a short period of time, or over years. It may occur in a single unit or across many hospitals. Evaluating and managing outbreaks is complex and multifaceted and often multiple steps occur concurrently. In any setting, the investigation should be efficient, thoughtful, and systematic so that appropriate infection prevention processes are implemented to protect patients and health care personnel quickly (**Box 1**).

Commonly, a potential outbreak is identified in one of three ways: (1) a vigilant clinician who notices an unusual pattern of infection, (2) the laboratory that notes an increase in an unusual organism, or (3) an increase in the frequency of an

---

Box 1
Outbreak investigation

1. Verify the diagnosis and notify laboratory.

2. Determine if this is an outbreak (baseline rates, assess changes in definition and changes in population).

3. Generate an epidemic curve and a line list (describe potential cases person, place, and time).

4. Perform a literature review, to guide risk factor assessment.

5. Develop a case definition.

6. Find cases.

7. "Shoe leather epidemiology," talk to staff, evaluate facility structure.

8. Implement appropriate infection prevention interventions.

9. Communicate with hospital leadership, public relations department, and risk department as indicated. Involve public health authorities.

10. Generate hypothesis and review cases for common epidemiologic links.

11. Test the hypothesis (case-controlled evaluation).

12. Perform additional environmental or personnel screening as indicated.

13. Evaluate impact of intervention.

---

organism or type of infection based on infection prevention surveillance data. The initial step is to verify the diagnosis and assess if there is a true increase in infection rates. A varicella rash may be confused with smallpox, a culture may have been misread or the organism misidentified, or a perceived increase in infections may not be greater than the expected number of infections because of a definition change or changes in how data are captured. Verification may require additional laboratory testing or clinical evaluation. Early in the investigation it is critical to communicate with the laboratory and ensure they save any and all isolates and specimens that may be related to the situation under investigation even before it is determined that there truly is an outbreak. Because routine microbiologic specimens are not saved indefinitely, this step is time-sensitive to preserve specimens that would have otherwise been discarded. These specimens can then be used to identify a common source, trace transmission patterns, or reveal that a perceived outbreak was a cluster of unrelated events.

Once the diagnosis has been confirmed, and the laboratory has been notified, a line list that describes potential cases with regards to person, place, and time is developed. This is used to help focus the investigation. Data collected may include demographic and exposure information, such as age, gender, unit or service, operating room, type of infection, organism, date of infection, and so forth. Simultaneously, it is important to determine if the baseline rate of the organism or infection of interest has changed over time, keeping in mind seasonal variation and comparing equivalent seasons. Such assessments must consider and ensure that other factors are not leading to the newly identified increase to accurately ascertain if there is a "true" increase in the rate of interest. A change in rates could result from altered surveillance, definitions, new or more frequent testing approaches (changes in the numerator), or changes in the patient population sampled (changes in the denominator). Outbreak investigation is an iterative process and as this assessment process is occurring, other cases should be identified, which may involve broadening the numbers and types of patients tested.

Once it has been determined that the observed infections represent a true increase above baseline, the next step in investigating an outbreak is to create a case definition. This definition should be broad enough to capture any potential cases that may have been missed on initial evaluation but not too broad to lose specificity in investigating any important epidemiologic links. Case finding should be performed systematically to avoid bias in data collection. Commonly this requires a review of the literature to understand incubation period, transmission dynamics, and common identified sources of a specific organism or syndrome (**Table 1**). Case definitions may need to be revised in the course of an investigation as new information becomes available. To identify cases, multiple data sources are available including medical records, microbiology reports, operating room notes, respiratory therapy and procedure logs, or pharmacy records. Whatever the source, it is important the cases be collected systematically from these sources using the same definition to ensure reliable information is collected and analyzed. Once case finding has been performed, generating an epidemic curve, which is a spatial presentation of the number of cases over time, aids in understanding transmission patterns. For example, these data may help differentiate a point source versus ongoing transmission and secondary transmission, and can help in assessing the phase of the epidemic.

These early steps are used to create and test a hypothesis by assessing if the suspected exposure differs in the cases from the uninfected patients (control subjects) to understand the relative contribution of risk factors to the outbreak. Depending on the situation (see **Table 1**), additional testing, such as environmental sampling from the patient's room or equipment, or testing of health care personnel and other patients may be undertaken to understand the extent of the outbreak. The epidemiologic review guides and supplements culture and clinical data in the investigative phase and is later used to evaluate the impact of the control measures implemented to control the outbreak.

Importantly and in reality, measures to stop the outbreak are put into place before the hypothesis can be confirmed. In such situations, a line list of the cases with a list of possible exposures is used to simultaneously investigate epidemiologic links between cases and to implement control measures, such as changing a practice; enhancing compliance with a practice, such as hand hygiene; enhancing isolation practices; testing personnel or patients; or closing a unit. These interventions should be performed thoughtfully and through multidisciplinary groups representing all of the vested parties.

Communication is a critical part of an outbreak investigation. It is essential to keep hospital or entity leadership informed of findings and interventions in a timely and regular manner. It is helpful to include the legal team to advise on medicolegal issues. Communication outside the institution is challenging and is best handled by an experienced individual who is credible, respected, and can speak to the issues and offer reassurance when appropriate. It may also be necessary and useful to communicate with the local health department depending on the specifics of the outbreak.

PSEUDO-OUTBREAKS

Pseudo-outbreaks are defined as an increase in identified organisms without evidence of infection. Sometimes, these are difficult to distinguish from "true" clusters or outbreaks. Pseudo-outbreaks generally represent contamination. Identification of the source is important to prevent inappropriate treatment and additional testing in

Table 1
Approach to investigation of common organisms

Organism Type of Infections Associated with Outbreaks	Process	Common Reservoirs	Potential Sources and/or Sites Associated with Outbreaks	Method of Detection	Comments
Acinetobacter spp Wounds, bloodstream, and respiratory tract	I/C	Wounds, respiratory tract and GU, PR area, skin	Instrumentation, burns, trauma, surgery, respiratory equipment, gloves, parenteral nutrition, water	P = microbiologic clinical (micro) cultures E = surface swabs and culture of potentially implicated items	Intensive care units, patients returning from war zones Immunocompromised population; post-COVID-19 Contaminates the environment extensively and is difficult to eradicate
Adenovirus Epidemic keratoconjunctivitis; disseminated infection, cystitis	I	Oral pharyngeal secretions, urinary tract	Equipment (tonometers) and health care workers	P = viral cultures, PCR E = not known to be useful	Ophthalmology patients, NICU patients, immunocompromised patients
Aspergillus spp Bloodstream, lower respiratory tract	I/C	Air, dust, mold	Building demolition, renovation or construction sites, ventilation systems, dust-generating activities	P = microcultures E = air sampling, surface samples	Often pathogenic in immunocompromised populations, and premature infants Can see increases after floods, severe weather events, such as hurricanes
Burkholdaria cepacia Bloodstream, respiratory tract	I/C	Oropharynx, skin	Water and soil, contaminated solutions and skin disinfectants, contaminated equipment	P = microcultures, stool E = cultures of potentially implicated items	Disinfectants (especially those containing iodine), water, solutions; common organism in patients with cystic fibrosis, chronic lung disease, and compromised immune systems

(continued on next page)

Table 1
(continued)

Organism Type of Infections Associated with Outbreaks	Process	Common Reservoirs	Potential Sources and/or Sites Associated with Outbreaks	Method of Detection	Comments
Candida spp Bloodstream, wounds	I	Skin (intertriginous areas)	Hands, oncholysis, devices	P = microcultures E = cultures of hands and nail beds and environmental surfaces	Immunocompromised population at increased risk *Candida auris* is an emerging species that contaminates the environment and associated with ICU and nursing homes and in patients who have COVID-19 infections
Campylobacter fetus GI tract	I/C	GI	Food	P = microcultures E = cultures of potentially implicated items/personnel	NICU patients at risk
Coronavirus (SARS-CoV-1; SARS-CoV-2 and MERS-CoV) Respiratory tract	I/prolonged shedding	Respiratory tract	Unrecognized patients or infected individuals; aerosol-generating procedures	PCR and antigen primary diagnostic tool E = air samples and surface samples in research settings	Nosocomial transmission described with inadequate personal protective equipment in health care personnel; unrecognized patients, inadequate ventilation, and lack of cohorting

Organism/Infection	I/C	Reservoir/Sites	Mode of Transmission	Cultures	Comments
Enterobacter species (some now renamed as *Klebsiella*, such as *aerogenes*) Urinary tract, bloodstream Infection, respiratory tract infections, catheter-associated UTI and colonization	I/C	PR, bloodstream, wounds	Contaminated IV fluids, TPN Hands/dermatitis	P = microcultures E = cultures of potentially implicated items	ICU, reuse of calibrated pressure transducers, can be resistant to β-lactam and carbapenem antimicrobials and emerge in settings with extensive antimicrobial use
Enterococcus faecalis and *faecium* including vancomycin-resistant strains Asymptomatic bacteriuria, catheter-associated UTI, catheter-associated bloodstream infections, surgical site infections, and rarely neonatal sepsis	I/C	GU, PR, GI, and urinary tracts, wounds	Surgical and transplant patients/neonates	P = stool, PR vaginal cultures; hand cultures E = used for vancomycin-resistant strains, primarily surface samples	Vancomycin-resistant strains do contaminate the environment and hands of health care personnel Environmental cultures are not used for susceptible strains
Escherichia coli Epidemic diarrhea, wounds and surgical incisions, urinary tract, bloodstream, neonatal sepsis or meningitis	I/C	GI tract, skin, urinary tract, wounds	Equipment or fluids contaminated with organisms from lower GI tract, contaminated fluids especially in lower income settings	P = microcultures, stool E = cultures of potentially implicated items	Common normal flora of the GI tract Can develop resistance to β-lactam antimicrobials and carbapenems Common cause of infection in neonates

(continued on next page)

Table 1
(continued)

Organism Type of Infections Associated with Outbreaks	Process	Common Reservoirs	Potential Sources and/or Sites Associated with Outbreaks	Method of Detection	Comments
E coli O157:H7 and other hemorrhagic species Diarrhea and hemorrhagic colitis	I	GI tract of animals	Contaminated water, and foods (meat, salads)	P = microcultures E = cultures of potentially implicated items	Hemolytic uremic syndrome and thrombotic thrombocytopenic purpura are sequelae, high mortality among elderly and extremely young, cross-contamination described
Hepatitis A Hepatobiliary tract	I	Liver, stool, blood	Hands/foods, transfusion	P = microcultures E = not known to be useful, cultures of potentially implicated personnel	Generally foodborne and associated with inadequately prepared food but cross-contamination described
Hepatitis B Hepatobiliary tract	I (chronic)	Liver, blood, and sterile body fluids	Blood and secretions, transfusions, improperly cleaned equipment, poor infection control practices	P = serology E = not known to be useful, cultures of potentially implicated personnel	Patients with diabetes, on dialysis, patients in psychiatric units with cross-contamination when devices are shared and contaminated with blood
Hepatitis C Hepatobiliary tract	I (chronic)	Liver, blood, and sterile body fluids	Blood and secretions, transfusions, improperly cleaned equipment, multidose vials, poor infection-control practices	P = serology E = not known to be useful although recently integrated into an outbreak investigation, cultures of potentially implicated personnel	Patients on dialysis, patients in psychiatric units, homeless individuals or those with substance use with cross-contamination when devices are shared and contaminated with blood

Organism/Infection		Reservoir	Source	P/E	Comments
Herpes virus infection; Skin, pneumonia, mucosal surfaces	I/C	Skin, saliva, respiratory secretions	Patients and health care workers	P = microcultures E = not known to be useful	Outbreaks reported when patients shed via respiratory secretions or other bodily fluids or with lesions in health care workers
HIV; Bloodstream and lymphocytes	I	Blood and sterile body fluids	Blood and secretions, transfusions, improperly cleaned equipment and reused needles	P = serology E = not known to be useful	Patients with substance use disorders, multiple sexual partners, and other high-risk behaviors Cross-contamination reported when devices are shared and contaminated with blood
Influenza A and B; Respiratory tract	I/prolonged shedding	Respiratory tract	Unrecognized patients or infected individuals; aerosol-generating procedures; nursing homes and NICU important settings	PCR and antigen primary diagnostic tool E = rarely used	Nosocomial transmission described with inadequate personal protective equipment in health care personnel; unrecognized patients, inadequate ventilation, and lack of cohorting
Klebsiella aerogenes; Urinary tract, pneumonia, bloodstream infections	I/C	PR, respiratory secretions, wounds, skin, blood, and urine	Urinary catheters, ventilators, IV catheters	P = microcultures E = cultures of potentially implicated items	Pathogen in patients in the ICU and with immunosuppression including burn units Can be resistant to extended β-lactamases and carbapenemase Cross-contamination described

(continued on next page)

Table 1
(continued)

Organism Type of Infections Associated with Outbreaks	Process	Common Reservoirs	Potential Sources and/or Sites Associated with Outbreaks	Method of Detection	Comments
Klebsiella pneumoniae Urinary tract, pneumonia, bloodstream, and neonatal infections	I/C	PR, respiratory secretions, urine wounds, skin, blood	Urinary catheters, hand lotions, contaminated fluids, ventilators, eczema Foodborne outbreaks recently reported	P = microcultures E = cultures of potentially implicated items	Pathogen in patients in the ICU and with immunosuppression including burn units and neonatal ICUs Can be resistant to extended β-lactamases and carbapenem antimicrobials Cross-contamination described Rarely contaminates the environment
Legionella pneumophila and other species Pneumonia	I	Water	Potable water, air conditioning units, cooling towers, ice machines, construction	P = microcultures E = cultures of potentially implicated items/ personnel	Can be associated with intense media scrutiny; 1 health care–associated case should trigger an investigation
Listeria monocytogenes Bloodstream and central nervous system infections	I	Food	Contaminated foods	P = microcultures E = cultures of potentially implicated items	Immunocompromised and mother-infant pairs at highest risk
Mycobacterium tuberculosis Respiratory	I	Respiratory tract and larynx, can disseminate	Airborne, improperly cleaned respiratory equipment (bronchoscopes)	P = culture and PCR E = not known to be useful, cultures of potentially implicated personnel	Health care transmission suggests poor infection control measures including inadequate ventilation and inadequate respiratory protection

Organism/Site		Source	Diagnosis	Comments
Nontuberculous Mycobacteria (Mycobacterium avium, M gordonae, M chimaera) Respiratory, skin, bloodstream	I/C	Contaminated potable and hospital water and water systems, ice and ice machines, improperly cleaned and sterilized equipment	P = microcultures E = cultures of potentially implicated items	Associated with pseudo-outbreaks but recently reported in hospital water systems and contaminated heating cooling devices in cardiac surgery Improperly cleaned dialyzers and other equipment/devices, contaminated ice machines and contaminated water
Pseudomonas aeruginosa Burns, wounds, urinary and respiratory tracts	I/C	Ventilators, whirlpools, sitz baths, solutions (mouthwash), any other water sources	P = microcultures, stool E = cultures of potentially implicated items	Primarily seen in immunocompromised patients and in burn unit patients and can be normal flora
Rastonia pickettii Bloodstream	I	Water including sterile, skin disinfectants, incubator water baths	P = microcultures, stool, E = cultures of potentially implicated items	Deliberate contamination of sterile fluids has been reported Neonates and immunocompromised hosts
Respiratory syncytial virus Respiratory	I with prolonged shedding	Unrecognized infected individuals; aerosol-generating procedures, environmental contamination	PCR and antigen primary diagnostic tool E = air samples and surface samples in research settings	Nosocomial transmission described with inadequate personal protective equipment in health care personnel; unrecognized patients, and lack of cohorting

(continued on next page)

Table 1
(continued)

Organism Type of Infections Associated with Outbreaks	Process	Common Reservoirs	Potential Sources and/or Sites Associated with Outbreaks	Method of Detection	Comments
Salmonella species GI infections, bloodstream	I/C	GI and biliary tracts	Contaminated food, dairy, eggs/poultry, contaminated blood products	P = stool, blood cultures E = not known to be useful	Not normal flora, cross-contamination reported
Serratia marcescens Urinary and respiratory tracts, bloodstream	I/C	GI and GU tracts	Solutions, inhalation therapy equipment, disinfectants, plasma, EDTA collection tubes, air conditioning vents, improperly cleaned equipment, chlorhexidine	P = microcultures E = cultures of potentially implicated items	Cross-contamination well described, reuse of calibrated pressure transducers
Staphylococcus aureus including methicillin-resistant Surgical site, bloodstream, respiratory tract, and skin infection and/or colonization	I/C	Anterior nares, skin, throat and nasopharynx, and PR	Nasal/skin carriage in health care workers Increased nurse to patient ratios, gaps in infection prevention practices	P = microcultures and PCR E = hand and anterior nares cultures; rarely environmental cultures are indicated including settle plates if looking for a cloud spreader	25% of individuals are *S aureus* nasal carriers Can result from either point source (usually a carrier) or from poor infection prevention practices Human carriers can shed from skin or respiratory track Increased shedding associated with skin diseases and respiratory tract infections Decolonization is used if carrier identified

Organism / Infection	I/C	Reservoir	Mode / Source	Prevention (P) / Environmental (E)	Comments
Staphylococcus spp (coagulase negative) Blood	I/C	Human skin	IV fluids, contaminated hands of health care workers, implanted devices	P = microcultures E = not known to be useful	Pathogenic in immunocompromised hosts and premature infants Commonly a bloodstream contaminant
Streptococcus pyogenes (Group A streptococcus) Deep wounds or intra-abdominal abscess, bloodstream infections	I/C	Upper respiratory tract, perianal area (rectum and vagina)	Carriage among health care workers	P = wound, stool cultures E = settle plates	Not commonly normal flora Threshold for a health care–associated investigation especially with surgical site infection: 1 case Can be associated with a human carrier (respiratory tract, GU tract)
Varicella zoster virus Disseminated or localized infection	I (local or disseminated)	Respiratory secretions and skin lesions	Poor ventilation, inadequate use of transmission-based precautions	P = viral cultures, PCR or serology E = not known to be useful	Children and immunocompromised patients at risk and unvaccinated exposed can develop disease
Yersinia enterocolitica Bloodstream, GI tract	I	Gastrointestinal tract	Foodborne and packed red blood cells	P = microcultures E = cultures of potentially implicated items	Foodborne illness associated with poor food preparation

Abbreviations: C, colonization; E, environmental source; GI, gastrointestinal; GU, genitourinary tract; HIV, human immunodeficiency virus; I, infection; ICU, intensive care unit; IV, intravenous; NICU, neonatal intensive care unit; P, patients; PCR, polymerase chain reaction; PR, perirectal; UTI, urinary tract infection.

patients that do not have a true infection. Contamination can occur in the laboratory, pharmacy, at the bedside, or in a compounding facility. For example, between 1965 and 2010, 72 clusters of pseudobacteremia, 22 cases of pseudomeningitis, and 49 cases of pseudopneumonia were published. In these instances, clinical specimens, such as blood, cerebral spinal fluid, or tracheal aspirates, grew organisms yet the patients did not have evidence of infections.[9] Most commonly, these pseudoinfections are identified from cultured blood. These pseudobacteremias have been traced to contaminated culture media, contaminated skin antiseptics, contaminated blood culture vials, or inadequate disinfection of the analyzer. Although less common, pseudomeningitis has significant sequelae and has been caused by contamination of procedure kits or culture media. Pseudopneumonias are often noted with mycobacterial species and related to contaminated bronchoscopes or inadequate sterilization processes.[9]

LABORATORY AND TESTING

The expertise and collaboration of the laboratory is critical in the investigation of an outbreak.[10] It is essential to notify the microbiology laboratory staff of a potential outbreak as soon as possible and ask them to save any potentially related specimens. Laboratory testing plays an important role in outbreak investigation. The reverse is also true and the microbiology laboratory often identifies unusual organisms or clusters of an organism and in turn notifies the infection prevention department so they can initiate an investigation.

Microbiologic and molecular testing is continually evolving (**Table 2**). In addition to culturing, determining susceptibility patterns, and using newer techniques to facilitate rapid case-finding techniques to compare strains are critical to determining sources of outbreaks, potential transmission dynamics, and whether or not there is an outbreak or a perceived cluster of unrelated groups of organisms. In the past, determining relatedness of organisms was dependent on phenotypic methods. These methods include biotyping, which is the identification of genus and species or organisms, comparison of antibiotic susceptibility patterns, serotyping, and phage typing.[11,12] Serotyping involves the use of antibodies to bind antigens on the bacterial surface and phage typing assesses the sensitivity of the bacteria to various bacteriophage viruses.[13,14] Biotyping and antibiotic susceptibility testing are inexpensive and readily available in most clinical laboratories but all of these phenotypic methods are limited in their sensitivity.

Over the last decade, many new genotypic approaches have become available and accessible and have allowed for greater resolution of specific strains. Plasmid typing was one of the first genotypic techniques used to type bacterial strains. Plasmids are extracted and a comparison of the number and types of plasmids is performed. The sensitivity of this technique is enhanced by using restriction endonucleases. This method is time-consuming and is limited in its ability to discriminate strain relatedness in some organisms because plasmids can be mobile between species. Still this process may aid in the evaluation of a specific plasmid or transposon outbreak, which is suspected when different strains present with similar resistance profiles.[11,13–15]

Pulse field gel electrophoresis has been considered the gold standard for molecular typing. Bacterial DNA is extracted and subsequently cleaved by specific restriction endonucleases, which are then separated in an agarose gel by a shifting electric field creating a pattern of bands known as restriction fragment length polymorphisms, which is used to compare strains.[14,16] A large proportion of the bacterial genome is assessed using this method, and there have been international fingerprinting

Table 2
Laboratory strain relatedness testing

Phenotypic testing methods	
Biotyping	Identifies the organism genus and species through morphology and biochemical reactions
Antimicrobial susceptibility testing	Determines antimicrobial susceptibility patterns including bacteria, fungi, and viruses
Serotyping	Uses specific antibodies against surface antigens for organism identification
Phage typing	Determines susceptibility to bacteriophage viruses
Genotypic testing methods	
DNA microarray hybridization	Uses probes attached to solid media, hybridized to labeled organism DNA
Plasmid typing	Isolates the plasmids; may use restriction endonucleases to enhance sensitivity of method
Pulse field gel electrophoresis	Uses infrequent cutting restriction endonucleases, bands of various lengths are separated in agarose gel by pulsed electrical fields
Ribotyping	Uses frequent-cutting restriction endonucleases, bands of various lengths are separated in agarose gel by pulsed electrical fields, hybridized to labeled rRNA
Random amplification of polymorphic DNA Arbitrarily primed polymerase chain reaction	Uses nonspecific primers to amplify at low temperature with high error rate, not used frequently
Repetitive element polymerase chain reaction	Uses polymerase chain reaction amplification of specific repeating sequence fragments
Single locus sequence typing	Uses polymerase chain reaction amplification of a single gene
Multilocus sequence typing	Uses polymerase chain reaction amplification of multiple genes
Optical mapping	Identifies embedded labeled bacterial DNA, microfluidic stretching, restriction endonuclease, fluorescence microscopy in sequence
Whole genomic sequencing	Sequences the entire organism genome

databases that allow for standardized comparisons.[12–14,16] Ribotyping uses a similar process with more frequent cutting restriction endonucleases. After electrophoresis, the gel is blotted onto a nitrocellulose or nylon membrane and labeled DNA or RNA probe is hybridized to the bacterial DNA. When rRNA is used as the probe, this technique is referred to as ribotyping.[13,14] Virtually all bacteria can be ribotyped because this gene is highly conserved, but this process is less able to discriminate between strains than pulse field gel electrophoresis.[13,14,17]

DNA microarray hybridization is another way to type bacterial strains. In this process, DNA probes are attached to a surface and the DNA of the bacteria is isolated, labeled, and then hybridized with the DNA probes to be analyzed. This approach also allows for the detection of plasmids.[16]

More recently, polymerase chain reaction (PCR) techniques have been used to amplify certain DNA segments. Random amplification of polymorphic DNA, also known as arbitrarily primed PCR, uses primers that are specific to the bacterial strain, but not directed at specific sequences. This is a process that allows for multiple mismatches, to amplify DNA segments that are then placed in agarose gel and electrophoresed. This process has been used frequently in outbreak investigations, because it is easy to perform and fast, yet there is significant interlaboratory and intralaboratory variability with this technique.[11,14,16] Repetitive element PCR is similar to the random amplification of polymorphic DNA process, but uses specific primers and more stringent amplification process. This process is advantageous in that it is semiautomated in commercial machines.[16]

PCR is used to amplify and sequence a specific gene as in the case of *emm* gene in group A streptococcus, or the protein A gene (*spa*) in *S aureus*. This process is referred to as single locus sequence typing.[12,14,16] In multilocus sequence typing, several specific housekeeping genes are amplified and sequenced. Each unique sequence is assigned a number and a sequence type is determined.[12,14,16,18] The most significant advantage of this method is standardization. It is, however, an expensive modality.

Optical mapping imbeds bacterial genomic DNA in agarose, which is then stretched in a microfluidic device. Restriction endonucleases are used to digest the bacterial DNA, which is stained with fluorescent dye and visualized by fluorescence microscopy. In this process, the individual genes remain in the order they are seen in vivo. A genomic optimal map is created using specialized software. This technique is evolving, but it's use is limited by cost and the need for specialized equipment.[16]

Whole genomic sequencing (WGS) is the newest tool in outbreak investigation in which the genome is sequenced and will likely become the gold standard.[16] This technique is becoming much more affordable, making it a viable option for outbreak investigation.[12,16,18] WGS has been used in outbreak investigations and has uncovered clusters of genetically related organisms that were unnoticed by phenotypic analysis alone, which has helped define previously unrecognized transmission patterns, as in the case of a *Klebsiella pneumoniae* carbapenemase outbreak at the National Institutes of Health. This technology has also demonstrated that, in some suspected outbreak settings such organisms as *Clostridioides difficile* and *S aureus*, thought to be related, were in fact, genetically distinct.[19–22] With newer high throughput technologies that have been developed and are more affordable, WGS is rapidly becoming the gold standard for comparing strains. This technique is used on bacterial, fungal, and viral organisms.[23]

SOURCES

It is important to recognize that rarely is a single source for an outbreak found. Most outbreaks are attributed to multiple conditions that occurred in a stressed environment. These conditions, such as failures in following policies, inadequate practices, or structural malfunctions, can all add up to the "perfect storm."

Health Care Personnel

Health care personnel have been implicated in the transmission of gram-negative pathogens; respiratory pathogens, such as influenza, respiratory syncytial virus (RSV), pertussis, SARS, Middle East respiratory syndrome, coronavirus disease 2019 (COVID-19; SARS coronavirus 2 [SARS-CoV-2]); and gastrointestinal pathogens, such as *Salmonella* spp, *Norovirus*, and *C difficile*.[24] The most common mechanism of spread in these outbreaks is contact transmission, which is most often related to poor compliance with hand hygiene practices.[7] Artificial nails, rings, and dermatitis are associated with higher rates of gram-negative carriage and can reduce the effectiveness of appropriate hand hygiene practices, which has also led to outbreaks.[25] *Streptococcus pyogenes* colonizes the throat, rectum, and vagina and caused outbreaks in health care settings.[26] Although health care personnel have been implicated as the primary source in less than 10% of *S pyogenes* nosocomial outbreaks, 60% of personnel may carry an outbreak strain.[27] Similarly, *S aureus* has a predilection for the anterior nares and outbreaks have been associated with caregivers who are carriers.[28]

Hospital Environment

The hospital environment has been increasingly appreciated as a reservoir of organisms, especially *C difficile*, *Norovirus*, and multidrug resistant organisms. Contamination of the environment and protective personal equipment (PPE) has been further described with bacterial and viral pathogens including viruses that cause COVID-19 and Ebola.[29–33] Many of these organisms persist in the environment for hours to days and sometimes even months and can persist on health care personnel's hands for several hours.[34] Health care personnel frequently touch room surfaces and their hands can transfer organisms to patients. In one study, over a single hour, 93 contact episodes occurred between the environment and patients housed in medical, surgical, and neurosurgical units.[35] Up to 52% of contacts with contaminated environment can result in a transfer of *S aureus*, vancomycin-resistant enterococcus, and gram-negative bacilli, which is similar to the rate of transfer after health care workers touch colonized patients.[36]

It is difficult to implicate environmental surfaces alone as a cause for transmission of infection, because of the uncertainty of the role that many concurrent events that occur with care individually play. Nonetheless, most experts acknowledge the role of the environment in outbreaks. Several elegant studies have provided data supporting the role the environment plays. For example, in a prospective cohort study in an intensive care unit (ICU), Hardy and colleagues[37] demonstrated that 11.5% of newly colonized patients become colonized with a preexisting environmental strain of methicillin-resistant *S aureus* (MRSA). They used molecular fingerprinting to demonstrate that the acquired and environmental strains were identical. Data from several studies show that room contamination by a prior occupant with *Acinetobacter*, *C difficile*, *Pseudomonas*, vancomycin-resistant enterococcus, and MRSA increases the risk that the subsequent occupant will be colonized by 1.5- to 3.3-fold.[36]

This risk is mitigated through thorough cleaning; disinfection; education and training around the use of and donning and doffing of PPE; use of appropriate disinfectants; good compliance with cleaning protocols; and the use of no-touch technologies, such as hydrogen peroxide vapor and ultraviolet light.[36,38–44]

Waterborne Sources

Over the last century, better public water sanitation methods have reduced community-onset waterborne illness.[45] Nevertheless, outbreaks are frequently recognized in hospital settings because of complex and antiquated water systems, repairs that leave blind pipe loops where organisms proliferate, poor understanding of the risks to patients, or inadequate water treatment of potable water systems. More recently electronic faucets, bath tub drains, and shower heads have been shown to be more likely to have a higher burden of organisms.[46] Many organisms have been implicated in pseudo and actual water-borne outbreaks. Geography, weather and climate, and existing infrastructure influence the types of organisms causing waterborne outbreaks in the community and individual health care settings. The most commonly reported waterborne infection in North America is reported to be *Legionella*.[47,48] Between 2011 and 2012, the Centers for Disease Control and Prevention waterborne illness surveillance system identified potable drinking water as the source of 66% percent of water-related outbreaks and in 26% of these, the associated organism was *Legionella*. Other implicated organisms were Shiga toxin producing *Escherichia coli*, *Shigella*, and *Pantoea agglomerans*.[49] Most recently, multidrug-resistant gram-negatives, fungi, and nontuberculous mycobacteria have been increasingly recognized and important contaminants of hospital water supplies.[46,50,51]

The transmission of waterborne pathogens to patients likely results from a buildup of organism containing biofilm in plumbing structures. This biofilm is dislodged into the water supply through increased use, changes or additions in the existing plumbing, or construction. Patients may become exposed to organisms when showering, flushing toilets, bathing, drinking water, sucking on ice, or through equipment that is rinsed in contaminated potable water. This contaminated water may be in direct contact with patients who may have mucosal disruption or by indirect contact through sinks and health care personnel, both of which can serve as fomites for transmission.[52,53] Wastewater drains have been specifically implicated in 30 carbapenem-resistant organism outbreaks. These outbreaks have been persistent and difficult to remediate, often involving replacement of wastewater systems (14/23).[54,55] In one outbreak of *Sphingomonas koreensis*, cases were linked to contaminated plumbing. WGS was used to demonstrate that patient, water, and plumbing isolates were identical.[50,56] Only one-third of responses to outbreaks were successful in eliminating the inciting organism from the environment.[55]

Legionella infections garner significant media attention, yet they are rare. In the United States, there were 3500 reported cases in 2005 and 2006.[57,58] *Legionella* spp are detected in 40% of water samples by culture and in 90% of water samples by PCR. Only 4% of these water samples were related to an outbreak.[57,59] This organism thrives in water temperatures at 35°C and most organisms are found within biofilms rather than in free-flowing water, making it particularly difficult to disinfect plumbing and the associated contaminated biofilm.[59] Although cooling towers and air conditioning units have been implicated as a common source for this organism, potable water, including hospital ice machines, accounts for most cases.[60] *Legionella* infection presents as a nonspecific pneumonia and requires a specific testing, such as the antigen test, which only identifies serogroup 1, or sophisticated culture media for diagnosis. Therefore this infection is likely underdiagnosed as a cause of nosocomial pneumonia.[61] A variety of disinfection methods have been used including copper-silver ionization, chlorine dioxide, monochloramine, ultraviolet light, and hyperchlorination.[62]

Nontuberculous mycobacteria have a predilection for water and frequently colonize potable water because of their ability to form biofilm. These organisms are difficult to culture, but modern techniques have demonstrated their importance in outbreaks and pseudo-outbreaks (discussed later).[46] Multiples species have been reported with *Malassezia mucogenicum*, *Malassezia gordonae*, *Malassezia simaie*, *Malassezia fortuitum*, *Malassezia chimaera*, and *Malassezia chelonae*.[52,63] These organisms have been shown to be responsible for outbreaks and pseudo-outbreaks in hospitals and in outpatient settings. Outbreaks have been traced to hospital water, dialysis water, fountains, ice machines and hospital water supplies, and disinfectant trays.[64]

Gram-negative organisms are emerging as important pathogens that can contaminate the water supply. Gram-negative organisms were cultured in 79% of sampled water from six hospital water supplies.[65] *Pseudomonas* spp is a common water contaminate in ICU settings and in one outbreak patient strains were linked to ICU water sources through molecular fingerprinting techniques.[52,66,67] Other organisms that can contaminate water-based supplies and equipment include other *Pseudomonas* spp, *Ralstonia* spp, *Serratia* spp, *Aeromonas* spp, *Burkholderia* spp, *Acinetobacter* spp, and *Klebsiella* spp.[52] These organisms have been associated with outbreaks traced to contaminated ventilators, sitz baths, distilled water, pulsed lavage equipment, incubators, and hand creams.[63] Most recently and worrisome, Walsh and colleagues[68] described the contamination of the environmental water supply in India with the carbapenem-resistant New Delhi metallo-β-lactamases (NDM-1)-producing strains. A recent systematic review highlights that wastewater from hospitals and water surrounding hospitals may be a source of antimicrobial-resistant organisms with extended spectrum β-lactamases and carbapenemase.[69]

Other unusual organisms may be associated with waterborne outbreaks. One of the great controversies surrounds the importance of water as a source of fungi, such as *Aspergillus* spp, *Exophiala jeanselmei*, and *Fusarium* spp.[52] Norovirus has also rarely been linked to health care–associated outbreaks and traced to water sources.[70]

ORGANISMS
Acinetobacter Spp

Acinetobacter is a gram-negative organism commonly identified in the setting of health care–associated outbreaks.[71] The genus consists of multiple species, many of which are found in soil and water.[72] This genus also acquires resistance genes quickly, thus contributing to the importance of this species in nosocomial infections and outbreaks.[71] *Acinetobacter* has the largest known resistance island harboring 45 resistance genes acquired from *Pseudomonas*, *Salmonella*, and *Escherichia* spp reflecting its propensity to collect such genes.[73] The most concerning of the myriad of resistance mechanisms this organism can acquire is the ability to hydrolyze carbapenems, which limits treatment with β-lactam-containing antimicrobials. Resistance is increasing worldwide and is clinically important.[74–76]

From 1977 to 2000, 51 *Acinetobacter* spp outbreaks were reported. Twenty-nine (56%) involved respiratory sites and 22 (43%) involved nonrespiratory sites including the bloodstream stream and wounds. In 26 (51%) of these outbreaks, a contaminated common source was found in respiratory equipment, humidifiers, and patient bedding.[77] Most outbreaks occur in ICUs and commonly among patients requiring mechanical ventilation and who have been treated extensively with antimicrobials.[78]

These organisms are isolated from up to 43% of healthy humans volunteers, 17% of sampled fresh fruits and vegetables, and in 21% of human body lice.[72] *Acinetobacter* spp resist desiccation and can survive for prolonged periods of time in the environment.[72] *Acinetobacter baumannii* is the most frequent species associated with health care outbreaks, yet is rarely isolated from the environment in nonoutbreak settings.[72] Because of its ability to survive in the environment, *Acinetobacter* frequently contaminates gowns and gloves used for isolation in health care settings.[79] Airborne dissemination of *Acinetobacter* has also been described.[80–82] Outbreaks caused by this organism, especially when the organism is resistant to multiple antimicrobials, is associated with mortality up to 50% and are costly to health systems.[78] Commonly, mitigation requires repeated and aggressive cleaning and disinfection strategies, use of barrier precautions, isolation, and cohorting of patients and health care providers.[83,84] *Acinetobacter* is increasingly being reported as an important pathogen among patients who have suffered traumatic wound injuries and in alternative health care settings, such as nursing homes and rehabilitation facilities.[85,86]

Carbapenem-Resistant Enterobacteriaceae

Carbapenem resistance among gram-negative organisms is an important and emerging phenomenon and occurs by a variety of mechanisms, including chromosomal resistance (increase in AmpC production), plasmid and mobile element-mediated resistance, and porin mutations.[87] Resistance genes that are coded on plasmids are readily transmissible across species[87] and this mechanism of resistance is concerning because of the potential to transfer to other organisms. Horizontal transfer of carbapenem resistance has been seen using WGS among different species in the hospital environment among others.[88] Since identified in 2001, problematic resistance determinants, such as NDM, continue to emerge and the prevalence of carbapenem-resistant Enterobacteriaceae (CREs) worldwide increased from 1.2% in 2001 to 4.2% in 2011 with an overall incidence in the United States of 2.93 per 100,000 population.[89,90] The increase in the United States is largely fueled by clonal spread of a single clone of *Klebsiella* spp ST258.[87]

Infection with these organisms is challenging to treat and is independently associated with increased mortality.[87,91] Cases tend to occur in individuals in ICUs with prior or indwelling devices who have received antibiotics, especially cephalosporins, fluoroquinolones, and carbapenems; been ventilated; or are receiving steroids.[92] Medical tourism and care in a country with endemic CRE has also been associated with CRE infection and long-term care facilities are becoming an important reservoir.[93,94]

Environmental reservoirs have been linked to CRE outbreaks and include patient room surfaces, equipment (eg, endoscopes, stethoscopes, tables), sinks, showers, and wastewater drainage systems.[92] Furthermore, many CRE outbreaks are associated with asymptomatic carriers and transmission from contaminated environmental sources, such as endoscopes and sinks.[95] Transmission is often silent and 50% of colonized patients are not detected through clinical cultures alone.[95] Commonly referred to as the iceberg effect, asymptomatic carriers are thought to be one of the mechanisms of spread in several outbreaks including one caused by NDM-producing organisms.[20,96] In an 18-person hospital outbreak investigated using WGS, complex and multiple modalities of transmission of CRE were found and linked to asymptomatic carriers and environmental reservoirs.[20]

Multiple strategies are used to control health care outbreaks including increased compliance with hand hygiene, use of barrier and contact precautions, separating patients to single rooms or cohorting colonized patients, active surveillance, and enhanced environmental cleaning.[92] These strategies are commonly bundled together to stop transmission in acute outbreak settings. Additional methods to control spread include chlorhexidine bathing and no-touch environmental disinfection.[97]

Fungus and Mold Including Aspergillus

Mold species are found in dirt and water and hence throughout the health care environment. Outbreaks with these organisms are common.[98] Mold infections cause significant morbidity and mortality in high-risk patients, especially those with impaired granulocyte function or altered or immature skin (ie, extreme prematurity or burns). Aspergillus spp outbreaks are the best described of the molds and have been associated with more than 60 published outbreaks in health care settings. Almost 50% of these have been attributed to construction, renovation, or demolition with airborne dissemination from primary sources.[99–101] Multiple studies demonstrate that the clinical and environmental isolates are clonal highlighting the role of the environment in acquisition of these organisms.[99] Fungal outbreaks have been associated with spread of organisms through nearby construction, vacuum cleaning, contaminated carpet, contaminated air ducts, humidifiers, fireproofing material, rotting wood cabinets, dressings, in-hospital plants, and tape.[98,99] Zygomycete outbreaks are rare, and adhesive bandage rolls, tongue depressors, and water-damaged areas are implicated more often than airborne sources in outbreaks caused by this type of organism.[102,103]

Installation of high-efficiency particle (HEPA) filtration and the use of fungicides have been shown to be instrumental in prevention and abatement of fungal environmental contamination and clinical outbreaks.[100] However, sealing and repairing leaky or open windows, assessing water leaks in ceilings, maintaining appropriate air pressure relationships in patient care areas, and dust removal remain key strategies to prevent and abate fungal outbreaks occurring in the presence of HEPA filtration.[99,101]

Weather may play a significant role in fungal outbreaks. Several studies have documented seasonal variation of fungal spores with higher levels in the fall; however, these results are inconsistent and indoor samples do not correlate with outdoor samples.[104,105] The seasonal variation in the prevalence of *Aspergillus* spores inside a hospital has been associated with rainfall and internal relative humidity and temperature.[105] Severe weather events, such as floods and hurricanes, have been associated with outbreaks of fungal (and bacterial) diseases.[106,107] Flooding in Thailand has been associated with fungal outbreaks and pseudo-outbreaks.[106] The 2005 tsunami in Sri Lanka resulted in an outbreak of *Aspergillus* meningitis because of contaminated supplies from poor post-flooding storage.[108]

Candida auris was first identified in 2009 and has caused hospital outbreaks worldwide over the last several years.[109] This organism, now considered by the Centers for Disease Control and Prevention a priority threat in the United States, is resistant to many antifungals. Spread of this organism is associated with failures in infection prevention practices and it is difficult to eradicate from the hospital environment with routine cleaning, making it challenging to mitigate outbreaks.[98] Importantly, the organism has distinct clades that harbor similar strains and are seen across multiple different countries.[110] It causes invasive infections in immunosuppressed hosts and are thus particularly difficult to treat because of poor host immune response and resistance to antifungal therapy.[98,111] Close to 75% of infections occurred in patients with central venous catheters.[98] High-risk patients become colonized with the organism, might remain asymptomatic, and can contaminate the environment for weeks.[112] This organism has also emerged as one of the pathogens that is associated with secondary infections in critically ill patients with COVID-19.[113,114] Contributing factors in these outbreaks are similar to those previously reported and include inadequate cleaning of the environment and use of multiple layers of PPE. Control strategies include enhancing cleaning and disinfection, transmission-based precautions, and cohorting of patients and screening patients in certain cases.[114]

Unusual causes of fungal infections and outbreaks are reported and continue to emerge. In 2012, *Exserohilum rostratum* contaminated steroids used for epidural injections causing a nationwide outbreak.[98] Other uncommon fungi reported to cause outbreaks include *Saprochaete clavata* described in three health care facilities in France; *Sarocladium kiliense* causing bloodstream infections; and *Malassezia furfur*, which caused bloodstream infections in neonates exposed to lipids and an outbreak associated with colonization of a health care worker from their pet.[98,115] Importantly in these latter outbreaks WGS was critical and identifying outbreak sources.[98]

Respiratory Infections

Respiratory tract infections, especially those caused by viruses, are some of the most common types of infections encountered in the health care setting and their importance and impact is being increasingly recognized.[116] Initially recognized as an important source of morbidity and mortality in pediatric settings, most of these types of infections are generally transmitted by large respiratory droplets. In some settings and situations, aerosolization is an important mode of transmission. Viral respiratory tract infections account for a large number of hospital admissions and complications and is a reason to close a hospital unit. Annual seasonal increases of respiratory infections during respiratory virus seasons can also lead to outbreaks within the health care setting.

Viruses account for the largest proportion of identified pathogens (22%) in hospitalized patients with respiratory infections.[117] Until 2020, influenza A and B accounted for the largest proportion of respiratory viral pathogens in patients older than 65 year old and RSV was the most prevalent pathogen in children and immunosuppressed patients.[118] However, parainfluenza, rhinovirus, and adenoviruses have commonly been associated with infection and transmission in health care settings. Influenza causes many health care–associated outbreaks and sporadic cases.[119] Attack rates in outbreak settings are 55% among health care personnel and 37% of patents.[120] Transmission-based precautions, hand hygiene, and surveillance are important to control these infections and outbreaks. Health care personnel vaccinations are a mainstay of prevention for influenza among health care workers and may reduce the incidence of nosocomial influenza.[121]

More recently, SARS and Middle East respiratory syndrome coronaviruses have been reported in health care settings. Risk factors for transmission of these viruses include aerosol-generating procedures and failure to comply with recommended infection control practices for contact and droplet precautions.[122] Both of these infections are associated with high mortality rates and dramatic illness in health care providers and patients.[122–124] Better understanding of the transmission dynamics of these organisms has reduced outbreaks in health care settings.

Pertussis is a bacterial infection caused by *Bordetella pertussis* that causes significant morbidity and mortality in young unvaccinated infants.[125] It is easily transmitted via droplets from unsuspecting adults with acute infection. Because of its communicability, it has led to outbreaks in primarily pediatric health care settings.[125] The sources of these infections are commonly adults and adolescents and include staff and family members. These outbreaks are difficult to manage because of the long latency period of pertussis, the infectiousness of the organism, and the activities and care rendered in pediatric settings.[125] In one report, a single case cost $75,000 to manage.[126] Pertussis cases have increased over the last 10 years[127] and outbreaks are likely to increase because of the decreased immunogenicity of the acellular vaccine compared with the whole-cell vaccine.[128]

Coronavirus disease 2019

SARS-CoV-2 was identified as the cause of unexplained pneumonia in Wuhan, China in December of 2019. Since then, SARS-COV-2, the novel coronavirus causing this infection, has spread worldwide and caused more than 125 million cases of COVID-19 and led to more than 2.7 million deaths in 1 year. The organism is transmitted via droplets and is aerosolized.[122] It is spread by asymptomatic and presymptomatic carriers in 50% of cases, making it challenging to control this disease.[129] In the early days of the pandemic, spread in hospital settings was largely through close contact with undiagnosed patients who were infected with SARS-CoV- 2.[130] In 2020, SARS-CoV-2 became the primary cause of respiratory viral infections and outbreaks. Whether this trend will continue remains to be seen. In the early days of the epidemic, transmission in health care settings was associated with inadequate supply of PPE and unfamiliarity with the equipment and PPE. After the institution of universal pandemic precautions including ensuring adequate supply of PPE at many health care facilities, nosocomial infections have occurred less frequently with sporadic small outbreaks.[131,132] In a robust evaluation of an outbreak at Brigham and Women's hospital, the authors demonstrate how small failures in infection prevention including placement of patients in semiprivate rooms (as opposed to single occupancy rooms), use of nebulized medications, and close contact with unmasked patients led to patient and health care worker transmission.[133]

Gastrointestinal Infections

Gastroenteritis is common and in settings where rotavirus vaccine is available, *Norovirus* is the leading cause of gastroenteritis epidemics across various health care settings and also in long-term care facilities, cruise ships, schools, and recreational activities. In a retrospective review of 90 gastrointestinal outbreaks reported to health departments, 96% of nonbacterial gastroenteritis was ultimately attributed to *Norovirus*.[134] *Norovirus* is a resilient, round virus that is spread through fecal oral contamination even before infected patients are symptomatic. Recently, genogroup II type 4 was reported to cause most outbreaks.[135]

Norovirus is highly infectious and a low inoculum of virus leads to asymptomatic or symptomatic infection.[136] Viral shedding persists for up to a week and the organism is viable in the environment for days to weeks.[136] Additionally, the virus has a high rate of genetic mutation and host immunity is transient, making humans continually susceptible hosts.[136] These factors lead to secondary attack rates of 30% and in addition, make control in outbreak settings challenging.[137] Infection control interventions that are effective include restricting movement, screening staff and visitors and isolating individuals who are ill, enhanced cleaning, and improved compliance with hand hygiene.[136,138] Cleaning of environmental surfaces with hypochlorite can reduce the attack rate for *Norovirus* because this organism is resistant to many disinfectants.[138] A new study found significantly less *Norovirus* outbreaks in nine states that implemented nonpharmaceutical interventions, such as universal masking, physical distancing, and increased hand hygiene to control COVID-19.[139]

C difficile is the most common pathogen identified in health care–associated infections in North America.[140] It is identified in the stool of 25% of hospitalized patients and in 2% to 3% of healthy adults.[141] To develop *C difficile* disease, two-steps are needed; acquisition of the pathogen and alteration of gastrointestinal microbiome primarily through antibiotic use. Patients with active disease shed up to 100 million *C difficile* spores per gram of stool. Hence the organism, which is resistant to many cleaning agents, has a predilection for the hospital environment.[142] Anywhere from 20% to 51% of hospital room surfaces in rooms of patients with active *C difficile* infection are contaminated.[142] Health care personnel hands are easily contaminated by spores after examining patients or even through contact with the patient's environment.[143] Daily cleaning reduces the risk of hand contamination.[144] Admission to a room where the previous occupant was diagnosed *C difficile* disease, or having a roommate with disease, increased the risk the current occupant developing *C difficile* infection.[36] These data suggest an important role of the environment in the development of *C difficile* infection.

The understanding of *C difficile* epidemiology has evolved with the use of better laboratory tests including WGS. Despite the heavy and frequent environmental contamination with *C difficile* only 25% of health care–acquired *C difficile* is epidemiologically and genetically traced to another symptomatic contact re-emphasizing the importance of combined antimicrobial stewardship, diagnostic stewardship, and infection prevention strategies to prevent outbreaks and pseudo-outbreaks.[145]

Gastroenteritis is extremely common in resource-limited settings and the epidemiology is different than in the United States. Less is known about the pathogens in these settings. Such organisms as rotavirus, *Salmonella*, and enterotoxigenic *E coli* should be considered as important pathogens in these settings.[146] Furthermore, recent outbreaks associated with contamination of food (or breast milk) because of extended-spectrum β-lactamase-producing and antimicrobial-resistant pathogens have also been reported as causes of gastroenteritis in various settings.[147,148]

HIGH-RISK SETTINGS
Neonatal Intensive Care Unit

The neonatal ICU (NICU) is a unique environment with significant risks for outbreaks because of immature immune systems of some of these babies, the use of incubators and other strategies to retain heat, and socialization and visitation processes unique to this setting. The prevalence of infections ranges from 5% to 24%; and is higher in premature infants than in full-term infants.[149] Studies evaluating the unique physical environment in the NICU demonstrate the importance of the facility design, and in fact, temporary facilities have been shown to have a higher rate of infection.[150] Modeling pathogen transmission in an NICU using surrogate DNA demonstrated rapid spread throughout the NICU.[149,151] For these reasons, NICUs account for 38% of ICU outbreaks and 18% of all published outbreaks.[152] Source was only identified in 51% of outbreaks.[152] *Klebsiella* spp, *S aureus*, *Serratia* spp, and *Enterobacter* spp are the most common outbreak organisms identified. Gram-negative bacteria accounted for 54% of outbreaks, many with extended-spectrum β-lactamase resistance.[153,154] Patients were the source of 20% of outbreaks, contaminated equipment accounted for 12%, personnel were the source in 11%, and the environment contributed to 9%.[152]

Viral infections including rotavirus (23%), RSV (17%), enterovirus (15%), and hepatitis A (11%) have been increasingly recognized as important pathogens among infants hospitalized in NICU settings.[155] Unsurprisingly, patients and personnel accounted for the source of transmission in 50% and 8% of viral outbreaks, respectively.[152]

S aureus and MRSA outbreaks are commonly reported in this unique setting.[152] Intravenous fluid may be a significant risk factor for infection acquired in an outbreak in this setting. Because of the common use of intravenous lipids, this is one of the settings that *M furfur* is commonly seen.[156] Additionally, in resource-limited settings, bloodstream infection outbreaks with gram-negative organisms may be traced to poor sterile practices associated with mixing intravenous medications.[157–159]

Multiple interventions have been implemented to control outbreaks in this setting, most commonly reinforcing hand hygiene practices, conducting active surveillance of patients, implementing barrier precautions, and cohorting of patients and in some cases of health care personnel. Personnel screening was performed in 44% of outbreaks (most often in *S aureus* outbreaks), and modifications of care processes and equipment was implemented in 39% of NICU outbreaks.[152]

Endoscopes and Endoscopy Suites

As more complex technology and sophisticated medical devices are introduced into health care settings to treat patients, these devices are increasingly recognized as sources of organisms that are transmitted from patient to patient. Endoscopes are a common example of such technology. These scopes have been found to be contaminated even after high-level disinfection in up to 50% to 70% of encounters depending on sampling method used.[160] With their myriad of crevices, channels, and ports, inappropriately cleaned and disinfected endoscopes are the source of microbiologic contamination and biofilm identified in these devices.[161]

Between 1966 and 2004, 19 outbreaks were linked to gastrointestinal endoscopy.[162] More than 90% of outbreaks linked to bronchoscopes and gastrointestinal endoscopes could have been prevented by using appropriate cleaning and disinfection processes.[162] Endoscopes have complex channels, ports, elevators, and cameras providing environments for water-based organisms, such as pseudomonas, multidrug-resistant *Klebsiella* spp, and nontuberculous mycobacteria (NTM), and these organisms have been associated with several outbreaks where the cause was related to insufficient reprocessing.[162,163] A recent highly publicized outbreak of NDM-producing CREs resulted in 29 cases of colonization or infection where no lapses in reprocessing were noted, suggesting that usual cleaning methods may not be effective in sterilizing complicated endoscopes with multiple moving pieces.[164] Similarly an outbreak involving 32 cases of an AmpC-producing carbapenem-resistant *E coli* with seven deaths was related to damaged endoscopes.[165,166]

Despite these reports and other challenges with determining how to safely reprocess endoscopes of all types, manual cleaning remains the cornerstone of good practice and can reduce the bioburden in colonoscopes up to five logs.[163] These recent outbreaks highlight the difficulties in cleaning and disinfecting novel and potentially important medical devices with designs that are not effectively disinfected by the current processes.[167]

Long-Term Care Settings

Long-term care facilities including nursing homes and rehabilitation centers are particularly susceptible to outbreaks with a vulnerable aging population that often requires close-contact care and living in close quarters for extended periods of time in facilities with variable air-handling and other facility design challenges. These types of facilities are where care is provided for an increasing number of individuals and are a hybrid of living quarters and hospital settings thus creating unique challenges in controlling the spread of infection.[168] Commonly, they have inadequate numbers of staff or inadequately trained staff to manage the complex patients they are caring for. Respiratory and gastrointestinal infections are the most common types of infections and outbreaks in these settings.[169] Influenza was reported in 49 of 206 published outbreaks, norovirus was associated with 25 outbreaks, and Group A streptococci caused 16 outbreaks. *Sarcoptes scabei* (70%), *Clostridium perfringens* (48%), norovirus (45%), *Chlamydia pneumoniae* (46%), adenovirus (42%), parainfluenza (41%), and RSV (40%) were associated with the highest attack rates and Group A *streptococci* (50%), *Legionella* (32%), and *Streptococcus pneumoniae* (27%) were associated with highest case fatality rates.[169,170]

Transplant Units

Infections are the leading cause of death in solid organ transplant recipients.[171] In the first 30 days after transplantation most bacterial health care–associated infections occur after medical procedures.[171] Bloodstream and urinary tract infections, especially associated with catheter use, are highest during the first month and then sharply decline after this period.[172] Multidrug-resistant organisms, particularly enterococcus and gram-negative organisms, are frequent causes of infection in solid organ transplant patients.[173] Respiratory viruses, such as influenza, RSV, adenovirus, and rhinovirus, are common reasons for medical consultation and hospitalization in transplant patients. These viruses are more likely to cause lower lung involvement in transplant recipients compared with normal hosts with high associated mortality rates. These viruses can lead to outbreaks in this patient population.[174]

Hematopoietic stem cell transplants are life-saving procedures for patients with leukemia and lymphoma. These procedures involve host bone marrow ablation, which results in profound immunosuppression until the autologous (host) or allogenic (donor) bone marrow engrafts. Engraftment can take several weeks.[175] Gram-positive infections (20%–30%), gram-negative infections (5%–10%), C difficile (5%–10%), and respiratory viruses (15%) are the most common causes of infection in the preengraftment period.[175] The hospital environment poses significant risks to patients in this vulnerable time period. In addition, transmission from hands of health care personnel, and such sources as creams, mouthwash, sitz baths, and sinks have been associated with infections in these patients.[176]

In addition to being at risk for catheter-associated bloodstream and other health care–associated infections, both these transplant patient populations are at risk for infections associated with disruption of the physical environment, such as fungal infections associated with construction or legionella infections after changes in plumbing. In addition to overall attention to infection prevention, optimal infection prevention for these patient populations may require additional interventions including the use of sterile water, universal masking, or a protective environment with HEPA filtration.

SUMMARY

Outbreaks should be considered a threat in any health care delivery site and can encompass a variety of pathogens and vectors of transmission. Epidemiologic and laboratory diagnostic tools can help guide a systematic investigation; however, often multiple evaluative steps occur simultaneously in complex situations.

Many interventions have been used to abort an ongoing outbreak. Most significantly, it is important to ensure that basic infection prevention practices, such as hand hygiene and isolation, are in place and that health care personnel are compliant with these practices. Beyond this, mitigation measures need to be tailored to the epidemiologic findings, the organism, and the patients. The goal is to remove the offending source and protect patients and health care personnel.

In most situations these interventions are applied in combination and simultaneously because there are limited data to empirically guide management. Specific interventions, such as enhanced patient screening and surveillance, are implemented 54% of the time. In 38% of outbreaks, personnel are screened and isolation or cohorting is implemented in 32% of outbreaks. Sterilization or disinfection practices are enhanced or revised in 24% of these situations, care of equipment is modified in 23%, increased use of PPE implemented in 19%, and wards are closed in 11% of outbreaks.[7]

Epidemiologic data is an important tool in identifying potential outbreak sources and guiding additional testing. It is important to quickly implement reasonable prevention strategies, and effectively communicate to leadership and public health authorities while refining further investigations. The goal is to abort further patient transmission or harm and provide a safe atmosphere for patient care while protecting the health care personnel and the institution. This harmonious balance requires engagement of all of the vested parties and access to necessary resources.

DISCLOSURE

The authors have nothing to disclose.

REFERENCES

1. Lee XJ, Elliott TM, Harris PNA, et al. Clinical and economic outcomes of genome sequencing availability on containing a hospital outbreak of resistant *Escherichia coli* in Australia. Value Health 2020;23(8):994–1002.

2. Gagnaire J, Gagneux-Brunon A, Pouvaret A, et al. Carbapenemase-producing *Acinetobacter baumannii*: an outbreak report with special highlights on economic burden. Med Mal Infect 2017;47(4):279–85.

3. Baggett HC, Duchin JS, Shelton W, et al. Two nosocomial pertussis outbreaks and their associated costs: King County, Washington, 2004. Infect Control Hosp Epidemiol 2007;28(5):537–43.

4. Dik JW, Dinkelacker AG, Vemer P, et al. Cost-analysis of seven nosocomial outbreaks in an academic hospital. PLoS One 2016;11(2):e0149226.

5. Hansen S, Stamm-Balderjahn S, Zuschneid I, et al. Closure of medical departments during nosocomial outbreaks: data from a systematic analysis of the literature. J Hosp Infect 2007;65(4):348–53.

6. Girerd-Genessay I, Bénet T, Vanhems P. Multidrug-resistant bacterial outbreaks in burn units: a synthesis of the literature according to the ORION statement. J Burn Care Res 2016;37(3):172–80.

7. Gastmeier P, Stamm-Balderjahn S, Hansen S, et al. How outbreaks can contribute to prevention of nosocomial infection: analysis of 1,022 outbreaks. Infect Control Hosp Epidemiol 2005;26(4):357–61.

8. Gastmeier P, Stamm-Balderjahn S, Hansen S, et al. Where should one search when confronted with outbreaks of nosocomial infection? Am J Infect Control 2006;34(9):603–5.

9. Cunha CB, Cunha BA. Pseudoinfections and pseudo-outbreaks. In: Mayhall CG, editor. Hospital epidemiology and infection control. 4th edition. Baltimore (MD): Lippincott Williams & Wilkins; 2012. p. 143–52.

10. Pfaller MA, Herwaldt LA. The clinical microbiology laboratory and infection control: emerging pathogens, antimicrobial resistance, and new technology. Clin Infect Dis 1997;25(4):858–70.

11. Weber S, Pfaller MA, Herwaldt LA. Role of molecular epidemiology in infection control. Infect Dis Clin North Am 1997;11(2):257–78.

12. MacCannell D. Bacterial strain typing. Clin Lab Med 2013;33(3):629–50.

13. Tenover FC, Arbeit RD, Goering RV. How to select and interpret molecular strain typing methods for epidemiological studies of bacterial infections: a review for healthcare epidemiologists. Molecular Typing Working Group of the Society for Healthcare Epidemiology of America. Infect Control Hosp Epidemiol 1997; 18(6):426–39.

14. Singh A, Goering RV, Simjee S, et al. Application of molecular techniques to the study of hospital infection. Clin Microbiol Rev 2006;19(3):512–30.

15. John JF, Twitty JA. Plasmids as epidemiologic markers in nosocomial gram-negative bacilli: experience at a university and review of the literature. Rev Infect Dis 1986;8(5):693–704.

16. Sabat AJ, Budimir A, Nashev D, et al. Overview of molecular typing methods for outbreak detection and epidemiological surveillance. Euro Surveill 2013;18(4): 20380.

17. Bingen EH, Denamur E, Elion J. Use of ribotyping in epidemiological surveillance of nosocomial outbreaks. Clin Microbiol Rev 1994;7(3):311–27.

18. Mirande C, Bizine I, Giannetti A, et al. Epidemiological aspects of healthcare-associated infections and microbial genomics. Eur J Clin Microbiol Infect Dis 2018;37(5):823–31.

19. Harris SR, Cartwright EJP, Török ME, et al. Whole-genome sequencing for analysis of an outbreak of methicillin-resistant *Staphylococcus aureus*: a descriptive study. Lancet Infect Dis 2013;13(2):130–6.

20. Snitkin ES, Zelazny AM, Thomas PJ, et al. Tracking a hospital outbreak of carbapenem-resistant *Klebsiella pneumoniae* with whole-genome sequencing. Sci Transl Med 2012;4(148):148ra16.

21. Eyre DW, Golubchik T, Gordon NC, et al. A pilot study of rapid benchtop sequencing of *Staphylococcus aureus* and *Clostridium difficile* for outbreak detection and surveillance. BMJ Open 2012;2(3):e001124.

22. Koser CU, Holden MT, Ellington MJ, et al. Rapid whole-genome sequencing for investigation of a neonatal MRSA outbreak. N Engl J Med 2012;366(24): 2267–75.

23. Reuter JA, Spacek DV, Snyder MP. High-throughput sequencing technologies. Mol Cell 2015;58(4):586–97.

24. Huttunen R, Syrjänen J. Healthcare workers as vectors of infectious diseases. Eur J Clin Microbiol Infect Dis 2014;33(9):1477–88.

25. Boyce JM, Pittet D, Healthcare Infection Control Practices Advisory Committee. Society for Healthcare Epidemiology of America. Association for Professionals in Infection Control. Infectious Diseases Society of America. Hand Hygiene Task Force. Guideline for hand hygiene in health-care settings: recommendations of the healthcare infection control practices advisory committee and the HIC-PAC/SHEA/APIC/IDSA hand hygiene task force. Infect Control Hosp Epidemiol 2002;23(12 Suppl):S3–40.

26. Kolmos HJ, Svendsen RN, Nielsen SV. The surgical team as a source of postoperative wound infections caused by *Streptococcus pyogenes*. J Hosp Infect 1997;35(3):207–14.

27. Daneman N, McGeer A, Low DE, et al. Hospital-acquired invasive group a streptococcal infections in Ontario, Canada, 1992-2000. Clin Infect Dis 2005; 41(3):334–42.

28. Albrich WC, Harbarth S. Health-care workers: source, vector, or victim of MRSA? Lancet Infect Dis 2008;8(5):289–301.

29. Ye G, Lin H, Chen S, et al. Environmental contamination of SARS-CoV-2 in healthcare premises. J Infect 2020;81(2):e1–5.

30. Ong SWX, Tan YK, Chia PY, et al. Air, surface environmental, and personal protective equipment contamination by severe acute respiratory syndrome coronavirus 2 (SARS-CoV-2) from a symptomatic patient. JAMA 2020;323(16):1610–2.

31. Poliquin PG, Vogt F, Kasztura M, et al. Environmental contamination and persistence of Ebola virus RNA in an Ebola Treatment Center. J Infect Dis 2016; 214(suppl 3):S145–52.

32. Casanova LM, Erukunuakpor K, Kraft CS, et al. Assessing viral transfer during doffing of Ebola-level personal protective equipment in a biocontainment unit. Clin Infect Dis 2018;66(6):945–9.

33. Rock C, Thom KA, Masnick M, et al. Frequency of *Klebsiella pneumoniae* carbapenemase (KPC)-producing and non-KPC-producing *Klebsiella* species contamination of healthcare workers and the environment. Infect Control Hosp Epidemiol 2014;35(4):426–9.

34. Kampf G, Kramer A. Epidemiologic background of hand hygiene and evaluation of the most important agents for scrubs and rubs. Clin Microbiol Rev 2004;17(4): 863–93, table of contents.

35. Cheng VC, Chau PH, Lee WM, et al. Hand-touch contact assessment of high-touch and mutual-touch surfaces among healthcare workers, patients, and visitors. J Hosp Infect 2015;90(3):220–5.

36. Otter JA, Yezli S, French GL. The role played by contaminated surfaces in the transmission of nosocomial pathogens. Infect Control Hosp Epidemiol 2011; 32(7):687–99.

37. Hardy KJ, Oppenheim BA, Gossain S, et al. A study of the relationship between environmental contamination with methicillin-resistant *Staphylococcus aureus* (MRSA) and patients' acquisition of MRSA. Infect Control Hosp Epidemiol 2006;27(2):127–32.

38. Fischer WA 2nd, Weber D, Wohl DA. Personal protective equipment: protecting health care providers in an Ebola outbreak. Clin Ther 2015;37(11):2402–10.

39. Chou R, Dana T, Buckley DI, et al. Epidemiology of and risk factors for coronavirus infection in health care workers: a living rapid review. Ann Intern Med 2020; 173(2):120–36.

40. Weber DJ, Fischer WA, Wohl DA, et al. Protecting healthcare personnel from acquiring Ebola virus disease. Infect Control Hosp Epidemiol 2015;36(10): 1229–32.

41. Anderson DJ, Moehring RW, Weber DJ, et al. Effectiveness of targeted enhanced terminal room disinfection on hospital-wide acquisition and infection with multidrug-resistant organisms and *Clostridium difficile*: a secondary analysis of a multicentre cluster randomised controlled trial with crossover design (BETR Disinfection). Lancet Infect Dis 2018;18(8):845–53.

42. Anderson DJ, Chen LF, Weber DJ, et al. Enhanced terminal room disinfection and acquisition and infection caused by multidrug-resistant organisms and *Clostridium difficile* (the Benefits of Enhanced Terminal Room Disinfection study): a cluster-randomised, multicentre, crossover study. Lancet 2017; 389(10071):805–14.

43. Marra AR, Schweizer ML, Edmond MB. No-touch disinfection methods to decrease multidrug-resistant organism infections: a systematic review and meta-analysis. Infect Control Hosp Epidemiol 2018;39(1):20–31.

44. Dong Z, Zhou N, Liu G, et al. Role of pulsed-xenon ultraviolet light in reducing healthcare-associated infections: a systematic review and meta-analysis. Epidemiol Infect 2020;148:e165.

45. Centers for Disease C, Prevention. Control of infectious diseases. MMWR Morb Mortal Wkly Rep 1999;48(29):621–9.

46. Kanamori H, Weber DJ, Rutala WA. Healthcare outbreaks associated with a water reservoir and infection prevention strategies. Clin Infect Dis 2016;62(11): 1423–35.

47. Craun GF, Brunkard JM, Yoder JS, et al. Causes of outbreaks associated with drinking water in the United States from 1971 to 2006. Clin Microbiol Rev 2010;23(3):507–28.

48. Agarwal S, Abell V, File TM Jr. Nosocomial (health care-associated) Legionnaire's disease. Infect Dis Clin North Am 2017;31(1):155–65.

49. Beer KD, Gargano JW, Roberts VA, et al. Surveillance for waterborne disease outbreaks associated with drinking water—United States, 2011-2012. MMWR Morb Mortal Wkly Rep 2015;64(31):842–8.

50. Chia PY, Sengupta S, Kukreja A, et al. The role of hospital environment in transmissions of multidrug-resistant gram-negative organisms. Antimicrob Resist Infect Control 2020;9(1):29.
51. Vincenti S, Quaranta G, De Meo C, et al. Non-fermentative gram-negative bacteria in hospital tap water and water used for haemodialysis and bronchoscope flushing: prevalence and distribution of antibiotic resistant strains. Sci Total Environ 2014;499:47–54.
52. Anaissie EJ, Penzak SR, Dignani MC. The hospital water supply as a source of nosocomial infections: a plea for action. Arch Intern Med 2002;162(13):1483–92.
53. Gestrich SA, Jencson AL, Cadnum JL, et al. A multicenter investigation to characterize the risk for pathogen transmission from healthcare facility sinks. Infect Control Hosp Epidemiol 2018;39(12):1467–9.
54. Carling PC. Wastewater drains: epidemiology and interventions in 23 carbapenem-resistant organism outbreaks. Infect Control Hosp Epidemiol 2018;39(8):972–9.
55. Kizny Gordon AE, Mathers AJ, Cheong EYL, et al. The hospital water environment as a reservoir for carbapenem-resistant organisms causing hospital-acquired infections: a systematic review of the literature. Clin Infect Dis 2017; 64(10):1435–44.
56. Johnson RC, Deming C, Conlan S, et al. Investigation of a cluster of *Sphingomonas koreensis* infections. N Engl J Med 2018;379(26):2529–39.
57. Centers for Disease C, Prevention. Legionellosis—United States, 2000-2009. MMWR Morb Mortal Wkly Rep 2011;60(32):1083–6.
58. Joseph CA, Ricketts KD, European Working Group for Legionella Infections. Legionnaires disease in Europe 2007-2008. Euro Surveill 2010;15(8):19493.
59. Fields BS, Benson RF, Besser RE. Legionella and Legionnaires' disease: 25 years of investigation. Clin Microbiol Rev 2002;15(3):506–26.
60. Sabria M, Yu VL. Hospital-acquired legionellosis: solutions for a preventable infection. Lancet Infect Dis 2002;2(6):368–73.
61. Cunha BA, Burillo A, Bouza E. Legionnaires' disease. Lancet 2016;387(10016): 376–85.
62. Lin YE, Stout JE, Yu VL. Controlling *Legionella* in hospital drinking water: an evidence-based review of disinfection methods. Infect Control Hosp Epidemiol 2011;32(2):166–73.
63. Ferranti G, Marchesi I, Favale M, et al. Aetiology, source and prevention of waterborne healthcare-associated infections: a review. J Med Microbiol 2014; 63(Pt 10):1247–59.
64. Brown-Elliott BA, Wallace RJ Jr. Nontuberculous mycobacteria. Hospital epidemiology and infection control. Philadelphia: Lippincott Williams & Wilkins; 2012. p. 594–610.
65. Stojek NM, Szymanska J, Dutkiewicz J. Gram-negative bacteria in water distribution systems of hospitals. Ann Agric Environ Med 2008;15(1):135–42.
66. Bukholm G, Tannaes T, Kjelsberg AB, et al. An outbreak of multidrug-resistant *Pseudomonas aeruginosa* associated with increased risk of patient death in an intensive care unit. Infect Control Hosp Epidemiol 2002;23(8):441–6.
67. Muscarella LF. Contribution of tap water and environmental surfaces to nosocomial transmission of antibiotic-resistant *Pseudomonas aeruginosa*. Infect Control Hosp Epidemiol 2004;25(4):342–5.
68. Walsh TR, Weeks J, Livermore DM, et al. Dissemination of NDM-1 positive bacteria in the New Delhi environment and its implications for human health: an environmental point prevalence study. Lancet Infect Dis 2011;11(5):355–62.

69. Hassoun-Kheir N, Stabholz Y, JU Kreft, et al. Comparison of antibiotic-resistant bacteria and antibiotic resistance genes abundance in hospital and community wastewater: a systematic review. Sci Total Environ 2020;743:140804.

70. Schvoerer E, Bonnet F, Dubois V, et al. A hospital outbreak of gastroenteritis possibly related to the contamination of tap water by a small round structured virus. J Hosp Infect 1999;43(2):149–54.

71. Fournier PE, Richet H. The epidemiology and control of *Acinetobacter baumannii* in health care facilities. Clin Infect Dis 2006;42(5):692–9.

72. Peleg AY, Seifert H, Paterson DL. *Acinetobacter baumannii*: emergence of a successful pathogen. Clin Microbiol Rev 2008;21(3):538–82.

73. Fournier PE, Vallenet D, Barbe V, et al. Comparative genomics of multidrug resistance in *Acinetobacter baumannii*. PLoS Genet 2006;2(1):e7.

74. Munoz-Price LS, Arheart K, Nordmann P, et al. Eighteen years of experience with *Acinetobacter baumannii* in a tertiary care hospital. Crit Care Med 2013; 41(12):2733–42.

75. Zilberberg MD, Kollef MH, Shorr AF. Secular trends in *Acinetobacter baumannii* resistance in respiratory and blood stream specimens in the United States, 2003 to 2012: a survey study. J Hosp Med 2016;11(1):21–6.

76. Kurihara MNL, Sales RO, Silva KED, et al. Multidrug-resistant *Acinetobacter baumannii* outbreaks: a global problem in healthcare settings. Rev Soc Bras Med Trop 2020;53:e20200248.

77. Villegas MV, Hartstein AI. *Acinetobacter* outbreaks, 1977-2000. Infect Control Hosp Epidemiol 2003;24(4):284–95.

78. Wieland K, Chhatwal P, Vonberg RP. Nosocomial outbreaks caused by *Acinetobacter baumannii* and *Pseudomonas aeruginosa*: results of a systematic review. Am J Infect Control 2018;46(6):643–8.

79. Morgan DJ, Liang SY, Smith CL, et al. Frequent multidrug-resistant *Acinetobacter baumannii* contamination of gloves, gowns, and hands of healthcare workers. Infect Control Hosp Epidemiol 2010;31(7):716–21.

80. Rock C, Harris AD, Johnson JK, et al. Infrequent air contamination with *Acinetobacter baumannii* of air surrounding known colonized or infected patients. Infect Control Hosp Epidemiol 2015;36(7):830–2.

81. Shimose LA, Doi Y, Bonomo RA, et al. Contamination of ambient air with *Acinetobacter baumannii* on consecutive inpatient days. J Clin Microbiol 2015;53(7): 2346–8.

82. Munoz-Price LS, Fajardo-Aquino Y, Arheart KL, et al. Aerosolization of *Acinetobacter baumannii* in a trauma ICU*. Crit Care Med 2013;41(8):1915–8.

83. Ben-Chetrit E, Wiener-Well Y, Lesho E, et al. An intervention to control an ICU outbreak of carbapenem-resistant *Acinetobacter baumannii*: long-term impact for the ICU and hospital. Crit Care 2018;22(1):319.

84. Ayraud-Thevenot S, Huart C, Mimoz O, et al. Control of multi-drug-resistant *Acinetobacter baumannii* outbreaks in an intensive care unit: feasibility and economic impact of rapid unit closure. J Hosp Infect 2012;82(4):290–2.

85. Mody L, Gibson KE, Horcher A, et al. Prevalence of and risk factors for multidrug-resistant *Acinetobacter baumannii* colonization among high-risk nursing home residents. Infect Control Hosp Epidemiol 2015;36(10):1155–62.

86. Cornejo-Juarez P, Cevallos MA, Castro-Jaimes S, et al. High mortality in an outbreak of multidrug resistant *Acinetobacter baumannii* infection introduced to an oncological hospital by a patient transferred from a general hospital. PLoS One 2020;15(7):e0234684.

87. Gupta N, Limbago BM, Patel JB, et al. Carbapenem-resistant Enterobacteri-aceae: epidemiology and prevention. Clin Infect Dis 2011;53(1):60–7.

88. Conlan S, Thomas PJ, Deming C, et al. Single-molecule sequencing to track plasmid diversity of hospital-associated carbapenemase-producing Enterobac-teriaceae. Sci Transl Med 2014;6(254):254ra126.

89. Guh AY, Bulens SN, Mu Y, et al. Epidemiology of carbapenem-resistant entero-bacteriaceae in 7 US Communities, 2012-2013. JAMA 2015;314(14):1479–87.

90. Centers for Disease C, Prevention. Vital signs: carbapenem-resistant Entero-bacteriaceae. MMWR Morb Mortal Wkly Rep 2013;62(9):165–70.

91. van Duin D, Arias CA, Komarow L, et al. Molecular and clinical epidemiology of carbapenem-resistant Enterobacterales in the USA (CRACKLE-2): a prospec-tive cohort study. Lancet Infect Dis 2020;20(6):731–41.

92. van Loon K, Voor In 't Holt AF, Vos MC. A systematic review and meta-analyses of the clinical epidemiology of carbapenem-resistant enterobacteriaceae. Anti-microb Agents Chemother 2018;62(1). e01730–17.

93. Aliyu S, Smaldone A, Larson E. Prevalence of multidrug-resistant gram-negative bacteria among nursing home residents: a systematic review and meta-anal-ysis. Am J Infect Control 2017;45(5):512–8.

94. McKinnell JA, Miller LG, Singh RD, et al. High prevalence of multidrug-resistant organism colonization in 28 nursing homes: an "iceberg effect". J Am Med Dir Assoc 2020;21(12):1937–43.e2.

95. Temkin E, Adler A, Lerner A, et al. Carbapenem-resistant Enterobacteriaceae: biology, epidemiology, and management. Ann N Y Acad Sci 2014;1323:22–42.

96. Epson EE, Pisney LM, Wendt JM, et al. Carbapenem-resistant *Klebsiella pneu-moniae* producing New Delhi metallo-beta-lactamase at an acute care hospital, Colorado, 2012. Infect Control Hosp Epidemiol 2014;35(4):390–7.

97. Munoz-Price LS, Quinn JP. Deconstructing the infection control bundles for the containment of carbapenem-resistant Enterobacteriaceae. Curr Opin Infect Dis 2013;26(4):378–87.

98. Bougnoux ME, Brun S, Zahar JR. Healthcare-associated fungal outbreaks: new and uncommon species, new molecular tools for investigation and prevention. Antimicrob Resist Infect Control 2018;7:45.

99. Weber DJ, Peppercorn A, Miller MB, et al. Preventing healthcare-associated *Aspergillus* infections: review of recent CDC/HICPAC recommendations. Med Mycol 2009;47(Suppl 1):S199–209.

100. Kanamori H, Rutala WA, Sickbert-Bennett EE, et al. Review of fungal outbreaks and infection prevention in healthcare settings during construction and renova-tion. Clin Infect Dis 2015;61(3):433–44.

101. Vonberg RP, Gastmeier P. Nosocomial aspergillosis in outbreak settings. J Hosp Infect 2006;63(3):246–54.

102. Antoniadou A. Outbreaks of zygomycosis in hospitals. Clin Microbiol Infect 2009;15(Suppl 5):55–9.

103. Walther G, Wagner L, Kurzai O. Outbreaks of *Mucorales* and the species involved. Mycopathologia 2020;185(5):765–81.

104. Panackal AA, Li H, Kontoyiannis DP, et al. Geoclimatic influences on invasive aspergillosis after hematopoietic stem cell transplantation. Clin Infect Dis 2010;50(12):1588–97.

105. Cavallo M, Andreoni S, Martinotti MG, et al. Monitoring environmental *Asper-gillus* spp. contamination and meteorological factors in a haematological unit. Mycopathologia 2013;176(5–6):387–94.

106. Apisarnthanarak A, Warren DK, Mayhall CG. Healthcare-associated infections and their prevention after extensive flooding. Curr Opin Infect Dis 2013;26(4): 359–65.

107. Sood G, Vaidya D, Dam L, et al. A polymicrobial fungal outbreak in a regional burn center after Hurricane Sandy. Am J Infect Control 2018;46(9):1047–50.

108. Gunaratne PS, Wijeyaratne CN, Chandrasiri P, et al. An outbreak of *Aspergillus* meningitis following spinal anaesthesia for caesarean section in Sri Lanka: a post-tsunami effect? Ceylon Med J 2006;51(4):137–42.

109. Rhodes J, Fisher MC. Global epidemiology of emerging *Candida auris*. Curr Opin Microbiol 2019;52:84–9.

110. Lone SA, Ahmad A. *Candida auris*: the growing menace to global health. Mycoses 2019;62(8):620–37.

111. Vallabhaneni S, Jackson BR, Chiller TM. *Candida auris*: an emerging antimicrobial resistance threat. Ann Intern Med 2019;171(6):432–3.

112. Corsi-Vasquez G, Ostrosky-Zeichner L. *Candida auris*: what have we learned so far? Curr Opin Infect Dis 2019;32(6):559–64.

113. Sabino R, Verissimo C, Pereira AA, et al. *Candida auris*, an agent of hospital-associated outbreaks: which challenging issues do we need to have in mind? Microorganisms 2020;8(2):181.

114. Prestel C, Anderson E, Forsberg K, et al. *Candida auris* outbreak in a COVID-19 specialty care unit—Florida, July-August 2020. MMWR Morb Mortal Wkly Rep 2021;70(2):56–7.

115. Tragiannidis A, Bisping G, Koehler G, et al. Minireview: *Malassezia* infections in immunocompromised patients. Mycoses 2010;53(3):187–95.

116. Wilson P, Zumla A. Transmission and prevention of acute viral respiratory tract infections in hospitals. Curr Opin Pulm Med 2019;25(3):220–4.

117. Jain S, Self WH, Wunderink RG, et al. Community-acquired pneumonia requiring hospitalization among U.S. adults. N Engl J Med 2015;373(5):415–27.

118. Gaunt ER, Harvala H, McIntyre C, et al. Disease burden of the most commonly detected respiratory viruses in hospitalized patients calculated using the disability adjusted life year (DALY) model. J Clin Virol 2011;52(3):215–21.

119. Evans ME, Hall KL, Berry SE. Influenza control in acute care hospitals. Am J Infect Control 1997;25(4):357–62.

120. Horcajada JP, Pumarola T, Martinez JA, et al. A nosocomial outbreak of influenza during a period without influenza epidemic activity. Eur Respir J 2003;21(2): 303–7.

121. Ahmed F, Lindley MC, Allred N, et al. Effect of influenza vaccination of healthcare personnel on morbidity and mortality among patients: systematic review and grading of evidence. Clin Infect Dis 2014;58(1):50–7.

122. Suwantarat N, Apisarnthanarak A. Risks to healthcare workers with emerging diseases: lessons from MERS-CoV, Ebola, SARS, and avian flu. Curr Opin Infect Dis 2015;28(4):349–61.

123. Maltezou HC, Tsiodras S. Middle East respiratory syndrome coronavirus: implications for health care facilities. Am J Infect Control 2014;42(12):1261–5.

124. Hui DS, Azhar EI, Kim YJ, et al. Middle East respiratory syndrome coronavirus: risk factors and determinants of primary, household, and nosocomial transmission. Lancet Infect Dis 2018;18(8):e217–27.

125. Maltezou HC, Ftika L, Theodoridou M. Nosocomial pertussis in neonatal units. J Hosp Infect 2013;85(4):243–8.

126. Calugar A, Ortega-Sanchez IR, Tiwari T, et al. Nosocomial pertussis: costs of an outbreak and benefits of vaccinating health care workers. Clin Infect Dis 2006; 42(7):981–8.

127. (CDC) CfDCaP. Pertussis—United States, 2001-2003. MMWR Morb Mortal Wkly Rep 2005;54(50):1283–6.

128. Sheridan SL, Frith K, Snelling TL, et al. Waning vaccine immunity in teenagers primed with whole cell and acellular pertussis vaccine: recent epidemiology. Expert Rev Vaccines 2014;13(9):1081–106.

129. Johansson MA, Quandelacy TM, Kada S, et al. SARS-CoV-2 transmission from people without COVID-19 symptoms. JAMA Netw Open 2021;4(1):e2035057.

130. Baker MA, Rhee C, Fiumara K, et al. COVID-19 infections among HCWs exposed to a patient with a delayed diagnosis of COVID-19. Infect Control Hosp Epidemiol 2020;41(9):1075–6.

131. Abbas M, Robalo Nunes T, Martischang R, et al. Nosocomial transmission and outbreaks of coronavirus disease 2019: the need to protect both patients and healthcare workers. Antimicrob Resist Infect Control 2021;10(1):7.

132. Rhee C, Baker M, Vaidya V, et al. Incidence of nosocomial COVID-19 in patients hospitalized at a large US Academic Medical Center. JAMA Netw Open 2020; 3(9):e2020498.

133. Klompas M, Baker MA, Rhee C, et al. A SARS-CoV-2 cluster in an acute care hospital. Ann Intern Med 2021. M20–7567.

134. Fankhauser RL, Noel JS, Monroe SS, et al. Molecular epidemiology of "Norwalk-like viruses" in outbreaks of gastroenteritis in the United States. J Infect Dis 1998;178(6):1571–8.

135. Iturriza-Gomara M, Lopman B. Norovirus in healthcare settings. Curr Opin Infect Dis 2014;27(5):437–43.

136. Kambhampati A, Koopmans M, Lopman BA. Burden of norovirus in healthcare facilities and strategies for outbreak control. J Hosp Infect 2015;89(4):296–301.

137. Robilotti E, Deresinski S, Pinsky BA. Norovirus. Clin Microbiol Rev 2015;28(1): 134–64.

138. Greig JD, Lee MB. A review of nosocomial norovirus outbreaks: infection control interventions found effective. Epidemiol Infect 2012;140(7):1151–60.

139. Kraay ANM, Han P, Kambhampati AK, et al. Impact of non-pharmaceutical interventions (NPIs) for SARS-CoV-2 on norovirus outbreaks: an analysis of outbreaks reported by 9 US States. J Infect Dis 2021. Available at: https://nam03.safelinks.protection.outlook.com/?url=https%3A%2F%2Fdx.doi.org%2F10.1093%252Finfdis%252Fjiab093&data=04%7C01%7Cr.mayakrishnan%40elsevier.com%7C9c8d5e0426c645264e5c08d9252cfa2a%7C9274ee3f94254109a27f9fb15c10675d%7C0%7C0%7C637581697401753979%7CUnknown%7CTWFpbGZsb3d8eyJWIjoiMC4wLjAwMDAiLCJQIjoiV2luMzIiLCJBTil6lk1haWwiLCJXVCI6Mn0%3D%7C1000&sdata=Oof5PrlxpmPYlfbn%2FloX28bJOmHzDRSw%2FtTpK9sDWsw%3D&reserved=0.

140. Magill SS, Edwards JR, Bamberg W, et al. Multistate point-prevalence survey of health care-associated infections. N Engl J Med 2014;370(13):1198–208.

141. Carroll KC, Bartlett JG. Biology of *Clostridium difficile*: implications for epidemiology and diagnosis. Annu Rev Microbiol 2011;65:501–21.

142. Barbut F. How to eradicate *Clostridium difficile* from the environment. J Hosp Infect 2015;89(4):287–95.

143. Otter JA, Yezli S, Salkeld JA, et al. Evidence that contaminated surfaces contribute to the transmission of hospital pathogens and an overview of

strategies to address contaminated surfaces in hospital settings. Am J Infect Control 2013;41(5 Suppl):S6–11.

144. Kundrapu S, Sunkesula V, Jury LA, et al. Daily disinfection of high-touch surfaces in isolation rooms to reduce contamination of healthcare workers' hands. Infect Control Hosp Epidemiol 2012;33(10):1039–42.

145. Eyre DW, Cule ML, Wilson DJ, et al. Diverse sources of C. difficile infection identified on whole-genome sequencing. N Engl J Med 2013;369(13):1195–205.

146. Lanata CF, Fischer-Walker CL, Olascoaga AC, et al. Global causes of diarrheal disease mortality in children <5 years of age: a systematic review. PLoS One 2013;8(9):e72788.

147. Rettedal S, Lohr IH, Natas O, et al. First outbreak of extended-spectrum beta-lactamase-producing Klebsiella pneumoniae in a Norwegian neonatal intensive care unit; associated with contaminated breast milk and resolved by strict cohorting. APMIS 2012;120(8):612–21.

148. Calbo E, Freixas N, Xercavins M, et al. Foodborne nosocomial outbreak of SHV1 and CTX-M-15-producing Klebsiella pneumoniae: epidemiology and control. Clin Infect Dis 2011;52(6):743–9.

149. Curtis C, Shetty N. Recent trends and prevention of infection in the neonatal intensive care unit. Curr Opin Infect Dis 2008;21(4):350–6.

150. Von Dolinger de Brito D, de Almeida Silva H, Jose Oliveira E, et al. Effect of neonatal intensive care unit environment on the incidence of hospital-acquired infection in neonates. J Hosp Infect 2007;65(4):314–8.

151. Oelberg DG, Joyner SE, Jiang X, et al. Detection of pathogen transmission in neonatal nurseries using DNA markers as surrogate indicators. Pediatrics 2000;105(2):311–5.

152. Gastmeier P, Loui A, Stamm-Balderjahn S, et al. Outbreaks in neonatal intensive care units: they are not like others. Am J Infect Control 2007;35(3):172–6.

153. Stapleton PJ, Murphy M, McCallion N, et al. Outbreaks of extended spectrum beta-lactamase-producing Enterobacteriaceae in neonatal intensive care units: a systematic review. Arch Dis Child Fetal Neonatal Ed 2016;101(1):F72–8.

154. Johnson J, Quach C. Outbreaks in the neonatal ICU: a review of the literature. Curr Opin Infect Dis 2017;30(4):395–403.

155. Civardi E, Tzialla C, Baldanti F, et al. Viral outbreaks in neonatal intensive care units: what we do not know. Am J Infect Control 2013;41(10):854–6.

156. Devlin RK. Invasive fungal infections caused by Candida and Malassezia species in the neonatal intensive care unit. Adv Neonatal Care 2006;6(2):68–77 [quiz: 8–9].

157. De Smet B, Veng C, Kruy L, et al. Outbreak of Burkholderia cepacia bloodstream infections traced to the use of Ringer lactate solution as multiple-dose vial for catheter flushing, Phnom Penh, Cambodia. Clin Microbiol Infect 2013; 19(9):832–7.

158. Kimura AC, Calvet H, Higa JI, et al. Outbreak of Ralstonia pickettii bacteremia in a neonatal intensive care unit. Pediatr Infect Dis J 2005;24(12):1099–103.

159. Macias AE, Munoz JM, Galvan A, et al. Nosocomial bacteremia in neonates related to poor standards of care. Pediatr Infect Dis J 2005;24(8):713–6.

160. Ofstead CL, Wetzler HP, Doyle EM, et al. Persistent contamination on colonoscopes and gastroscopes detected by biologic cultures and rapid indicators despite reprocessing performed in accordance with guidelines. Am J Infect Control 2015;43(8):794–801.

161. Pajkos A, Vickery K, Cossart Y. Is biofilm accumulation on endoscope tubing a contributor to the failure of cleaning and decontamination? J Hosp Infect 2004; 58(3):224–9.

162. Seoane-Vazquez E, Rodriguez-Monguio R, Visaria J, et al. Exogenous endoscopy-related infections, pseudo-infections, and toxic reactions: clinical and economic burden. Curr Med Res Opin 2006;22(10):2007–21.

163. Rutala WA, Weber DJ. ERCP scopes: what can we do to prevent infections? Infect Control Hosp Epidemiol 2015;36(6):643–8.

164. Epstein L, Hunter JC, Arwady MA, et al. New Delhi metallo-beta-lactamase-producing carbapenem-resistant *Escherichia coli* associated with exposure to duodenoscopes. JAMA 2014;312(14):1447–55.

165. Wendorf KA, Kay M, Baliga C, et al. Endoscopic retrograde cholangiopancreatography-associated AmpC *Escherichia coli* outbreak. Infect Control Hosp Epidemiol 2015;36(6):634–42.

166. Ross AS, Baliga C, Verma P, et al. A quarantine process for the resolution of duodenoscope-associated transmission of multidrug-resistant *Escherichia coli*. Gastrointest Endosc 2015;82(3):477–83.

167. Rutala WA, Kanamori H, Sickbert-Bennett EE, et al. What's new in reprocessing endoscopes: are we going to ensure "the needs of the patient come first" by shifting from disinfection to sterilization? Am J Infect Control 2019;47S:A62–6.

168. Katz MJ, Roghmann MC. Healthcare-associated infections in the elderly: what's new. Curr Opin Infect Dis 2016;29(4):388–93.

169. Utsumi M, Makimoto K, Quroshi N, et al. Types of infectious outbreaks and their impact in elderly care facilities: a review of the literature. Age Ageing 2010; 39(3):299–305.

170. Lee MH, Lee GA, Lee SH, et al. A systematic review on the causes of the transmission and control measures of outbreaks in long-term care facilities: back to basics of infection control. PLoS One 2020;15(3):e0229911.

171. Singh N, Limaye AP. Infections in solid-organ transplant recipients. In: Bennett JE, Dolin R, Blaser MJ, editors. Mandell, Douglas, and Bennett's principles and practice of infectious diseases. 8th edition. Philadelphia: Churchill Livingstone Elsevier; 2015. p. 3440–52.

172. Al-Hasan MN, Razonable RR, Eckel-Passow JE, et al. Incidence rate and outcome of gram-negative bloodstream infection in solid organ transplant recipients. Am J Transplant 2009;9(4):835–43.

173. Cervera C, van Delden C, Gavaldà J, et al. Multidrug-resistant bacteria in solid organ transplant recipients. Clin Microbiol Infect 2014;20(Suppl 7):49–73.

174. Manuel O, López-Medrano F, Keiser L, et al. Influenza and other respiratory virus infections in solid organ transplant recipients. Clin Microbiol Infect 2014; 20(Suppl 7):102–8.

175. Young J-AH, Weisdorf DJ. Infections in recipients of hematopoietic stem cell transplants. In: Bennett JE, Dolin R, Blaser MJ, editors. Mandell, Douglas, and Bennett's principles and practice of infectious diseases. 8th edition. Philadelphia: Churchill Livingstone Elsevier; 2015. p. 3425–39.

176. Paitoonpong L, Neofytos D, Cosgrove SE, et al. Infection prevention and control in hematopoietic stem cell transplant patients. In: Mayhall CG, editor. Hospital epidemiology and infection control. 4th edition. Baltimore: Lippincott Williams & Wilkins; 2012. p. 837–71.

Water Safety and Health Care

Preventing Infections Caused by Opportunistic Premise Plumbing Pathogens

Shantini D. Gamage, PhD, MPH[a,b,*], Meredith Ambrose, MHA[a,1],
Stephen M. Kralovic, MD, MPH[a,b,c,1], Gary A. Roselle, MD[a,b,c,1]

KEYWORDS

- Water-associated infections • Health care premise plumbing
- Water management program • Risk assessment
- Opportunistic premise plumbing pathogens • *Legionella*
- Nontuberculous mycobacteria

KEY POINTS

- There is increasing evidence of the contribution of opportunistic premise plumbing pathogens, such as *Legionella* and nontuberculous mycobacteria, to water-related infections in the United States.
- In recent years, regulatory and guidance bodies have issued multiple documents based on growing consensus for water management programs to control pathogens in premise plumbing, especially in health care settings.
- Many health care facilities do not have specific plans to address prevention of opportunistic premise plumbing pathogens, despite numerous case studies and outbreaks in the literature highlighting the importance of prioritizing comprehensive and sustained prevention practices.

INTRODUCTION

The remarkable advances in water safety in the United States (US), with regulations such as the Safe Drinking Water Act, prioritized prevention of contaminated potable water from fecal pathogens in the environment.[1] Fecal pathogens that are not killed

Funding Statement: No funding was received for this work.

[a] National Infectious Diseases Service, Specialty Care Services, Veterans Health Administration, Department of Veterans Affairs (VA), Washington, DC, USA; [b] Division of Infectious Diseases, Department of Internal Medicine, University of Cincinnati College of Medicine, Cincinnati, OH, USA; [c] Cincinnati VA Medical Center, Cincinnati, OH, USA
[1] Present address: 312 Elm Street, Suite 1475, Cincinnati, OH 45202
* Corresponding author. 312 Elm Street, Suite 1475, Cincinnati, OH 45202.
E-mail address: Shantini.Gamage@va.gov

by proper implementation of treatment at the community level and then enter building water systems are low in number, do not proliferate, and are unlikely to cause disease.[2] In contrast, some water-based pathogens are naturally present in the environment in low numbers and, if not killed by water treatment, can enter and colonize building water systems by establishing complex biofilms in pipes that provide nutrients and protection from control measures. These organisms are often referred to as opportunistic premise plumbing pathogens (OPPPs) because exposure to these pathogens that have amplified in pipes can cause disease in susceptible hosts.[2–4] Importantly, in the US in general, federal regulations for water quality and treatment to control pathogens pertain to water in the municipal distribution system up to a premise property line; conditions in premise water for inhibiting the growth of pathogens in the pipes are under the management of the property owner.[1]

Many cases of disease caused by OPPPs are considered to be sporadic (with no known exposure source). However, when a source is known, it is often large buildings such as hospitals and hotels that are implicated. These types of structures have complex water systems and multiple occupants, which can enhance factors influencing pathogen growth and exposure potential. Furthermore, outbreaks with numerous cases in these setting are more likely to trigger investigations to confirm source attribution.

Previously, the authors wrote in detail about the priorities and practices for water usage and safety in health care settings, particularly as they related to disease caused by *Legionella*.[5] In particular, the article addressed the challenges with balancing water safety (ie, preventing water-associated infections) with other water priorities such as meeting water demand, implementing water conservation, and ensuring water security. Here, this article builds on that work, describing OPPPs and practical considerations for prevention. There are numerous OPPPs that have been associated with waterborne diseases, including, but not limited to, *Legionella* species, nontuberculous mycobacteria (NTM), *Pseudomonas* species, *Acinetobacter* species, *Elizabethkingia meningosepticum* (*Flavobacterium meningosepticum*), *Stenotrophomonas maltophilia*, *Fusarium* species and *Naegleria* species,.[5,6] Although each contributes to the overall concept and burden of OPPPs, this article focuses on 2, *Legionella* and NTM, which serve as examples to highlight the many facets of this topic, and which in certain ways provide unique challenges.

Epidemiology of Opportunistic Premise Plumbing Pathogens in the United States

Recently, and for the first time, the US Centers for Disease Control and Prevention (CDC) has estimated the burden of 17 waterborne diseases in the nation, including respiratory illnesses caused by OPPPs (*Legionella*, NTM, and *Pseudomonas*), from data that encompassed both natural and engineered sources of exposure.[7] In 2014, there were an estimated 7.15 million cases of domestically acquired waterborne illness; although enteric diseases had a higher proportion of the estimated burden (2.3 million cases) compared with respiratory diseases (96,000 cases), the 3 respiratory pathogens named earlier resulted in the most hospitalizations and deaths. They also accounted for 72% ($2.39 billion) of all health care costs for domestically acquired waterborne illnesses. The report substantiates the significant impact of OPPPs on water-associated illness and health care systems in the US. Importantly, the report also highlights the limitations to determining incidence estimates, such as underdiagnosis and the lack of notifiable surveillance for diseases caused by some pathogens. Surveillance data specifically for *Legionella* and NTM are discussed later and summarized in **Table 1**.

Table 1
Characteristics of *Legionella* and nontuberculous mycobacteria

Pathogen Genus and Key Species[a]	Diseases	Cases in US	Modes of Exposure	Comments	References
Legionella pneumophila (predominantly serogroup 1) *Legionella longbeachae* *Legionella bozemanii* *Legionella micdadei*	Acute pneumonia (conventionally known as legionnaires disease);Pontiac fever (a mild, flulike illness); extrapulmonary infection (rare)	9933 reported cases (2018) 52,000–70,000 estimated cases each year *Legionella* associated with the largest proportion of drinking water outbreaks 24out of 42 (57%) in 2013–2014	Inhalation or aspiration No confirmed person-to-person transmission; 1 documented report of probable person-to-person transmission	>50 species of *Legionella*, but *L pneumophila* accounts for 90% of *Legionella* pneumonia cases in the US; other species have been associated with illness in people with compromised immune systems; *Legionella* pneumonia attack rate approximately 5%; seasonal variation; nationally notifiable disease in the US Survives in free-living amebae; grows best in warm water (25–42°C); some reported resistance to chlorine; documented health care–associated cases occurring over many months or years in absence of comprehensive intervention	5,11,27,33,71

(continued on next page)

Table 1
(continued)

Pathogen Genus and Key Species[a]	Diseases	Cases in US	Modes of Exposure	Comments	References
Nontuberculous Mycobacteria *Mycobacterium avium-intracellulare* complex *Mycobacterium chelonae* *Mycobacterium fortuitum* *Mycobacterium chimaera* *Mycobacterium abscessus* *Mycobacterium kansasii*	Pulmonary disease (both bronchiectatic and fibronodular disease); cervical lymphadenitis (children); skin/soft tissue infection; disseminated infection	Prevalence of 11.70 cases per 100,000 persons (2015) Estimated 68,900 annual waterborne NTM cases	Inhalation or aspiration; ingestion; direct inoculation Person-to-person transmission not known to occur, except suspicion of transmission between patients with cystic fibrosis	Opportunistic pathogens, especially affecting immunocompromised persons; slowly progressive disease that can become chronic and/or disseminated; slight, elderly women identified as a risk group; not nationally notifiable in the US Survives in free-living amebae; greater resistance to chlorine and monochloramine compared with other premise pathogens	1,4,7,45,72

[a] Major known pathogenic species are included for each genus. Other pathogenic species may exist.

Adapted from Gamage SD, Ambrose M, Kralovic SM, Roselle GA. Water Safety and Legionella in Health Care: Priorities, Policy, and Practice. Infect Dis Clin North Am. 2016 Sep;30(3):689-712; with permission.

Guidelines and Practices for Opportunistic Premise Plumbing Pathogen Prevention

Although the presence of pathogens in premise plumbing, especially *Legionella*, has been recognized for decades, attention in the US to the implementation of water management programs for buildings to control pathogen growth and prevent illness has been gaining traction in the last 5 to 10 years. A building water management program is a process for the methodical assessment and management of risks in the building water system.[8] Components of a comprehensive water management program include formation of a multidisciplinary team and development of a plan that addresses (1) description of the water systems, (2) identification of hazards (eg, OPPPs), (3) risk assessment and prioritization, (4) identification and implementation of control measures, (5) definition of corrective actions, and (6) verification of the implementation of the program. **Table 2** lists some of the decision points to consider when developing a water management program.

Control measures to prevent the growth of OPPPs (eg, inhibitory hot water temperatures, maintaining residual disinfectant levels) in building water systems have been described extensively in our prior article[5] and by others.[1,9–11] These measures are a primary aspect of water management programs. However, experience shows that, although buildings may have written plans, routine and sustained implementation and verification of the program can be challenging. Recent reports[12–14] that compiled data from multiple *Legionella* outbreak investigations or on-site consultative reviews have found that process challenges (ie, the ability to implement water management controls) are a major barrier to an effective program. From a practical perspective, key control measure implementation questions for the building water management team to address include:

- How consistently are the control measures in the water management plan being implemented as expected in the water distribution system and to user end points (eg, faucets and showers)?
- What monitoring data are collected to understand implementation of controls?
- How does the team determine that control measures are sufficient to inhibit OPPP growth and occupant exposure to them?
- Who will be responsible for reviewing control measure data, identifying potential issues, and implementing corrective actions?
- For health care facilities, how are risk assessments and clinical surveillance data factored into these decisions? The responsibilities for identifying and mitigating issues related to OPPPs necessitate collaboration between clinical disciplines (eg, infection prevention and control) and environmental disciplines (eg, engineering or facilities management).

Despite the growing consensus on the importance of reducing risk of OPPPs, there is no national law in the US requiring their control in buildings. Different entities (eg, federal agencies or state governments, standards organizations, and professional societies) have published various regulations, standards, or guidelines addressing water management programs in general or targeted to *Legionella* control. Some entities, such as US states, have enacted regulations for specific stakeholders subject to their oversight.[11,15,16] **Table 3** provides a list of select US and international guidelines, which have also been reviewed and described in detail by others.[11,15]

Validating the Effectiveness of Water Management Programs

Many guidelines and standards promote the routine assessment of the effectiveness of water management programs, which can then inform whether adjustments to the

Table 2
Examples of decision points for health care facility water management programs

Component	Decision Points
Decision making	Involvement of facility leadership Chair and membership of water management team Water management team responsibilities Prioritization of actions
Scope	Potable and process water systems to be included in the program Water safety focus and/or other water priorities (eg, water security, conservation) Special water uses to be included (eg, dialysis, dental) Microbiological focus or all-hazards approach (eg, chemical, scald injury) For microbiological component: *Legionella* focus or other potential water pathogens as well Types of buildings included (eg, inpatient facilities, outpatient clinics, long-term care facilities/residential buildings, administrative buildings)

Management plan	Knowledge and understanding
	    Water distribution system infrastructure
	    Staff education/training: competency requirements
	Use of water management consultant
	Risk assessment mechanism and criteria
	Selection of control measures (eg, water temperature, disinfection residual)
	    Prevention of scald injury
	    Mechanism to ensure implementation of controls
	Determination of necessity for supplementary disinfectant treatment system and, if so, which one
	    Ensure appropriate permits if necessary
	Triggers for corrective actions
	Corrective actions that will be taken
	Safety considerations
	    Patients and long-term care residents
	    Employees and visitors

Data collection	Surveillance for disease: which infections and tracking mechanism Monitoring of engineering controls: which ones, mechanism, and frequency Environmental testing on a routine basis for microbial pathogens or indicators: which ones, if any; mechanism; and frequency

Adapted from Gamage SD, Ambrose M, Kralovic SM, Roselle GA. Water Safety and Legionella in Health Care: Priorities, Policy, and Practice. Infect Dis Clin North Am. 2016 Sep;30(3):689-712; with permission.

program's plans or implementation are needed. In the past, the occurrence of an OPPP case or an outbreak was the first indication that water management actions were needed, or needed to be improved. However, this misses potential opportunities to improve water systems before even 1 case.[17] There are varying perspectives on the best mechanisms for validating program effectiveness at controlling OPPPs. One area of thought is to test physical characteristics such as water temperature, residual disinfectant, and pH at certain outlets in the water distribution system to ensure they are at levels that inhibit OPPPs. However, data show that this type of testing may not correlate well with presence of OPPPs in the water system.[18] Similarly, although testing building water systems for nonpathogenic indicator organisms such as heterotrophs

Table 3
Select regulations, standards, and guidelines for the control of premise plumbing pathogens in building water systems

Location	Organization	Publication Name (Year)	Scope (*Legionella* or Water Management) and Type of Publication[a]	Hyperlink
US	CDC	Prevention with Water Management Programs (Web site, last reviewed 2018)	Water management guidance	https://www.cdc.gov/Legionella/wmp/index.html
US	CDC	Guidelines for the environmental infection control in health-care facilities (2003)	Water management and *Legionella* guidance	https://www.cdc.gov/mmwr/preview/mmwrhtml/rr5210a1.htm
US	CDC	Guidelines for preventing health care–associated pneumonia (2004)	Water management and *Legionella* guidance	https://www.cdc.gov/mmwr/preview/mmwrhtml/rr5303a1.htm
US	CDC	Tools to Reduce Risk from Water (Web site, last reviewed 2019) • Water Infection Control Risk Assessment for Healthcare Settings • Tap Water Quality and Infrastructure Discussion Guide for Investigation of Potential Water-Associated Infection in Healthcare Facilities • Healthcare Facility Water Management Program Checklist	Water management guidance	https://www.cdc.gov/hai/prevent/environment/water.html
US	CDC	Toolkit: Developing a Water Management Program to Reduce *Legionella* Growth and Spread in Buildings (2017)	*Legionella* guidance	https://www.cdc.gov/Legionella/wmp/toolkit/index.html
US	Centers for Medicare and Medicaid (CMS)	Requirement to Reduce *Legionella* Risk in Healthcare Facility Water Systems to Prevent Cases and Outbreaks of Legionnaires' Disease (LD) (2018)	Water management memorandum	https://www.cms.gov/Medicare/Provider-Enrollment-and-Certification/SurveyCertificationGenInfo/Downloads/QSO17-30-HospitalCAH-NH-REVISED-.pdf

(continued on next page)

Table 3
(continued)

Location	Organization	Publication Name (Year)	Scope (*Legionella* or Water Management) and Type of Publication[a]	Hyperlink
US	Department of Veterans Affairs, Veterans Health Administration	VHA Directive 1061: Prevention of Healthcare-associated *Legionella* Disease and Scald Injury from Potable Water Distribution Systems (2014)	*Legionella* directive	https://www.va.gov/vhapublications/ViewPublication.asp?pub_ID=3033
US	Occupational Safety and Health Administration	Legionellosis (Legionnaires' Disease and Pontiac Fever) (Web site)	*Legionella* guidance	https://www.osha.gov/legionnaires-disease
US	ASHRAE[b]	Standard 188–2018, Legionellosis: Risk Management for Building Water Systems (2018)	*Legionella* standard	https://www.techstreet.com/ashrae/standards/ashrae-188-2018?product_id=2020895
US	ASHRAE[b]	Guideline 12–2020, Managing the Risk of Legionellosis Associated with Building Water Systems (2020)	*Legionella* guidance	https://www.techstreet.com/ashrae/standards/guideline-12-2020-managing-the-risk-of-legionellosis-associated-with-building-water-systems?product_id=2111422
US	Cooling Tower Institute	Guideline 159: Practices to Reduce the Risk of Legionellosis from Evaporative Heat Rejection Equipment Systems (2020)	*Legionella* guidance	https://www.coolingtechnology.org/product-page/legionellosis-guideline-gld-159
US	New York State	New York Codes, Rules and Regulations: Part 4 – Protection Against *Legionella* (2016)	*Legionella* regulation	https://regs.health.ny.gov/content/part-4-protection-against-Legionella
US	WHO	*Legionella* and the Prevention of Legionellosis (2007)	*Legionella* guidance	https://apps.who.int/iris/handle/10665/43233
United Nations	WHO	Water Safety in Buildings (2011)	Water management guidance	https://www.who.int/water_sanitation_health/publications/2011/9789241548106/en/

Country	Organization	Title	Type	URL
European Union	European Centre for Disease Prevention and Control	ESGLI European Technical Guidelines for the Prevention, Control and Investigation of Infections Caused by *Legionella* species (2017)	*Legionella* guidance	https://www.ecdc.europa.eu/en/publications-data/european-technical-guidelines-prevention-control-and-investigation-infections
Australia	NSW Ministry of Health	NSW Water – Requirements for the Provision of Cold and Heated Water (2015)	Water management directive	https://www1.health.nsw.gov.au/pds/Pages/doc.aspx?dn=PD2015_008
Australia	Government of South Australia	Guidelines for *Legionella* Control in the Operation and Maintenance of Water Distribution Systems in Health and Aged Care Facilities(2015)	*Legionella* guidance	https://www1.health.gov.au/internet/main/publishing.nsf/Content/A12B57E41EC9F326CA257BF0001F9E7D/$File/Guidelines-*Legionella*-control.pdf
Canada	Public Works and Government Services Canada	D 15,161–2013 Control of *Legionella* in Mechanical Systems (2013)	*Legionella* standard	https://www.tpsgc-pwgsc.gc.ca/biens-property/documents/*Legionella*-eng.pdf
Germany	German Technical and Scientific Association for Gas and Water	Technical Rule: Code of Practice W551. Drinking water heating and drinking water piping systems; technical measures to reduce *Legionella* growth; design, construction, operation and rehabilitation of drinking water installations (2004)	*Legionella* code of practice	http://www.monachos.gr/forum/attachment.php?attachmentid=191&d=1371566673
Ireland	Health Protection Surveillance Centre	National Guidelines for the Control of Legionellosis in Ireland (2009)	*Legionella* guidance	https://www.hpsc.ie/a-z/respiratory/legionellosis/guidance/nationalguidelinesforthecontroloflegionellosisinireland/File,3936,en.pdf

(continued on next page)

Table 3
(continued)

Location	Organization	Publication Name (Year)	Scope (*Legionella* or Water Management) and Type of Publication[a]	Hyperlink
New Zealand	Ministry of Health	The Prevention of Legionellosis in New Zealand: Guidelines for the control of *Legionella* bacteria (2012)	*Legionella* guidance	https://www.health.govt.nz/publicat on/prevention-legionellos's-new-zealand-guidelines-control-*Legionella*-bacteria
Singapore	Institute of Environmental Epidemiology Ministry of the Environment	Code of Practice for the Control of *Legionella* Bacteria in Cooling Towers (2001)	*Legionella* code of practice	https://www.nea.gov.sg/docs/default-source/resource/practices-/-code-of-practice-for-contrcl-of-*Legionella*-bacteria-'n-cooling-towers.pdf
United Kingdom	Health and Safety Executive	Legionnaires' Disease: The Control of *Legionella* Bacteria in Water Systems (2013)	*Legionella* guidance	https://www.hse.gov.uk/pubns/books/l8.htm

Abbreviations: ESGLI, ESCMID Study Group for Legionella Infections; NSW, New South Wales; WHO, World Health Organization.
[a] The type of publication is designated as it is referenced by the publication. For publications that have requirements or regulations (ie, not just guidance), specifics on the entities subject to the rules are as described within the documents.
[b] ASHRAE is the current name in use for the American Society of Heating, Refrigerating, and Air-conditioning Engineers.

may inform overall water quality, these results also do not correlate well with presence of OPPPs.[18,19]

Growing attention is being given to routinely testing building water systems for OPPPs, especially *Legionella*, to evaluate water management programs. This trend is particularly true for health care buildings, and OPPP testing in these settings is addressed later in this article. The key barrier to widespread use of routine environmental testing for OPPPs is the lack of information on which OPPP testing should be implemented to best indicate program effectiveness, which sampling and testing methods to use, and how results should be used because building design, water use, and control measures can vary greatly between buildings and in their impact on different OPPPs.[20]

OPPORTUNISTIC PREMISE PLUMBING PATHOGENS AND HEALTH CARE
Nature of the Problem

Water-related pathogens are a significant issue in health care,[21] with reports often pertaining to health care–associated (HCA) Legionella infections. However, other pathogens in water are significant risks to patient safety as well. A report of non-*Legionella* water-related CDC investigations found that NTM was the most common cause involved (40 out of 134, 29%).[22] The growth of OPPPs and potential risks are not limited to health care, but there are characteristics of these settings that contribute to increased propensity for both pathogen growth and occupant risk:

- Health care buildings can be large with many miles of pipes, and on sprawling campuses with extensive water distribution piping and on-site water storage tanks. These factors can affect water age in the system, resulting in low disinfectant residual, and complicate the ability to implement OPPP control measures throughout the water distribution systems to user end points.
- There are multiple uses of water in different health care settings, including the use of devices that can optimize exposure of patients or residents to aerosolized water[22] (**Table 4** provides a list of water uses in health care and examples of HCA cases or outbreaks).
- Health care facilities, by their nature, cohort occupants (patients, long-term care residents) at higher risk for opportunistic infections, including those with compromised or suppressed immune systems, older age, and comorbidities such as chronic obstructive pulmonary disease.
- The ability to deliver hot water temperatures at outlets at a level that inhibits pathogen growth (at least 55°C) is compromised by the need to avoid scald injury in building occupants. This need is especially critical in long-term care.
- Frequent construction and renovation projects are common in health care settings, which can cause disturbances to building water systems. Construction-related activities have been associated with HCA cases of disease caused by OPPPs.[23] Routine practice is to perform an infection control risk assessment before initiating the work to prevent causing exposure to pathogens, but these exercises often focus on airborne exposures, and inclusion of water-related exposures are often neglected.

In the US, a significant development in OPPP prevention in health care was the 2017 requirement by the Centers for Medicare and Medicaid Services (CMS) that all CMS-certified hospitals, critical access hospitals, and long-term care facilities "have water management policies and procedures to reduce the risk of growth and spread of *Legionella* and other opportunistic pathogens in building water systems."[24] The

Table 4
Water uses in health care settings and infection risks

Water Use	Infection Risks and/or Considerations	Case/Outbreak Example	References
Fixtures on potable water system (eg, faucets, showers)	Location in health care buildings where patients come in contact with water; may be difficult to deliver hot water consistently to distal locations; may have thermostatic mixing valves to prevent scald injury; water can stagnate in low-use fixtures, resulting in reduced hot water temperature and disinfection residual	Cases of *Pseudomonas aeruginosa* linked to water from electronic faucets in a neonatal intensive care unit Case of *Mycobacterium fortuitum* breast infection from contamination of surgical site with hospital shower water during postoperative care	Yapicioglu et al,[73] 2012 Jaubert et al,[74] 2015
Ice from plumbed ice machines	Aspiration risk; cold water in piping can become warmed by heat from condenser and/or compressor; water stagnation when not in use; charcoal filter colonized by bacteria; lack of routine maintenance, cleaning, and disinfection	Legionellosis from aspiration of water from ice chips Clusters of NTM infections from intensive care unit ice machines	Bencini et al,[75] 2005 Oda et al,[64] 2020
Respiratory equipment (eg, nebulizers, continuous positive airway pressure devices)	Bacterial growth in devices without sufficient maintenance and cleaning; aerosolization of water Use sterile water only; follow CDC guidelines for cleaning/disinfecting equipment	*P aeruginosa* infection caused by contaminated nebulizers Hospital-associated *Legionella* infection from use of tap water in a nebulizer	Cobben et al,[76] 1996 Kyritsi et al,[77] 2018
Food preparation	Appropriate washing and disinfection procedures; use of sterilizers	Outbreak of *P aeruginosa* infection in a neonatal intensive care unit was linked to the feeding bottle preparation room	Sánchez-Carrillo et al,[78] 2009

Dialysis	Chemical or bacterial contamination, or modifications to potable water system (eg, supplementary treatment) can affect dialysis water. Dialysis water must meet specific ANSI/AAMI/ISO requirements to prevent illness as a result of contaminants in the water (eg, endotoxin, disinfection byproducts)	Outbreak of Mycobacterium chelonae at a hemodialysis outpatient clinic caused by use of high-flux dialyzers that were manually reprocessed	Lowry et al,[79] 1990
Pharmacy: medication preparation	Water for pharmaceutical use should meet drinking water standards. Water used for specific pharmaceutical purposes (eg, water for injections, water for compounding) should meet pharmacopeial specifications for chemical and microbiological purity	Outbreak of Exophiala jeanselmei fungemia, most likely linked to deionized water from the hospital pharmacy for preparation of antiseptic solutions. Outbreak of Pantoea agglomerans blood stream infections caused by preparation of infusates near a contaminated pharmacy sink	WHO[80], Nucci et al,[81] 2002 Yablon et al,[82] 2017
Hydrotherapy	Aerosolization of water; water stagnation because of intermittent use; contaminated pumps and hoses; insufficient cleaning and disinfection	Folliculitis among patients and staff that used a pool in a physiotherapy unit. A case of legionnaires disease associated with a respiratory hydrotherapy system	Schlech et al,[83] 1986 Leoni et al,[84] 2006
Dental	Aerosolization of water; water stagnation; plastic tubing conducive to biofilm and bacterial growth; water temperatures in ranges that allow bacterial growth; patient oral microorganisms can contaminate the unit during procedure. The CDC recommends that water used in nonsurgical dental units should meet drinking water standards; surgical procedures should use only sterile solutions	Legionella infection from contaminated dental unit water lines. Mycobacterium abscessus infections in pediatric patients after pulpotomies at a dental practice	Ricci et al,[85] 2012; CDC,[86] 2003 Peralta et al,[87] 2016

(continued on next page)

Table 4
(continued)

Water Use	Infection Risks and/or Considerations	Case/Outbreak Example	References
Heater-cooler devices	Aerosolization of water from the device's exhaust vent The Food and Drug Administration recommends the use of sterile or filtered water and other practices to reduce risk to patients	*Mycobacterium chimaera* infections diagnosed in cardiothoracic surgery patients	Sax et al,[88] 2015
Cooling towers used for air conditioning	Cooling tower systems can promote bacterial growth, including pathogens such as *Legionella*, if not cleaned and maintained; water can contain nutrients that can support bacterial growth; aerosols from cooling towers can disperse *Legionella* over a large area	Outbreak of legionella infection in a long-term care facility associated with a cooling tower using an automated disinfection system	Quinn et al,[89] 2015

Abbreviations: AAMI, Association for the Advancement of Medical Instrumentation; ANSI, American National Standards Institute; ISO, International Organization for Standardization.

Adapted from Gamage SD, Ambrose M, Kralovic SM, Roselle GA. Water Safety and Legionella in Health Care: Priorities, Policy, and Practice. Infect Dis Clin North Am. 2016 Sep;30(3):689-712; with permission.

expectations for the facility plans are in alignment with the components of water management plans described earlier: a risk assessment to identify where OPPPs could grow and spread in the water system, a water management program, and protocols for control measures. The CMS requirement indicates consideration of American Society of Heating, Refrigerating, and Air-conditioning Engineers (ASHRAE) Standard 188[25] and the CDC Toolkit[26] when developing water management programs, although both of these documents are *Legionella* specific and the CMS requirement is not limited to addressing just this pathogen. The practices to reduce the risk of *Legionella* in building water systems can also target the other pathogens, but facilities may need to consult other resources (eg, as listed in **Table 3**) for comprehensive water management programs and risk assessment tools. Listed next are seminal characteristics of *Legionella* and NTM, and considerations for preventing infections in health care settings.

Legionella

Description
The bacterial genus *Legionella* comprises more than 50 species, with *Legionella pneumophila* responsible for about 90% of reported infections in North America.[12] Diseases caused by *Legionella*, collectively known as legionellosis, usually manifest as respiratory illness including *Legionella* pneumonia (L-PNA), traditionally known as legionnaires disease. See **Table 1** for key characteristics of *Legionella* and legionellosis. A comprehensive *Legionella* review, and recommendations, addressing clinical topics, ecology, control in buildings, quantification of legionellosis and *Legionella*, and regulations and guidelines is presented in the recent Consensus Study Report of the National Academies of Science, Engineering, and Medicine (NASEM).[11]

Information on the occurrence of *Legionella* in premise plumbing is minimal, especially for non–health care buildings. The National Academies found that studies of *Legionella* in buildings typically yielded sample positivity rates of 30% to 80% (3% to 20% positivity for *L pneumophila*).[11] Less is known about when the presence of *Legionella* in plumbing will result in cases, although evidence is accumulating for the use of quantitative microbial risk assessments to guide knowledge and actions.[11] At present, prevention centers on maintaining building water systems that are inhospitable to *Legionella* proliferation and monitoring the control efforts, with recognition of the areas of the water systems where *Legionella* exposure may occur.[10,25,26] Sources of exposure include, but are not limited to, aerosolized water from showering, heated spas, decorative fountains, and cooling towers, or ice that is consumed and water that is inadvertently aspirated.[21] A CDC review of 23 L-PNA outbreak investigations showed that all buildings had deficiencies in water system maintenance, reinforcing the need for well-managed water management programs.[12]

Legionellosis epidemiology
The most comprehensive information on the incidence of diagnosed OPPP illnesses pertains to diseases caused by *Legionella*. Legionellosis is a notifiable disease in the US and the CDC has reported about a 10-fold increase in cases between 2000 and 2018 from approximately 1000 cases to almost 10,000 cases.[27] Incidence of reported cases in the US has also increased from 0.42 per 100,000 persons in 2000 to 2.27 per 100,000 persons in 2017.[28] National data from the US Department of Veterans Affairs (VA) reported similar increasing rates of legionellosis for veterans enrolled in VA health care (1.5–2.0 cases per 100,000 enrolled veterans for 2014–2016),[29] and potential long-term health effects of L-PNA.[30] Legionellosis is underdiagnosed and it is estimated that the annual case burden is up to 70,000 cases.[11] The estimated true

incidence of L-PNA in Connecticut between 2000 and 2014 was calculated to be 11.6 cases per 100,000 persons, a 10-fold difference from the observed incidence of 1.2 cases per 100,000 persons.[31] Legionella was also associated with the largest number of drinking water outbreaks in the US in 2013 to 2014 (24 out of 42 outbreaks, or 57%) based on the most recent reporting to the CDC waterborne disease surveillance system.[32] However, outbreaks of L-PNA account for only about 5% of reported cases, and the source of the remaining 95% is often not determined.[33]

Legionella and Health Care Settings

Epidemiology of health care–associated Legionella pneumonia

Of the OPPPs, HCA cases of L-PNA have the most surveillance data available, although information is still sparse. Attribution of the source of exposure is facilitated by L-PNA being an acute pneumonia. In the US, health care association is determined to be presumptive or possible based on temporal definitions of exposure to health care settings in the 14-day period before symptom onset (**Box 1**).[34] Before those updated definitions were adopted by the CDC in January 2020, the exposure window was a narrower 10 days[35] and the term definite was used instead of presumptive. Surveillance studies in the US have shown that about 3% of L-PNA cases were definite HCA L-PNA.[36] A European study also showed a definite HCA L-PNA rate of about 3%, although definitions were not standard among the included countries.[37] Surveillance for L-PNA that is possibly HCA is more variable, with a CDC-reported rate of 17%.[36] Limitations of HCA L-PNA surveillance data are the likely underdiagnosis of L-PNA in patients with HCA pneumonia and absent or inconclusive epidemiologic investigations into sources of Legionella exposure. The fatality rate for definite HCA L-PNA cases is about 25%,[29,36] which is substantially higher than the fatality rate for non-HCA cases (about 9%).

Clinical and infection prevention considerations

Legionella pneumonia is indistinguishable clinically from other pneumonias and requires specific confirmatory diagnostic testing. The Legionella urine antigen test, which targets detection of disease caused by L pneumophila serogroup 1, is the primary L-PNA diagnostic test used in the US and likely contributes to the high rate of this species and serogroup in L-PNA surveillance. Microbiological culturing of respiratory specimens can detect other Legionella species and serogroups as well as providing a clinical isolate for comparison with available environmental Legionella isolates by

---

Box 1
Health care–associated Legionella pneumonia (HCA L-PNA) definitions

Presumptive HCA L-PNA
 A case of L-PNA in which the person had continuous contact with a health care facility[a] for at least 10 days in the 14 days immediately preceding L-PNA symptom onset

Possible HCA L-PNA
 A case of L-PNA in which the person had some contact with a health care facility[a] for a portion of the 14 days immediately preceding L-PNA, but not 10 or more consecutive days

Details on these definitions for health care–associated legionella pneumonia (also known as legionnaires disease) are available from the Council of State and Territorial Epidemiologists.[34]

 [a] A health care facility is any setting where medical or nursing care is delivered and includes, but is not limited to, hospitals, long-term care facilities, ambulatory surgical centers, and outpatient clinics.

molecular methods. However, pneumonia is often treated empirically with antibiotics and an L-PNA diagnosis is not made. A 2011 retrospective review of L-PNA cases at 1 hospital found that 41% (15 out of 37) did not meet the professional guideline criteria for Legionella testing of community-acquired pneumonia.[38] With respect to hospital-acquired pneumonia (HAP), an active surveillance study in Spain identified L pneumophila as the causal agent in non–intensive care unit (ICU), nonoutbreak settings in 4.2% (7 out of 165) of HAP cases; the investigators suggest that the Legionella urinary antigen test be used for all HAP cases, especially because outcomes were worse for patients with HAP receiving inappropriate antibiotics.[39] Operationalizing such a comprehensive testing system is possible,[40] and especially in facilities with past cases or outbreaks of HCA L-PNA. In general, in health care settings, not diagnosing L-PNA can result in (1) treatment with inappropriate antibiotics and poorer outcomes, (2) a lack of recognition of environmental health care exposure, and (3) a missed opportunity for an epidemiologic investigation and water system remediation to prevent further cases.

The designation of an L-PNA case as HCA is clearest when a person has been at a health care setting continuously for multiple weeks before L-PNA symptom onset (eg, long-term care facility residents). The attribution to health care is more complicated when the Legionella infection occurs in a person who was at a health care facility for only a portion of the 2 weeks before symptom onset. However, determining the likelihood of even 1 possible HCA L-PNA case being exposed at the health care facility can alert the facility to a water management situation that needs corrective actions to prevent additional cases.[41]

Outbreak investigations have shown that Legionella strains associated with HCA L-PNA cases can persist in hospital plumbing and result in cases of disease decades later if allowed to proliferate.[42] The occurrence of HCA L-PNA cases can be prolonged over many months or years (a creeping outbreak),[5] which presents certain challenges for infection prevention and control:

- HCA L-PNA cases, especially those epidemiologically classified as possibly linked to the health care facility, may be viewed as sporadic occurrences rather than the potential to be a prolonged outbreak. Less impetus is placed on epidemiologic investigations or adjustments to the implementation of engineering controls.
- Documentation of HCA L-PNA cases needs to be sustained and available for the duration of the existence of the health care facility to account for staff turnover. One practical recommendation is to include any HCA L-PNA cases in the facility risk assessment document; this risk assessment should be reviewed annually as part of the water management program and serves as a reminder of past cases.

Routine testing of health care facility water for Legionella
Numerous studies substantiate that health care facility water systems can harbor Legionella, with varying percentages of buildings testing positive and varying levels of positivity within buildings.[11,43] However, the extent that Legionella routine testing, in the absence of cases, is implemented in the US to inform water management programs is not well characterized. In some entities, such as the VA health care system and in New York state, routine testing is required for health care facilities that are under the purview of their respective regulations.[16,44] For other facilities, such testing is voluntary.[24] In a significant indication of consensus, the NASEM report recommends that CMS expand its health care water management program requirements to include Legionella testing of water samples.[11]

Guidance is available for health care facilities that choose to implement routine *Legionella* testing to evaluate a water management program.[10,20] The following factors should be determined by the water management team considering such testing:

- The frequency of the routine *Legionella* testing and the sampling method
- The qualifications of the laboratory that will perform the sample analysis
- The type of analysis that will be done to determine whether *Legionella* is detected in the environmental sample (eg, culture and/or molecular methods)
- The type of *Legionella* that will be tested (eg, all *Legionella* species or *L pneumophila*)
- The type of results (eg, type of *Legionella* species detected, *Legionella* concentration, sample positivity rate) that will trigger a review of the water management program and assess the need for corrective actions

The CDC makes no recommendation for or against routine *Legionella* testing in health care, except for recommending such testing in high-risk settings (eg, hematopoietic stem cell transplant units and protective environments).[45] For facilities that do routine testing, there is no standard method for determining when results should trigger corrective actions. Some health care systems require actions when any *Legionella* is detected in any sample at any level.[29,44] Other entities have implemented a threshold of 30% sample positivity to trigger corrective actions for hospitals and long-term care facilities,[16,46] based on early work showing less association of water systems with L-PNA cases if positivity was less than 30%.[47,48] Some organizations have also recommended various *Legionella* concentration levels as indications for decision making. For example, ASHRAE supports a concentration level of 1 colony-forming unit (CFU) per milliliter as a threshold for action.[10] The NASEM consensus study found that a *Legionella* concentration greater than 50 CFU/mL was a breakpoint that differentiated *Legionella* concentrations in outbreaks compared with sporadic cases and offers an action level for immediate remediation.[11] Many of these entities reinforce that action could be taken without reaching suggested thresholds based on situational factors (eg, recent cases of L-PNA, or buildings that house higher-risk occupants. such as health care facilities).

Case study: health care–associated Legionella pneumonia

Castellino and colleagues[49] described a case of HCA L-PNA that was designated as possibly associated with the hospital because the patient was in a residential rehabilitation program and left the facility for a weekend in the 10 days before L-PNA symptom onset (**Fig. 1**). The patient was initially thought to have aspiration pneumonia and was treated with vancomycin and piperacillin/tazobactam. Because the health care facility performed routine testing of the water system for *Legionella*, and heightened awareness for L-PNA cases when water was *Legionella* positive, the patient had a urinary antigen test done that diagnosed the respiratory illness as L-PNA. Treatment was switched to an antibiotic that covered *Legionella* infection. A sputum sample grew *L pneumophila*, and this isolate was genetically similar to an *L pneumophila* isolate from the water system. Because of this similarity, the case was reclassified as definite HCA L-PNA and the water distribution system was remediated to address *Legionella* growth.

Lessons from this case study:

- Test patients with HCA pneumonia for *Legionella* infection. Avoid assuming that HCA pneumonia is not L-PNA because of a suspicion of aspiration pneumonia, or because the facility has not had cases of HCA L-PNA previously.

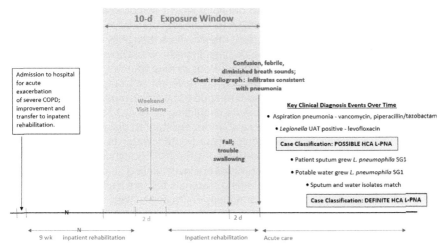

Fig. 1. The sequence of events for a case of HCA L-PNA. COPD, chronic obstructive pulmonary disease; SG1, serogroup 1; UAT, urine antigen test. (*Data from* Castellino LM, Gamage SD, Hoffman PV, Kralovic SM, Holodniy M, Bernstein JM, Roselle GA. Healthcare-associated Legionnaires' disease: Limitations of surveillance definitions and importance of epidemiologic investigation. J Infect Prev. 2017 Nov;18(6):307-310.)

- Performing routine testing of water systems for *Legionella* provides knowledge of potential risks and can alert clinical staff to have increased awareness for L-PNA in patients with HCA pneumonia.
- Consider *Legionella* clinical testing when symptoms first present, rather than empiric treatment and only testing for *Legionella* if treatment failure is evident. Early *Legionella* testing can optimize early treatment with an appropriate antibiotic and better prevent a severe clinical outcome.
- Identification of a single possible HCA L-PNA case should trigger a detailed review of the likelihood that the *Legionella* exposure was in the health care facility.
- Clinical culture for *Legionella* infection should be done in addition to *Legionella* urinary antigen testing. Isolation of a clinical strain can be used to determine linkage to the health care setting if environmental isolates are available.

Nontuberculous Mycobacteria

Description

The approximately 200 species of mycobacteria are generally categorized as the *Mycobacterium tuberculosis* complex (about 10 species), NTM (most of the species in the genus), and *Mycobacterium leprae* (causative agent of leprosy).[50,51] NTM are diverse and ubiquitous in soil and natural water bodies, as well as being present in engineered water systems. Most species are nonpathogenic and saprophytes. Of the pathogenic species (see **Table 1**), *Mycobacterium avium* complex account for about 80% of infections.[52] NTM infection is opportunistic. Most illness is pulmonary, although infections of other sites do occur (eg, skin and soft tissue, lymph nodes) as well as systemic infection.

There is little information on the prevalence of NTM in premise plumbing. Donohue and colleagues[53] sampled cold water from taps at 40 sites across the US for a period of 2 years and detected NTM in 78% (202 out of 258) of the samples. Of the 66 taps sampled, all but 1 had NTM detected during at least 1 sampling event, and 52% had NTM detected at all 4 sampling events. Other studies in the US have also found NTM in samples from outlets to varying degrees, often in more than 50% of the samples,[54,55] indicating that the presence of these bacteria in premise plumbing is not rare.

Exposure to NTM in buildings can occur from various sources, including showers, sinks, and ice machines. NTM are relatively resistant to control measures, even compared with other OPPPs. They can tolerate hot water temperatures up to about 55°C, a level higher than the temperature circulating in many health care facility hot water distribution systems. They are also more resistant to disinfectants than other OPPPs, with evidence that monochloramine-treated water is less successful at inhibiting NTM growth than chlorine-treated water.[53,55] Because of this resistance to traditional control measures, researchers are investigating other means to prevent OPPP growth or exposure, such as piping materials that are less conducive to bacterial adherence and biofilm formation, ultraviolet light disinfection, and filtration.[1,4,56]

Nontuberculous mycobacteria epidemiology

An increasing incidence in NTM has been recognized since at least the 1970s when clinical specimens sent for *M tuberculosis* testing were instead positive for NTM.[57] Disease caused by NTM is not reportable in the US and is underdiagnosed,[7] but most incidence studies indicate that the NTM rate continues to increase.[50] A review of NTM cases between 2008 and 2015 in a large managed care health plan in the US found an increase in annual incidence from 3.13 cases to 4.73 cases per 100,000 person-years and an increase in annual prevalence from 6.78 to 11.70 per 100,000 persons.[58] For persons more than 65 years of age, the same review reported an increase in annual incidence from 12.70 to 18.37 per 100,000 person-years and an increase in prevalence from 30.27 cases to 47.48 cases per 100,000 persons. A different review of NTM pulmonary disease nationally in Medicare beneficiaries (persons >65 years old) showed a similar increase in prevalence from 20 cases per 100,000 persons in 1997 to 47 cases per 100,000 persons in 2007, and this increase was observed in all geographic regions.[52] Prevalence increased for both women and men, with 65% of the cases in women. Two studies published in 2018 using health record data for veterans enrolled in VA health care across the US examined NTM prevalence and incidence in the context of patients with chronic obstructive pulmonary disease (COPD), a respiratory condition with higher prevalence in the VA patient population than in the general US population.[59,60] Jones and colleagues[59] studied NTM cases in the VA patient population from 2009 to 2012, and Pyarali and colleagues[60] examined NTM cases in VA patients with COPD from 2001 to 2015. Both found variability in geographic distribution, with a higher incidence rate[59] or period prevalence[60] in the southeastern US. Jones and colleagues[59] determined an incidence of 12.6 cases per 100,000 patient years; there was decreasing incidence of pulmonary NTM, in contrast with other reports for the US, and increasing extrapulmonary NTM. Of the patients with pulmonary NTM, 68% had COPD. Pyarali and colleagues[60] examined NTM rates in the subset of VA patients that had a diagnosis of COPD. Incidence of NTM was fairly stable from 2001 (34.2 cases per 100,000 patients with COPD) to 2012 (25.4 cases per 100,000 patients with COPD), followed by an inflection point and sharp increase in incidence from 2012 to 2015 (70.3 cases per 100,000 patients with COPD).

Reasons for the increasing incidence of NTM cases include host factors (eg, aging populations, increased numbers of people who are immunosuppressed or who have respiratory conditions such as cystic fibrosis or COPD) and improved culturing techniques, but changes in environmental prevalence or pathogen virulence may play a role as well.[61,62] With respect to NTM cases specifically attributed to water sources, the recent CDC infectious waterborne disease burden study estimates annual NTM cases in the US to be 68,900.[7]

Nontuberculous Mycobacteria and Health Care Premise Plumbing

Epidemiology of health care–associated nontuberculous mycobacteria

Determining the rate of NTM infections resulting from health care water exposures is complicated by the underdiagnosis of cases, the long incubation period, the challenge with source attribution, and the lack of a reporting requirement to public health authorities. Instead, understanding the impact of water-related HCA NTM depends on case and outbreak reports. Li and colleagues[63] reviewed 21 reports of water-related NTM infections from health care facility water systems. Results were highly variable with respect to NTM species, exposure sources (showers, sinks), patient susceptibility to infection from water colonized with mycobacteria (central venous catheters, postsurgical wounds), attack rate (2% to 60%), and water management deficiencies (eg, use of nonsterile water during procedures, colonization of water reservoirs). Recently, a retrospective investigation over 5 years at 3 VA medical centers in the same geographic region identified 41 patients colonized or infected (17%) with *Mycobacterium conceptionense*.[64] Most of the clinical isolates from these patients (93%) matched an environmental isolate from the ice machine in one of the hospitals. Although some of the patients diagnosed at other hospitals had visited the facility with the positive ice machine, not all patients did, and a definitive source of exposure could not be identified. This report is one of a growing body of evidence of ice machines as an exposure source for NTM in health care.[51]

Clinical and infection prevention considerations

Diagnosis of pulmonary NTM disease requires clinical, radiographic, and microbiological diagnostic criteria to be met as well as exclusion of other diagnoses, such as tuberculosis.[62,65–67] Because pulmonary infection can be present for months before diagnosis, attributing a prior health care visit as the exposure source is often not possible without clinical and environmental isolates to compare. Pseudo-outbreaks have also been documented,[63] in which NTM is isolated from patients' clinical specimens in the absence of disease. Environmentally, these pseudo-outbreaks can indicate a reservoir for NTM growth and/or a mechanism for exposure in the water distribution system and provide an opportunity to mitigate the situation before symptomatic cases occur.

Health care facility water is not typically routinely tested for NTM, and water management programs, if present, are often targeted to and validated by inhibition of *Legionella* growth. The general assumption is that practices to control *Legionella* growth in building water systems also reduce NTM prevalence. However, as described earlier, NTM can be more resistant to control measures than *Legionella*, and OPPPs differ in physiology and ecology.[20] NTM cases have been identified in health care facilities with rigorous water management plans targeting *Legionella*.[64] In practice, NTM infection prevention practices are often implemented in response to an identified issue. Because of this, diagnostic testing for NTM and epidemiologic surveillance for and awareness of NTM-positive cultures in patients with potential health care–associated disease are especially important to alert the facility water team of a possible issue needing corrective actions.

Case study: 2-phase outbreak of health care–associated nontuberculous mycobacteria
Baker and colleagues[68] described a 2-phase outbreak of *Mycobacterium abscessus*
complex over almost a 3-year period at a large hospital.

- After recognizing an increase in patients with *M abscessus*–positive cultures, the
  facility retrospectively identified hospitalized patients with an *M abscessus*
  isolate (excluding cultures obtained within 2 days of admission) for a period of
  about 18 months prior.
  - In the first 7 months of the review (preoutbreak baseline period) the incidence
    of *M abscessus* was 0.7 per 100,000 person-days (1.4 cases/mo).
  - In the next 10 months (phase 1 of the outbreak), the incidence increased to 3.0
    cases per 100,000 person-days (7.1 cases/mo). Fifty-five percent of these pa-
    tients were lung transplant recipients and the remaining patients were cardiac
    surgery patients or other types of patients.
  - The increased incidence of NTM cases coincided with the opening of a new
    hospital addition. Although the new addition, the existing hospital, and the
    community surrounding the hospital all had NTM detected in biofilms of water
    sources in the environmental investigation at 79%, 56%, and 42% positivity,
    respectively, only the new addition had detection of *M abscessus*.
  - A sterile water protocol was implemented[69] for heart and lung transplant recip-
    ients, ICU patients, and patients with disrupted gastrointestinal tracts to avoid
    contact with tap water; the incidence of NTM reduced to preoutbreak levels.
- A couple of months later, 2 cardiac surgery patients had cultures positive for *M
  abscessus*. The ensuing investigation found 13 cases in the following 7 months in
  cardiac surgery patients (phase 2 of the outbreak). All but 1 had extrapulmonary
  invasive disease.
  - A review of the entire investigation period (preoutbreak, phase 1, and phase 2)
    found 22 cardiac surgery cases with extrapulmonary NTM infection, the first
    case occurring in mid–phase 1.
  - All 22 patients had their surgeries in the new hospital addition and 21 out of 22
    cases had required cardiopulmonary bypass (for the other patient, the cardio-
    pulmonary bypass machine was on standby during the surgery). A review of
    maintenance and cleaning practices for heater-cooler units showed that unfil-
    tered tap water was being used in the devices instead of filtered tap water per
    manufacturer's recommendation. Environmental sampling found *M abscessus*
    in the biofilm of the tap used to fill the devices.

Lessons from this outbreak:

- New buildings and additions can be sources for transmission of OPPPs, despite
  assumptions that older buildings are more of a concern. In this situation, it was
  suspected that design elements in the new addition to conserve energy and
  reduce water usage unintentionally facilitated pathogen growth and persistence
  by reducing water flow rates, which resulted in lower residual disinfectant level,
  reduced hot water circulation, and less frequent replenishing of water in the system with chloraminated water from the municipal supply.
- Mitigation of NTM outbreaks can take several months of investigation and implementation of multiple interventions. Evidence of a mycobacteria-colonized water
  system that leads to clinical disease in one setting could manifest as disease
  cases in other settings in the hospital depending on how water is used and the
  host susceptibility.

- Devices that use water can be prone to biofilm formation and transmission of OPPPs to patients. With NTMs, regular cleaning schedules or procedures may not be sufficient to reduce risk. Some have recommended that ice machines not be used in high-risk areas and instead sterile ice should be supplied to patients.[70] With devices such as heater-coolers, ensuring use of filtered water, implementation of proper cleaning and disinfection protocols, and directing exhaust away from the sterile field can reduce risk. In this outbreak, new heater-cooler units were purchased so that the updated protocols were implemented on devices without biofilm from previous use.
- In facilities with a recognized NTM issue, and especially if immunosuppressed patients are treated, sterile water protocols and/or use of point-of-use filters may be needed to avoid exposure to tap water, at least until engineering solutions can be implemented to address NTM growth. After this outbreak, the facility flushed the water system and took measures to increase the water flow rate to improve residual disinfection and hot water delivery to outlets.

SUMMARY

With the growing recognition of the increasing burden of OPPP disease from building water systems, health care facilities must include prevention practices to reduce the incidence of HCA infections caused by these pathogens in their facility protocols. Guidance for water management programs that bring together clinical, engineering, and environmental factors for OPPP control is becoming more widely available, as are reports on implementing these programs to optimize success. With a well-engaged, multidisciplinary water management team, health care facilities can prioritize and sustain OPPP prevention and increase safety for their building occupants.

CLINICS CARE POINTS

- Consider OPPPs in the differential for health care–associated pneumonia, or other illnesses where water is suspected to be a source, and perform diagnostic testing as appropriate.
- Conduct epidemiologic investigations when health care water is suspected of being the source of exposure for a health care–associated infection.
- Implement a water management program that includes a risk assessment and a record of past health care–associated infections caused by OPPPs.

DISCLOSURE

All authors have no commercial or financial interests to disclose. All authors are employees of the US federal government. The views expressed in this work are those of the authors and do not necessarily reflect an official position of the VA.

REFERENCES

1. Pruden A, Edwards MA, Falkinham JO. State of the science and research needs for opportunistic pathogens in premise plumbing. Denver, Colorado: Water Research Foundation; 2013. Available at: https://www.waterrf.org/resource/state-science-and-research-needs-opportunistic-pathogens-premise-plumbing. Accessed January 12, 2021.

2. Falkinham JO, Pruden A, Edwards M. Opportunistic premise plumbing pathogens: increasingly important pathogens in drinking water. Pathogens 2015;4(2): 373–86.

3. Williams MM, Armbruster CR, Arduino MJ. Plumbing of hospital premises is a reservoir for opportunistically pathogenic microorganisms: a review. Biofouling 2013;29(2):147–62.

4. Falkinham JO. Living with Legionella and other water pathogens. Microorganisms 2020;8(12):2026.

5. Gamage SD, Ambrose M, Kralovic SM, et al. Water safety and Legionella in health care: priorities, policy, and practice. Infect Dis Clin North Am 2016; 30(3):689–712.

6. Centers for Disease Control and Prevention (CDC). Reduce risk from water. Available at: https://www.cdc.gov/hai/prevent/environment/water.html. Accessed January 13, 2021.

7. Collier SA, Deng L, Adam EA, et al. Estimate of burden and direct healthcare cost of infectious waterborne disease in the United States. Emerg Infect Dis 2021; 27(1):140–9.

8. World Health Organization. Water safety in buildings. 2011. Available at: http:// apps.who.int/iris/bitstream/10665/76145/1/9789241548106_eng.pdf. Accessed January 12, 2021.

9. Environmental Protection Agency. Technologies for Legionella control in premise plumbing systems: scientific literature review. 2016. Available at: https://www. epa.gov/sites/production/files/2016-09/documents/Legionella_document_master_ september_2016_final.pdf. Accessed January 12, 2021.

10. ASHRAE. Guideline 12-2020. Managing the risk of legionellosis associated with building water systems. Atlanta, Georgia, USA. 2020. Available at: https:// www.techstreet.com/ashrae/standards/guideline-12-2020-managing-the-risk-of-legionellosis-associated-with-building-water-systems?product_id=2111422. Accessed May 27, 2021.

11. National Academies of Sciences, Engineering, and Medicine. Management of Legionella in water systems. Washington, DC: The National Academies Press; 2020.

12. Garrison LE, Kunz JM, Cooley LA, et al. Vital signs: deficiencies in environmental control identified in outbreaks of Legionnaires' disease - North America, 2000-2014. MMWR Morb Mortal Wkly Rep 2016;65(22):576–84.

13. Ambrose M, Kralovic SM, Roselle GA, et al. Implementation of Legionella prevention policy in health care facilities: the United States Veterans Health Administration experience. J Public Health Manag Pract 2020;26(2):E1–11.

14. Clopper BR, Kunz JM, Salandy SW, et al. A methodology for classifying root causes of outbreaks of Legionnaires' disease: deficiencies in environmental control and water management. Microorganisms 2021;9(1):E89.

15. Parr A, Whitney EA, Berkelman RL. Legionellosis on the rise: a review of guidelines for prevention in the United States. J Public Health Manag Pract 2015; 21(5):E17–26.

16. New York State. New York Codes, Rules and Regulations. Part 4 – Protection Against Legionella. Available at: https://regs.health.ny.gov/content/part-4-protection-against-legionella. Accessed May 27, 2021.

17. Gamage SD, Kralovic SM, Roselle GA. The case for routine environmental testing for Legionella bacteria in healthcare facility water distribution systems-reconciling CDC position and guidance regarding risk. Clin Infect Dis 2015;61(9):1487–8.

18. Pierre D, Baron JL, Ma X, et al. Water quality as a predictor of Legionella positivity of building water systems. Pathogens 2019;8(4):295.

19. Duda S, Baron JL, Wagener MM, et al. Lack of correlation between *Legionella* colonization and microbial population quantification using heterotrophic plate count and adenosine triphosphate bioluminescence measurement. Environ Monit Assess 2015;187(7):393.

20. Wang H, Bédard E, Prévost M, et al. Methodological approaches for monitoring opportunistic pathogens in premise plumbing: a review. Water Res 2017;117: 68–86.

21. Kanamori H, Weber DJ, Rutala WA. Healthcare outbreaks associated with a water reservoir and infection prevention strategies. Clin Infect Dis 2016;62(11): 1423–35.

22. Perkins KM, Reddy SC, Fagan R, et al. Investigation of healthcare infection risks from water-related organisms: summary of CDC consultations, 2014-2017. Infect Control Hosp Epidemiol 2019;40(6):621–6.

23. Scanlon MM, Gordon JL, McCoy WF, et al. Water management for construction: evidence for risk characterization in community and healthcare settings: a systematic review. Int J Environ Res Public Health 2020;17(6):2168.

24. Centers for Medicare and Medicaid Services. Requirement to reduce *Legionella* risk in healthcare facility water systems to prevent cases and outbreaks of Legionnaires' disease (LD). June 2, 2017. Available at: https://www.cms.gov/Medicare/Provider-Enrollment-and-Certification/SurveyCertificationGenInfo/Downloads/QSO17-30-HospitalCAH-NH-REVISED-.pdf. Accessed December 15, 2020.

25. ASHRAE. ANSI/ASHRAE Standard 188-2018 Legionellosis: risk management for building water systems. Atlanta, Georgia, USA. 2018. Available at: https://www.techstreet.com/ashrae/standards/ashrae-188-2018?gateway_code=ashrae&product_id=2020895. Accessed May 27, 2021.

26. CDC. Toolkit - Developing a Water Management Program to Reduce *Legionella* Growth and Spread in Buildings. 2017. Available at: https://www.cdc.gov/*Legionella*/wmp/toolkit/index.html. Accessed January 12, 2021.

27. CDC. Nationally notifiable infectious diseases and conditions, United States: annual tables. 2018. Available at: https://wonder.cdc.gov/nndss/static/2018/annual/2018-table2h.html. Accessed January 7, 2021.

28. CDC. Legionnaires' disease surveillance summary report, 2016-2017. Available at: https://www.cdc.gov/*Legionella*/health-depts/surv-reporting/2016-17-surv-report-508.pdf. Accessed December 15, 2020.

29. Gamage SD, Ambrose M, Kralovic SM, et al. Legionnaires disease surveillance in US Department of Veterans Affairs medical facilities and assessment of health care facility association. JAMA Netw Open 2018;1(2):e180230.

30. Gamage SD, Ross N, Kralovic SM, et al. Health after Legionnaires' disease: a description of hospitalizations up to 5 years after *Legionella* pneumonia. PLoS One 2021;16(1):e0245262.

31. Cassell K, Gacek P, Rabatsky-Ehr T, et al. Estimating the true burden of Legionnaires' disease. Am J Epidemiol 2019;188(9):1686–94.

32. Benedict KM, Reses H, Vigar M, et al. Surveillance for waterborne disease outbreaks associated with drinking water - United States, 2013-2014. MMWR Morb Mortal Wkly Rep 2017;66(44):1216–21.

33. Cunha BA, Burillo A, Bouza E. Legionnaires' disease. Lancet 2016;387:376–85.

34. Council of State and Territorial Epidemiologists (CSTE). Revision to the case definition for national legionellosis surveillance, 19-ID-04. Available at: https://cdn.ymaws.com/www.cste.org/resource/resmgr/2019ps/final/19-ID-04_Legionellosis_final.pdf. Accessed January 12, 2021.

35. CSTE. Public health reporting and national notification for legionellosis. Position statement no. 09-ID-45. June 2010. Available at: https://cdn.ymaws.com/www.cste.org/resource/resmgr/PS/09-ID-45.pdf. Accessed May 27, 2021.

36. Soda EA, Barskey AE, Shah PP, et al. Vital signs: health care-associated Legionnaires' disease surveillance data from 20 states and a large metropolitan area - United States, 2015. *MMWR* Morb Mortal Wkly Rep 2017;66(22):584–9.

37. Beauté J, Plachouras D, Sandin S, et al. Healthcare-associated Legionnaires' disease, Europe, 2008-2017. Emerg Infect Dis 2020;26(10):2309–18.

38. Hollenbeck B, Dupont I, Mermel LA. How often is a work-up for *Legionella* pursued in patients with pneumonia? a retrospective study. BMC Infect Dis 2011; 11:237.

39. Sopena N, Sabrià M, Neunos. 2000 Study Group. Multi-center study of hospital-acquired pneumonia in non-ICU settings. Chest 2005;127(1). 213-209.

40. Decker BK, Harris PL, Muder RR, et al. Improving the diagnosis of *Legionella* pneumonia within a healthcare system through a systematic consultation and testing program. Ann Am Thorac Soc 2016;13(8):1289–93.

41. Ambrose M, Roselle GA, Kralovic SM, et al. Healthcare-associated *Legionella* disease: a multi-year assessment of exposure settings in a national healthcare system in the United States. Microorganisms 2021;9(2):264.

42. Demirjian A, Lucas CE, Garrison LE, et al. The importance of clinical surveillance in detecting legionnaires' disease outbreaks: a large outbreak in a hospital with a *Legionella* disinfection system-Pennsylvania, 2011-2012. Clin Infect Dis 2015; 60(11):1596–602.

43. Springston JP, Yocavitch L. Existence and control of *Legionella* bacteria in building water systems: a review. J Occup Environ Hyg 2017;14(2):124–34.

44. Veterans Health Administration. Prevention of health care-associated *Legionella* disease and scald injury from water systems. Washington, DC: VHA Directive 1061. 2021. Available at: https://www.va.gov/vhapublications/ViewPublication. asp?pub_ID=9181. Accessed May 27, 2021.

45. Sehulster L, Chinn RYW. Guidelines for environmental infection control in healthcare facilities. Recommendations of CDC and the Healthcare Infection Control Practices Advisory Committee (HICPAC). MMWR Morb Mortal Wkly Rep 2003; 52(RR10):1–42.

46. Nagy DJ, Dziewulski DM, Codru N, et al. Understanding the distribution of positive *Legionella* samples in healthcare-premise water systems: using statistical analysis to determine a distribution for *Legionella* and to support sample size recommendations. Infect Control Hosp Epidemiol 2021;42(1):63–8.

47. Best M, Yu VL, Stout J, et al. *Legionellaceae* in the hospital water supply – epidemiological link with disease and evaluation of a method of control of nosocomial Legionnaires' disease and Pittsburgh pneumonia. Lancet 1983;2:207–310.

48. Stout JE, Muder RR, Mietzner S, et al. Role of environmental surveillance in determining the risk of hospital-acquired legionellosis: a national surveillance study with clinical correlations. Infect Control Hosp Epidemiol 2007;28(7):818–24.

49. Castellino LM, Gamage SD, Hoffman PV, et al. Healthcare-associated Legionnaires' disease: limitations of surveillance definitions and importance of epidemiologic investigation. J Infect Prev 2017;18(6):307–10 [published correction appears in J Infect Prev. 2017;18(6):NP2].

50. Johansen MD, Herrmann JL, Kremer L. Non-tuberculous mycobacteria and the rise of *Mycobacterium abscessus*. Nat Rev Microbiol 2020;18(7):392–407.

51. Millar BC, Moore JE. Hospital ice, ice machines, and water as sources of nontuberculous mycobacteria: description of qualitative risk assessment models to

determine host-nontuberculous mycobacteria interplay. Int J Mycobacteriol 2020; 9(4):347–62.

52. Adjemian J, Olivier KN, Seitz AE, et al. Prevalence of nontuberculous mycobacterial lung disease in U.S. Medicare beneficiaries. Am J Respir Crit Care Med 2012;185(8):881–6.

53. Donohue MJ, Mistry JH, Donohue JM, et al. Increased frequency of nontuberculous mycobacteria detection at potable water taps within the United States. Environ Sci Technol 2015;49(10):6127–33.

54. Covert TC, Rodgers MR, Reyes AL, et al. Occurrence of nontuberculous mycobacteria in environmental samples. Appl Environ Microbiol 1999;65(6):2492–6.

55. Loret JF, Dumoutier N. Non-tuberculous mycobacteria in drinking water systems: a review of prevalence data and control means. Int J Hyg Environ Health 2019; 222(4):628–34.

56. Norton GJ, Williams M, Falkinham JO 3rd, et al. Physical measures to reduce exposure to tap water-associated nontuberculous mycobacteria. Front Public Health 2020;8:190.

57. du Moulin GC, Sherman IH, Hoaglin DC, et al. *Mycobacterium avium* complex, an emerging pathogen in Massachusetts. J Clin Microbiol 1985;22(1):9–12.

58. Winthrop KL, Marras TK, Adjemian J, et al. Incidence and prevalence of nontuberculous mycobacterial lung disease in a large U.S. managed care health plan, 2008-2015. Ann Am Thorac Soc 2020;17(2):178–85.

59. Jones MM, Winthrop KL, Nelson SD, et al. Epidemiology of nontuberculous mycobacterial infections in the U.S. Veterans Health Administration. PLoS One 2018; 13(6):e0197976.

60. Pyarali FF, Schweitzer M, Bagley V, et al. Increasing non-tuberculous mycobacteria infections in veterans with COPD and association with increased risk of mortality. Front Med (Lausanne) 2018;5:311.

61. Stout JE, Koh W-J, Yew WW. Update on pulmonary disease due to nontuberculous mycobacteria. Int J Infect Dis 2016;45:123–34.

62. Baldwin SL, Larsen SE, Ordway D, et al. The complexities and challenges of preventing and treating nontuberculous mycobacterial diseases. PLoS Negl Trop Dis 2019;13(2):e0007083.

63. Li T, Abebe LS, Cronk R, et al. A systematic review of waterborne infections from nontuberculous mycobacteria in health care facility water systems. Int J Hyg Environ Health 2017;220(3):611–20.

64. Oda G, Winters MA, Pacheco SM, et al. Clusters of nontuberculous mycobacteria linked to water sources at three Veterans Affairs medical centers. Infect Control Hosp Epidemiol 2020;41(3):320–30.

65. Griffith DE, Aksamit T, Brown-Elliott BA, et al. An official ATS/IDSA statement: diagnosis, treatment, and prevention of nontuberculous mycobacterial diseases. Am J Respir Crit Care Med 2007;175(4):367–416.

66. Daley CL, Iaccarino JM, Lange C, et al. Treatment of nontuberculous mycobacterial pulmonary disease: an official ATS/ERS/ESCMID/IDSA clinical practice guideline. Clin Infect Dis 2020;71(4):905–13.

67. Daley CL, Winthrop KL. *Mycobacterium avium* Complex: addressing gaps in diagnosis and management. J Infect Dis 2020;222(Supplement_4):S199–211.

68. Baker AW, Lewis SS, Alexander BD, et al. Two-phase hospital-associated outbreak of *Mycobacterium abscessus*: investigation and mitigation. Clin Infect Dis 2017;64(7):902–11.

69. Baker AW, Stout JE, Anderson DJ, et al. Tap water avoidance decreases rates of hospital-onset pulmonary nontuberculous mycobacteria. Clin Infect Dis 2020;ciaa1237. https://doi.org/10.1093/cid/ciaa1237.

70. Crist MB, Perz JF. Modern healthcare versus nontuberculous mycobacteria: who will have the upper hand? Clin Infect Dis 2017;64(7):912–3.

71. Correia AM, Ferreira JS, Borges V, et al. Probable person-to-person transmission of Legionnaires' disease. N Engl J Med 2016;374(5):497–8.

72. Bryant JM, Grogono DM, Greaves D, et al. Whole-genome sequencing to identify transmission of *Mycobacterium abscessus* between patients with cystic fibrosis: a retrospective cohort study. Lancet 2013;381(9877):1551–60.

73. Yapicioglu H, Gokmen TG, Yildizdas D, et al. *Pseudomonas aeruginosa* infections due to electronic faucets in a neonatal intensive care unit. J Paediatr Child Health 2012;48(5):430–4.

74. Jaubert J, Mougari F, Picot S, et al. A case of postoperative breast infection by *Mycobacterium fortuitum* associated with the hospital water supply. Am J Infect Control 2015;43(4):406–8.

75. Bencini MA, Yzerman EPF, Koornstra RHT, et al. A case of Legionnaires' disease caused by aspiration of ice water. Arch Environ Occup Health 2005;60(6):302–6.

76. Cobben NA, Drent M, Jonkers M, et al. Outbreak of severe *Pseudomonas aeruginosa* respiratory infections due to contaminated nebulizers. J Hosp Infect 1996;33:63–70.

77. Kyritsi MA, Mouchtouri VA, Katsiafliaka A, et al. Clusters of healthcare-associated Legionnaires' disease in two hospitals of central Greece. Case Rep Infect Dis 2018;2018:2570758.

78. Sánchez-Carrillo C, Padilla B, Marin M, et al. Contaminated feeding bottles: the sources of an outbreak of *Pseudomonas aeruginosa* infections in a neonatal intensive care unit. Am J Infect Control 2009;37:150–4.

79. Lowry PW, Beck-Sague CM, Bland LA, et al. *Mycobacterium chelonae* infection among patients receiving high-flux dialysis in a hemodialysis clinic in California. J Infect Dis 1990;161(1):85–90.

80. World Health Organization. WHO good manufacturing practices: water for pharmaceutical use. WHO Technical Report Series, No. 970. 2012. Annex 2. Available at: https://www.who.int/medicines/areas/quality_safety/quality_assurance/GMPWatePharmaceuticalUseTRS970Annex2.pdf. Accessed January 12, 2021.

81. Nucci M, Akiti T, Barreiros G, et al. Nosocomial outbreak of *Exophiala jeanselmei* fungemia associated with contamination of hospital water. Clin Infect Dis 2002;34(11):1475–80.

82. Yablon BR, Dantes R, Tsai V, et al. Outbreak of *Pantoea agglomerans* bloodstream infections at an oncology clinic-Illinois, 2012-2013. Infect Control Hosp Epidemiol 2017;38(3):314–9.

83. Schlech WF, Simonsen N, Sumarah R, et al. Nosocomial outbreak of *Pseudomonas aeruginosa* folliculitis associated with a physiotherapy pool. CMAJ 1986;134(8):909–13.

84. Leoni E, Sacchetti R, Zanetti F, et al. Control of *Legionella pneumophila* contamination in a respiratory hydrotherapy system with sulfurous spa water. Infect Control Hosp Epidemiol 2006;27(7):716–21.

85. Ricci ML, Fontana S, Pinci F, et al. Pneumonia associated with a dental unit waterline. Lancet 2012;379:684.

86. CDC. Guidelines for infection control in dental health-care settings—2003. MMWR Morb Mortal Wkly Rep 2003;52(RR-17):1–61. Available at: http://www.cdc.gov/mmwr/preview/mmwrhtml/rr5217a1.htm. Accessed January 12, 2021.

87. Peralta G, Tobin-D'Angelo M, Parham A, et al. Notes from the field: *Mycobacterium abscessus* infections among patients of a pediatric dentistry practice–Georgia, 2015. MMWR Morb Mortal Wkly Rep 2016;65(13):355–6.

88. Sax H, Bloemberg G, Hasse B, et al. Prolonged outbreak of *Mycobacterium chimaera* infection after open-chest heart surgery. Clin Infect Dis 2015;61(1):67–75.

89. Quinn C, Demirjian A, Watkins LF, et al. Legionnaires' disease outbreak at a long-term care facility caused by a cooling tower using an automated disinfection system–Ohio, 2013. J Environ Health 2015;78(5):8–13.

Reimagining Construction and Renovation of Health Care Facilities During Emergence from a Pandemic

Russell N. Olmsted, MPH, CIC, FAPIC

KEYWORDS

- COVID-19 pandemic • Construction • Renovation • Health care facilities
- Risk assessment • Aspergillosis • Waterborne and airborne pathogen
- Health care design

KEY POINTS

- The coronavirus disease 2019 (COVID-19) pandemic response has had a tremendous impact on society and delivery of health care around the world. Learnings during response have rapidly increased the use of remote communication strategies such as telehealth and challenged long-standing concepts of airborne transmission.
- Outbreaks of disease are associated with construction and renovation when planning and risk mitigation is ignored or not effective.
- The infection control risk assessment (ICRA) and mitigation recommendations are essential components of infection prevention and patient safety programs.
- Infection preventionists/health care epidemiologists need to be aware and have access to guidelines for design and construction of health care facilities as well as new investigations of interventions to prevent transmission from the environment of care.
- Policies and procedures that address ICRA and the newly adapted water ICRA, safe work practices, training, monitoring, contingencies, and authority should be optimized.

INTRODUCTION

As this article was being published it coincided with the approximate 1-year anniversary of declaration of the coronavirus disease 2019 (COVID-19) pandemic emergency in the United States.[1] Its cause, severe acute respiratory syndrome coronavirus-2 (SARS-CoV-2), has and continues to have dramatic and long-lasting impact on the lives of all people around the world.[2] According to Dr Keith Wailoo, Henry Putnam University Professor of History and Public Affairs at Princeton,

Integrated Clinical Services (ICS), Trinity Health, Mailstop W3B, 20555 Victor Parkway, Livonia, MI 48152, USA
E-mail address: olmstedr@trinity-health.org

Infect Dis Clin N Am 35 (2021) 697–716
https://doi.org/10.1016/j.idc.2021.06.001
0891-5520/21/© 2021 Elsevier Inc. All rights reserved.

This pandemic is right up there as a world-changing event. It has already had a profound impact on society, on basic questions like the nature of our social interactions. It's already shaped and reshaped this particular generation, and the ripple effects are likely to play out for years, perhaps even decades to come.[3]

Beyond humans, the pandemic also has had a dramatic impact on construction and renovation of health care facilities and likely will lead to increased use of engineering controls, designs, and planning to mitigate risk of exposures between those with possible infection and susceptibles and use of telehealth. This article includes examples of the impact of the COVID-19 pandemic on design and construction of health care facilities and reinforces core strategies that have been shown to be effective in protecting patients, health care personnel, visitors, and others when in these facilities.

The built environment encompasses a broad range of physical design elements, including spaces for care of patients; support services; electronics; patient care and major technical equipment; building systems that provide air, water, and surfaces; and finishes. This spectrum of spaces and surfaces collectively is referred as the environment of care (EOC). In general, these are less frequently a source of microorganisms causing health care–associated infection (HAI) compared with other sources, such as the patient's endogenous microflora, especially when an invasive device is present, or a from surgical procedure.[4] Carriage of microbes on hands of health care personnel also is a more likely mechanism of exposure to potential pathogens. Even so, the proportional contribution of the EOC as a reservoir of pathogens is estimated at 20%.[5] Over the past several years there have been several studies that find the EOC is a significant source of multidrug-resistant organisms (MDROs), *Clostridioides difficile*, and norovirus.[6] In addition, investigation of the role of EOC has found admission to a patient room previously occupied by a patient with an MDRO or *C difficile* is a risk factor for their acquisition by the next occupant.[7,8]

Fig. 1 shows the connection between occupants and the EOC. This complex ecosystem influences risk of transmission of infection between occupants, and the EOC serves as a constant reservoir of microorganisms.[9]

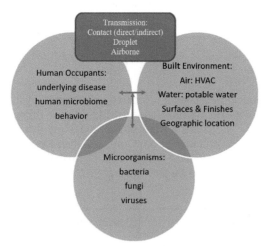

Fig. 1. Interrelationship between occupants, environment, and microorganisms. HVAC, heating, ventilation, and air conditioning. (*Adapted from* National Academies of Sciences. Microbiomes of the Built Environment: A Research Agenda for Indoor Microbiology, Human Health, and Buildings. The National Academies Press; 2017:20.)

Specific pathogens can suggest an environmental source; for example, from demolition of drywall or gaps in maintenance of key mechanical systems, which include *Aspergillus* spp, *Fusarium* spp, *Rhizopus* spp, *Bacillus cereus*, *Legionella* spp, a wide range of gram-negative bacteria, and nontuberculous mycobacteria.[4] When HAIs are caused by opportunistic pathogens it is important to apply key principles such as chain of transmission and the following criteria to determine whether reservoirs are present in the environment and help guide implementation of mitigation strategies, if applicable.

CRITERIA FOR EVALUATING THE STRENGTH OF EVIDENCE FOR ENVIRONMENTAL SOURCES OF INFECTION

1. The organism can survive after inoculation onto the fomite.[4]
2. The organism can be cultured from in-use fomites.
3. The organism can proliferate in or on the fomite.
4. Some measure of acquisition of infection cannot be explained by other recognized modes of transmission.
5. Retrospective case-control studies show an association between exposure to the fomite and infection.
6. Prospective case-control studies may be possible when more than 1 similar type of fomite is in use.
7. Prospective studies allocating exposure to the fomite to a subset of patients show an association between exposure and infection.
8. Decontamination of the fomite results in the elimination of infection transmission.

Coincident with this 1-year anniversary of the pandemic, the American Society for Healthcare Engineering (ASHE) 2020 Survey of Hospital Construction found increased use of building information modeling and cloud-based collaboration to improve efficiency, control costs, and provide a more nimble design process.[10] Other significant findings included prefabrication of elements of the built environment and using artificial intelligence to assist with design and construction.

From this ASHE survey, funding for new construction decreased slightly from 25% to 19%, investment in infrastructure increased from 18% to 20%, and renovation held steady at about 28%. Most projects involve renovations and expansions (74%) compared with new construction (31%), a trend likely to continue in 2020.[10] Investment in ambulatory care also remained very strong as a reflection of new payment models from agencies such as the Centers for Medicare and Medicaid Services (CMS) and to enhance convenience and access to care. This trend is reflected in the survey that finds more than 26% of hospitals are building or planning to build medical office buildings over the next 3 years, and roughly 22% have ambulatory facilities in the pipeline. Further, the pandemic has logarithmically increased use of telehealth, an essential administrative control measure to remotely triage patients with possible infection and direct them to a secure care location that mitigates risks.[11] CMS's support of response to the pandemic has also prompted the agency to encourage more efficient and safer care using strategies such as so-called hospital at home, when appropriate, and staffing flexibility to allow ambulatory surgical centers to provide greater inpatient care when needed.[12] The goal of the return of patients to continue their recovery at home relieves demand for inpatient beds and likely lessens risks of exposure to pathogens associated with prolonged hospitalization.

The 2020 ASHE survey also found important adherence to infection prevention and control; notably, 62% of projects underway required contractors to complete infection control risk assessments (ICRAs). Twenty-six percent of projects also require contractors to have Certified Healthcare Constructor credentials, whereas 6% require ASHE's newest certification program, Certified Health Care Physical Environment Worker.[10]

A core strategy to incorporate infection prevention and control into construction and renovation from planning and design through occupancy is through use of an ICRA.[13] It includes tactical decisions to ensure sufficient handwashing stations; alignment of functional planning of involved spaces with heating, ventilation, and air conditioning (HVAC) requirements (eg, number and location of airborne-infection isolation rooms [AIIRs]); and use of physical barriers to contain and confine dust, soil, and contaminants. ICRA has been incorporated into design standards issued by the American Society of Heating, Refrigerating and Air Conditioning Engineers (ASHRAE), and guidelines issued by the Centers for Disease Control and Prevention (CDC) Healthcare Infection Control Practices Advisory Committee (HICPAC) and Facility Guidelines Institute.[4,14,15]

A YEAR IN REVIEW: COVID-19 PANDEMIC AND IMPLICATIONS FOR THE FUTURE OF DESIGN AND CONSTRUCTION

The American Hospital Association published a retrospective on the impact of the pandemic on hospitals.[16] The highlights listed here capture some of the unprecedented impact on health care delivery in the United States:

- Nearly 30 million cases of the virus were identified, with approximately 1.5 million people hospitalized, and more than 530,000 deaths, which have driven a 15% increase in the death rate, making 2020 the deadliest year in US history.
- In 2020, hospitals were projected to lose an estimated $323 billion, leaving nearly half of America's hospitals and health systems with negative operating margins by the end of 2020.
- Emergency department visits also have experienced a nearly 25% decline from the same time last year, because many Americans remain skeptical of going to the hospital for critical care, such as heart attacks and strokes.

The pandemic triggered activation of emergency operations, most often using the Hospital Incident Command System. SARS-CoV-2 is not the only newly emergent pathogen, nor will it be the last. Rebmann[17] has provided a helpful review of this topic and the essential infrastructure to respond to pandemics and newly emergent pathogens. CDC's National Institute of Occupational Safety and Health (NIOSH) offers an effective framework for prevention and control of hazards, including emergent diseases, that can inform the design and construction of the EOC. This framework, referred to as a hierarchy of controls, is shown in **Fig. 2**. The concept is to give priority to control methods that are potentially more effective and protective than sole reliance on personal protective equipment (PPE).[18]

Reappraisal of Airborne Transmission from the COVID-19 Pandemic

The emergence of SARS-CoV-2 and its modes of transmission has prompted a reappraisal of transmissibility of pathogens through the air.[19,20] In particular the preexisting categorization of transmissibility based solely on the size of the pathogen is imprecise and misleading. Further, the epidemiology of this virus has been particularly difficult to control given that between 30% and 40% of those with infection may be presymptomatic or asymptomatic.[21]

SARS-CoV-2 is thought to spread mainly through close contact from person to person, including between people who are physically near each other (within about 2 m [6 feet]) by respiratory droplets containing the virus that are released by persons with

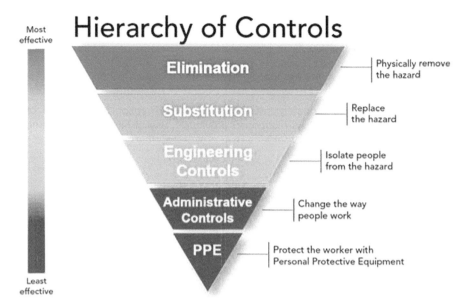

Fig. 2. Hierarchy of controls for safer systems of care. PPE, personal protective equipment. (*From* Center for Disease Control and Prevention (CDC). NIOSH. Hierarchy of controls. Available at: https://www.cdc.gov/niosh/topics/hierarchy/. Accessed 1/15/2021.)

infection when they talk, breathe, sing, cough, or sneeze. There is evidence that, under certain conditions, people with COVID-19 seem to have infected others who were more than 2 m away. These instances often occurred within enclosed spaces that had inadequate ventilation. Contaminated respiratory droplets can also land on surfaces and objects. It is possible that people could get COVID-19 by touching a surface or object that has the virus on it and then touching their own mouth, nose, or eyes. Transmission from touching surfaces is not thought to be a common way that COVID-19 spreads, but it is possible. Scientists from a broad range of disciplines have therefore recommended the following to prevent transmission of this virus, and these also are applicable to other emerging respiratory infections yet to be identified[19]:

- Provide enough and effective ventilation (supply clean outdoor air, minimize recirculating air), particularly in public buildings, workplace environments, schools, hospitals, and aged-care homes.
- Supplement general ventilation with airborne infection controls such as local exhaust, high-efficiency air filtration, and germicidal ultraviolet lights.
- Avoid overcrowding, particularly in public transport and public buildings.

The experience with this pandemic has also prompted some to recommend expansion of standard precautions to include universal pandemic precautions, which will have implications for design and operation of the built environment.[22] For the EOC, for example, it is likely there will be increased consideration to design patient care spaces with capability to activate negative pressure mode in response to presentation of patients with symptoms of undiagnosed respiratory infection. Other strategies under universal pandemic precautions described by Weber and others include source control (masks for all), addition of eye protection for health care personnel during direct care of all patients, increased level of respiratory protection for aerosol-generating procedures, and screening of all for symptoms of acute respiratory protection before entering facilities.[22]

Implications of Severe Acute Respiratory Syndrome Coronavirus-2 on the Environment of Care

CDC has published and frequently updated its infection prevention and control recommendations for this virus.[23] As mentioned previously, use of telehealth and remote triage are effective strategies to minimize exposure to others (under the hierarchy, this would be an example of eliminating the hazard). Examples of administrative controls include screening everyone (patients, health care personnel, and visitors) entering the facility for symptoms of COVID-19 or exposure to others with suspected or confirmed SARS-CoV-2 infection, physical distancing, and source control (wearing masks). All of these have and will influence how the built environment is designed and operated. Highlighted next are engineering controls to contain and remove this virus from the air and that are likely to be effective against other respiratory pathogens.

Engineering Controls for Severe Acute Respiratory Syndrome Coronavirus-2

ASHRAE has published several resources, positions, standards, and guidance that involve use of engineering controls and mechanically engineered systems to help prevent and control transmission of this virus. The following points summarize select recommendations from ASHRAE's Epidemic Taskforce[24]:

- Ventilation, filtration, and air cleaning
  - Provide and maintain at least the required minimum outdoor airflow rates (eg, 2 air changes per hour [ACH] of outdoor air) for ventilation specified in applicable codes and standards.
  - Use combinations of filters and air cleaners to achieve minimum efficiency reporting value (MERV) 13 or better for recirculated air.
  - Use only air cleaners for which evidence of effectiveness and safety is clear.
- Air distribution
  - Where directional airflow is not specifically required, or not recommended as the result of a risk assessment, promote mixing of space air without causing strong air currents that increase direct transmission from person to person.
- HVAC system operation
  - Maintain temperature and humidity design set points.
  - Maintain equivalent clean air supply required for design occupancy whenever anyone is present in the space served by the system.
  - When necessary to flush spaces (eg, time to clear contaminants from spaces such as an inpatient room or AIIR after administering an aerosol-generating procedure [AGP]) between occupied periods, operate systems for a time required to achieve 3 air changes of equivalent clean air supply.
  - Limit reentry of contaminated air that may reenter the building from energy recovery devices, outside air intakes, and other sources to acceptable levels.

Soon after the onset of the pandemic, ASHRAE also updated its Position Document on Infectious Aerosols,[25] which calls for the following when designing and operating facilities under a range of occupancy types, including health care:

- Mitigation of infectious aerosol dissemination should be a consideration in the design of all facilities, and, in those identified as high-risk facilities, the appropriate mitigation design should be incorporated.

- The design and construction team, including HVAC designers, should engage in an integrated design process in order to incorporate the appropriate infection control bundle in the early stages of design.
- Based on risk assessments, buildings and transportation vehicles should consider designs that promote cleaner airflow patterns for providing effective flow paths for airborne particulates to exit spaces to less clean zones and use appropriate air-cleaning systems.
- Where a significant risk of transmission of aerosols has been identified by ICRAs, design of AIIRs should include anterooms.
- Based on risk assessments, the use of specific HVAC strategies supported by the evidence-based literature should be considered, including the following:
  ○ Enhanced filtration (higher-MERV filters, better than code minimums, in occupant-dense and/or higher-risk spaces) (evidence level A)
  ○ Upper-room ultraviolet germicidal irradiation (UVGI) (with possible in-room fans) as a supplement to supply airflow
  ○ Local exhaust ventilation for source control
  ○ Personalized ventilation systems for certain high-risk tasks
  ○ Portable, free-standing high-efficiency particulate air (HEPA) filters
  ○ Temperature and humidity control
- Health care buildings should consider design and operation to do the following:
  ○ Capture expiratory aerosols with headwall exhaust, tent or snorkel with exhaust, floor-to-ceiling partitions with door supply and patient exhaust, local air HEPA-grade filtration
  ○ Exhaust toilets and bed pans (essential)
  ○ Maintain temperature and humidity as applicable to the infectious aerosol of concern
  ○ Deliver clean air to caregivers
  ○ Maintain negatively pressurized intensive care units where infectious aerosols may be present
  ○ Maintain rooms with infectious aerosol concerns at negative pressure
  ○ Provide 100% exhaust of patient rooms
  ○ Use UVGI
  ○ Increase the outdoor air change rate (eg, increase patient rooms from 2 to 6 ACH)
  ○ Establish HVAC contributions to a patient room turnover plan before reoccupancy

Because of the potential for increased contamination of the surrounding air and surfaces during care of patients with COVID-19, CDC has recommended placing patients for whom AGPs are needed into AIIRs, if available. Commensurate with this recommendation and response to surges of patients with COVID-19, health care facilities implemented both temporary negative pressure rooms and spaces. This change has also led to more permanent changes to the HVAC system to provide wider availability of AIIRs as well as an ability to run other inpatient rooms in net negative pressure with respect to the adjacent public corridor.[26]

ASHE has recently published guidance on use of HVAC engineering controls to prevent transmission.[27] These controls encompass stations or zones to screen those with symptoms of possible COVID-19, containment in emergency departments, dedicated whole units to care for large cohorts of patients with infection, use of operating rooms during the pandemic, and options for both running temporary AIIRs and converting other rooms or spaces to negative pressure.

Figs. 3–5 are included in this ASHE resource to enhance containment and removal of infectious aerosols from the patient care area. **Fig. 4** is an outdoor view of a deployment of the configuration in **Fig. 3**, wherein a HEPA unit is deployed inside the room with directed exhaust directly outdoor.

Headwall Ventilation: an Engineering Controls Whose Time has Arrived

CDC's NIOSH has been working tirelessly to support nationwide response to this pandemic, especially related to respiratory protection of healthcare personnel (HCP) and engineering controls. Notably, NIOSH researchers have published guidance on design and just-in-time deployment of a headwall ventilation system that uses a special inlet system just behind the patient's head for supplemental exhaust at the source that is then removed and filtered with a HEPA fan/filter unit.[28] The ventilated headboard and HEPA system can provide surge isolation capacity in either traditional health care facilities or alternative care sites. The ventilated headboard's improved inlet adopts a local control technique that provides near-instant capture of patient-generated aerosol. The retractable canopy allows for hands-on health care

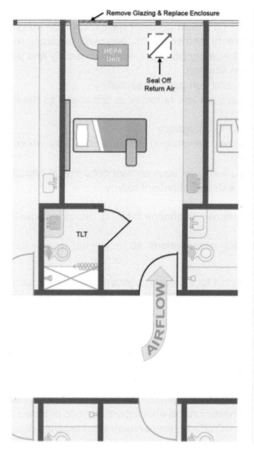

Fig. 3. Use of portable HEPA device to create negative pressure patient room TLT, toilet. (*From* ASHE. Current/Updated Health Care Facilities Ventilation Controls and Guidelines for Management of Patients with Suspected or Confirmed SARS-CoV-2 (COVID-19), 2021; with permission.)

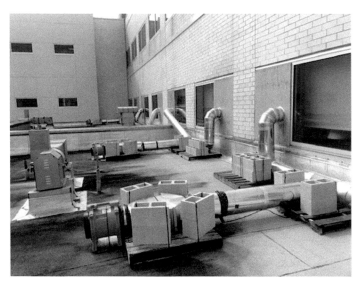

Fig. 4. Single-patient room negative air configuration through exterior windows.

procedures while still offering protection to attending health care personnel (**Fig. 6**). This system builds on prior investigations using a design called personal ventilation, which is containment and filtration as close to the source as possible.[29] Although the NIOSH guide is intended for just-in-time deployment, it may be used in the future

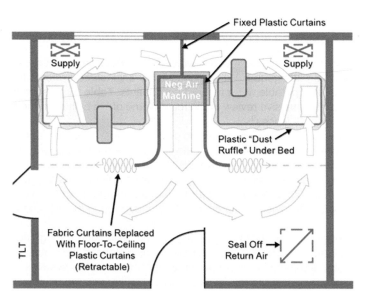

Fig. 5. Multibed zone-within-zone room. For this configuration, the negative air machine, which filters air in the room with HEPA filter, is recirculating filtered air in the same space. This system would be used when it is not feasible to discharge air to outdoors. (*From* ASHE. Current/Updated Health Care Facilities Ventilation Controls and Guidelines for Management of Patients with Suspected or Confirmed (SARS-CoV-2 (COVID-19).2021; with permission.)

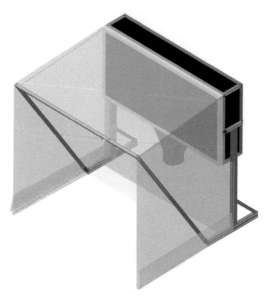

Fig. 6. Headwall ventilation. *(Courtesy of* Ken Mead, PhD, PE, Cincinnati, OH.)

as a more permanent engineering control that designers can use for new construction or renovation of patient care areas. Some aspects that will need to be investigated if this does occur are the location of the ventilated headwall in relation to standard headwall that provides medical gas, suction, monitors and so forth. Also, there will be a need to capture potential contaminants as the bed is lowered or raised for various clinical needs.

DISEASE TRANSMISSION RISKS FROM CONSTRUCTION AND RENOVATION

Both new construction and renovation involving the built environment can disrupt and release potential pathogens into the mechanically engineered systems that provide conditioned air and potable water to facility occupants. **Table 1** lists sources of these based on a comprehensive review of the microbiome of the built environment by National Academy of Sciences[9]:

Kanamori and colleagues[30] summarized outbreaks caused by fungi associated with construction and renovation published between 1974 and 2014. *Aspergillus* spp were the most common pathogens. The investigators described 28 definite outbreaks, with most involving invasive pulmonary aspergillosis, which also carries a high mortality of between 38% and 75%. Sixty percent of these outbreaks coincided with new construction projects, followed by renovation (30%), demolition (6.3%), and excavation (4.7%).

Water supplied to the health care facility is then distributed through an extensive network of plumbing to fixtures such as handwashing stations, ice machines, medical equipment (eg, automated endoscope reprocessors), and utility systems. This distribution network readily supports development of biofilm, and the microbial contaminants embedded in this matrix of extracellular polymeric substances mainly composed of exopolysaccharides, proteins, and nucleic acids protects microorganisms from disinfectants that are otherwise effective against planktonic forms. Stagnant water in this network, often from renovation of areas in the facility that results in redundant lengths of pipework that are left in place and capped, also enhances

Table 1
Sources and reservoirs of potential pathogens in the built environment

Air	Water
• Mechanical HVAC systems • Airborne particles that have been aerosolized via HVAC operation, from occupant activities, such as direct patient care or room cleaning, or removal of drywall that has prior damage from water intrusion • Outdoor air that enters through infiltration and natural or mechanical ventilation • Reservoirs in unfinished spaces, such as crawl spaces, basements, and attics, and concealed spaces that are linked to occupied spaces via a range of airflow pathways	• Municipal or well water supplies, harvested rainwater, recycled water, and drinking fountain water • Roof, foundation, and plumbing leaks • Condensation on or in walls and on cold water pipes • Mechanical equipment drain pans, coils, insulation, and filters • Cooling towers and natural or manufactured surface ponds • Hot water storage tanks, with subsequent aerosolization through plumbing fixtures • Aerosolized water from personal hygiene practices (eg, showering, bathing), splash from sink drain, and toilet flushing • Water features, including fountains, pools, hot tubs, whirlpool baths, and spas

Data from National Academies of Sciences. Microbiomes of the Built Environment: A Research Agenda for Indoor Microbiology, Human Health, and Buildings. 2017. The National Academies Pres; 2017.

development of biofilm. In addition, disruption of water utility systems during construction or renovation can disrupt biofilm and release contaminants into the water delivery network, posing a possible risk to patients, including those far away from the work area. This connection between occupants of health care facilities and water is shown in **Fig. 7**:

A recent, extensive review of waterborne disease outbreaks finds that the more susceptible patient populations, such as critically ill, neonates, transplant recipients, surgical patients, and those with hematological disease, are often the sentinel signal of a new cluster.[31] Of late, the types of devices and architectural features that were a source of infections is growing in complexity. That review calls out these outbreak investigations and emphasizes the need to be vigilant for their detection and mitigation:

> ...*Waterborne healthcare-associated outbreaks and infections continue to occur and were mostly associated with well-recognized water reservoirs as previously described. Moreover, recent studies document electronic faucets (Pseudomonas aeruginosa, Legionella spp, Mycobacterium mucogenicum), decorative water wall fountains (Legionella), and heater-cooler devices used for cardiac surgery (M. chimaera) as water reservoirs...*[13]

Of 620 consultations involving water as a reservoir of pathogens conducted by CDC investigators, 134 (21.6%) resulted in water-related HAIs or infection control lapses.[32] Nontuberculous mycobacteria were involved in the greatest number of investigations (n = 40, 29.9%). Most frequently, investigations involved medical products (n = 48, 35.8%), and most of these products were medical devices (n = 40, 83.3%). A variety of plausible water-exposure pathways were identified, including medication

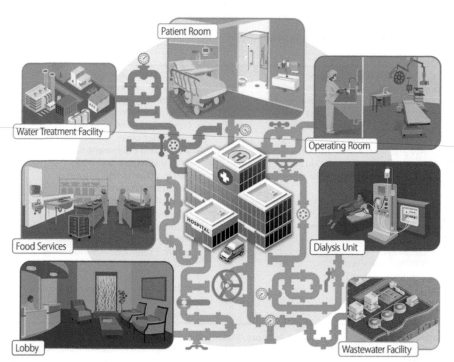

Fig. 7. Reservoirs and complex interconnectivity of waterborne pathogens. (*From* Center for Disease Control and Prevention (CDC). Reduce Risk from Water. 9/11/2019. Available at: https://www.cdc.gov/hai/prevent/environment/water.html. Accessed 3/20/2021.)

preparation near water splash zones and water contamination at the manufacturing sites of medications and medical devices.

Certain fixtures, such as handwashing stations, although essential for accomplishing hand hygiene, have also been associated with disease outbreaks. Parkes and Hota[33] reviewed reports of outbreaks of hospital sink-related infections, finding that this fixture can be a source of a diverse range of microorganisms that include *P aeruginosa* (most common), Enterobacterales (including those that are multidrug resistant), and nonfermenting gram negatives (eg, *Stenotrophomonas maltophilia, Acinetobacter baumanii, Elizabethkingia meningoseptica, Burkholderia* spp), as well as others such as *Fusarium* and *Mycobacterium mucogenicum*.[33] Design of sinks is an important aspect because some are more likely to disseminate water droplets contaminated with these organisms and there is increasing awareness that the biofilm is present in drains that capture wastewater and contaminate adjacent surfaces and hands of HCP during clinical care. The importance of the microbiome of the drain has been highlighted in a review by Carling[34] of 23 investigations of infection transmission associated with wastewater drains. Most involved multidrug-resistant gram-negative bacteria, and control strategies included attempts to disinfect the drain and its biofilm. Many of these were not successful and this led to replacement of the fixture.

A discussion of water and infection transmission would not be complete without highlighting the risk of water fixtures as a source of exposure to *Legionella* spp. According to the CDC, the number of cases of legionnaires disease in the United States is increasing, and associated mortality is substantial.[35] Gaps in maintenance that could be addressed with a water management program to prevent legionnaires disease outbreaks were described in 23 (85%) of 27 investigated outbreaks. Outbreaks resulted from a combination of deficiencies, most frequently classified as process failures and human errors. In most outbreaks, inadequate water disinfectant levels and temperatures in the optimal range for *Legionella* growth were observed; implementing a functional water management program consistent with CDC's *Legionella* toolkit and ASHRAE Standard 188 could address these deficiencies.[36,37]

PREVENTION BY DESIGN: STRATEGIES TO PROTECT OCCUPANTS AND MITIGATE DISEASE TRANSMISSION

Infection Control Risk Assessment and Infection Control Risk Assessment Mitigation Recommendations

ICRA is the core framework of design and construction and renovation of health care facilities. It is a key element of Facility Guidelines Institute (FGI) guidelines, which are adopted and enforced by authorities having jurisdiction in 42 states in the United States. An ICRA calls for design recommendations and infection control risk mitigation recommendations (ICRMRs) that are applied to the construction, renovation, and facility maintenance projects. Key aspects that ICRA needs to address include:

- Design elements that support infection prevention and control
- Proactive planning for mitigating sources of infection both within and external to the construction project that will be affected
- Identify potential risk for transmission of airborne and waterborne pathogens during construction, renovation, and commissioning
- Develop ICRMRs to mitigate identified risks

The details and steps of ICRA, including a risk assessment matrix and associated risk mitigation tactics, are available elsewhere.[38]

As highlighted earlier, there have been important learnings from published investigations of infection transmission involving the EOC in health care facilities. Some of these elements that benefit from specific focus are highlighted next.

Water Infection Control Risk Assessment

A water ICRA (WICRA) is a new adaptation of the traditional ICRA. The cumulative number of outbreaks of waterborne infection has identified the need for and benefit from careful attention and monitoring of water safety both for construction and renovation and as part of ongoing operation of health care facilities. The CDC describes WICRA as a process to assess water sources, modes of transmission, patient susceptibility, patient exposure, and program preparedness to prevent transmission of infection. A tool for conducting the WICRA is available from CDC.[39]

Scanlon and colleagues[40] recently analyzed the literature on risks associated with construction and waterborne infection. They describe that activity "associated with the most waterborne disease cases and deaths was inadequate commissioning of the building during beneficial occupancy (i.e., while preparing for the building opening to the public)." In addition, gaps in prevention strategies were identified, and they identified several risk factors that can be modified when construction or renovation is undertaken.

Specific Elements of Designing in Prevention

Handwashing station design features

- Basins should reduce risk of splashing and be made of porcelain, stainless steel, or other solid-surface material.[15]

- Basin size and depth of no less than 929.08 cm^2 (144 square inches) with 22.86-cm (9-inch) width or length is recommended.
- Sealed to prevent water intrusion into supporting cabinet, wall, and countertop.
- Install barriers (eg Plexiglas) to prevent splashes of contaminated water droplets to adjacent surfaces, especially if these are used for aseptic work such as medication preparation.
- Discharge of water from faucet spout is at least 25.4 cm (10 inches) above the bottom of the basin to prevent water stream from dropping directly into drain. In addition, the drain location should be offset so that it is not directly below the water outlet.
- Water pressure in station fixture is regulated.
- Allows controls for sink fixture to be wrist blade, single lever, or sensor activated.

Water feature: not allowed[15]

Decorative water features have been a popular element of design. These features are also referred to as decorative fountains and have an open reservoir through which water is recirculated on a continuous basis by a submerged pump. However, there have been several outbreaks of legionnaires disease associated with them. The FGI guidelines strongly recommend against inclusion of this element in any planning phase. In lieu of the difficulty in mitigating contaminants in water features, even with preventive cleaning and disinfection, facilities teams are advised to decommission this architectural feature.

Inpatient room design, surfaces, and finishes

There is a significant risk of acquisition of pathogens such as MDROs or *C difficile* related to infection or colonization in the room's prior occupant as after as long as 3 weeks.[8] However, this contamination can be removed with attention and focus on thorough cleaning and disinfection of surfaces in the room that are touched with high frequency when combined with real-time feedback.[41,42]

The evidence that MDROs can persist in the environment for prolonged time, as described earlier, in combination with observed efficiency of cross-transmission of these in multibed rooms, has led to a preference for single-patient rooms. This design also enhances safety related to a variety of other potential harms, supports patient privacy, and lessens disruption from ambient noise.[43] Newer models of room design have identified opportunities to lessen risk of transmission of *C difficile* and other MDROs. These designs include introduction of improved handwashing stations, and expanded HVAC infrastructure to increase the area of relative humidity control and increase the number of negative pressure rooms.[44,45]

Heating, ventilation, and air conditioning. HVAC is a building system that is designed to provide comfort, support aseptic procedures, remove contaminants from air, and deliver an acceptable indoor air quality. FGI 2018 guidelines include the ASHRAE 170 standard for design of HVAC for health care facilities.[14,15] This standard provides a wide range of parameters for HVAC systems that supply patient care, procedural (eg, surgery suite), and support areas. Parameters included in ASHRAE 170 include air changes per hour, design temperature and relative humidity ranges, and pressure relationships to adjacent areas.[14]

Universal or acuity-adaptable and single-occupancy patient care rooms. FGI commissioned a systematic review of available evidence on the value of single-patient rooms,[43] which found suggestive, albeit low-quality, evidence that this prevents infection and improves overall patient safety and experience of care. The addition of adaptability of these based on the patient's need also is worth considering. Additional elements for adult intensive care units have been described elsewhere and support this need for flexibility to accommodate changes in care practices and advances in technology.[46]

Airborne-infection isolation room. Planning for AIIR has increasingly taken center stage under the pandemic of COVID-19, and earlier in this article there are examples of new design features, including ventilated headwalls, that are likely to be incorporated into new construction and renovation.

Protective environment room. Protective environment (PE) rooms are designed to provide HEPA-filtered air to rooms used to care for patients who are severely immunocompromised (eg, solid organ transplant patients or allogeneic neutropenic patients). These rooms need to be designed to ensure that they are well sealed by maintaining ceilings that are smooth and free of fissures, open joints, and crevices; sealing walls above and below the ceiling; and, once occupied, to monitor for leakage. Additional details are available elsewhere.[4]

OPERATIONAL ASPECTS OF PRECONSTRUCTION AND INTRACONSTRUCTION PROJECTS
Environmental Containment at Point of Work

Figs. 8 and **9** provide examples of containment within the facility. Buchanan and colleagues[47] recently investigated the efficacy of this type of containment and found this containment significantly reduced the potential for aerosolization of pathogenic fungi, especially in above-ceiling spaces with high levels of fungi.

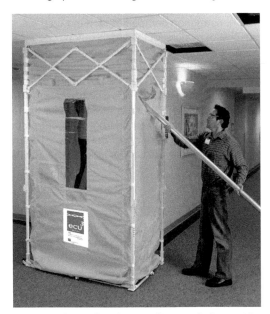

Fig. 8. Portable containment device for above-ceiling work. (*From* Olmsted RN. Prevention by Design: Construction and Renovation of Health Care Facilities for Patient Safety and Infection Prevention. Infect Dis Clin North Am. 2016 Sep;30(3):713-28; with permission.)

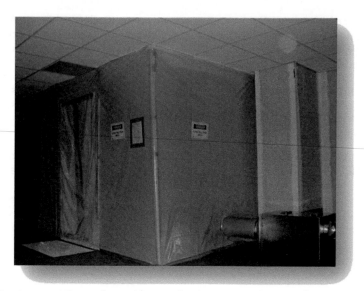

Fig. 9. Barrier separation and containment of active construction zone from occupied areas. (*From* Olmsted RN. Prevention by Design: Construction and Renovation of Health Care Facilities for Patient Safety and Infection Prevention. Infect Dis Clin North Am. 2016 Sep;30(3):713-28; with permission.)

TRAINING OF CONTRACTORS

Orientation and training of contractors and subcontractors that provide the talent to fulfill designs is an important and critical element of the ICRA process. Mousavi and colleagues[48] surveyed construction companies working on projects in health care facilities and found that 52% of owners (of the organizations contracting for the projects) always or often required the contractor's personnel to receive training. However, the recipients of these training modules most often were upper management personnel, not the employees providing the direct labor to install and build the work. Fifty-nine percent of respondents indicated that ICRA training was provided before the construction project and then every 6 (7%) or 12 (21%) months thereafter. Clearly these findings highlight the need for training to reach front-line contractors and subcontractors who are implementing ICRMRs throughout the project. There are several organizations that provide comprehensive training for contractors (see the resources listed later).

SUMMARY

The COVID-19 pandemic has left, and continues to leave, an indelible impact on delivery of care. Its prolonged trajectory will significantly influence design and construction of health care facilities. Some notable developments to date include dramatic increase in use of telehealth, innovative alternative models of care such as hospital at home, and emphasis on source control and physical distancing. Mechanical systems for delivery of conditioned air will increasingly be relied on to remove contaminants from patient care areas, and there are many projects in progress that are designed to increase use of negative pressure.

Infection prevention and control is an essential component of the built environment. When absent or there are disruptions, risk of exposure of patients and disease outbreaks often result. However, there are well-established, evidence-based guidelines to assist infection preventionists and health care epidemiologists with identifying strategies for prevention in collaboration with the multiple disciplines involved in construction and renovation.[4,15] The ICRA remains the keystone of designing in prevention at the inception of the concept of a project through the completion and commissioning phases. Future trends in care delivery in the United States. are going to have a significant impact on construction and renovation of health care facilities; however, involvement and subject matter expertise provided by infection preventionists/health care epidemiologists will remain a core component now and into the future.

CLINICS CARE POINTS

- The SARS-CoV-2 pandemic has affected, and will continue to affect, construction and design of health care facilities. As such, the role of infection preventionists and health care epidemiologists has grown in importance in planning for construction and renovation of the built environment in health care facilities to design the environment for an ability to ensure adequate ventilation and containment of emerging respiratory infections.

- Infection preventionists and health care epidemiologists are key stakeholders in planning for construction or renovation; notably, this engagement needs to be early and often because it is common to encounter unexpected work in progress that involves changes in the EOC.

- Establish effective awareness for routine operations work by facility maintenance, information technology, and contracted personnel; for example, work orders for repairs, running cables above dropped ceilings.

- Ask about ICRA training for contractors and subcontractors to ensure this training has not been limited to supervisory personnel.

- Expand risk assessment to include focus on the potable water system because this engineering also is an important reservoir of potential pathogens.

REFERENCES

1. Holshue M, DeBolt C, Lindquist S, et al. First Case of 2019 Novel Coronavirus in the United States. N Engl J Med 2020;382:929–36.
2. World Health Organization (WHO).Pneumonia of unknown cause – China. 1/5/2020. Available at: https://www.who.int/csr/don/05-january-2020-pneumonia-of-unkown-cause-china/en/. Accessed December 29, 2020.
3. Stein R. The Future Of The Pandemic In The U.S.: Experts Look Ahead. Health News from National Public Radio. March 24, 2021. Available at: Could The Worst Of The Pandemic Be Over In The United States? : Shots - Health News : NPR .Available at: https://www.npr.org/sections/health-shots/2021/03/24/976146368/the-future-of-the-pandemic-in-the-u-s-experts-look-ahead. Accessed March 25, 2021.
4. Centers for Disease Control & Prevention (CDC). Guidelines for environmental infection control in health-care facilities: recommendations of CDC and the Healthcare Infection Control Practices Advisory Committee (HICPAC). MMWR 2003;52(No. RR-10):1–48. Available at: https://www.cdc.gov/infectioncontrol/guidelines/environmental/index.html. Accessed February 1, 2021.
5. Weinstein RA. Epidemiology and control of nosocomial infections in adult intensive care units. Am J Med 1991;91(suppl 3B):179S–84S.

6. Weber DJ, Rutala WA. Understanding and Preventing Transmission of Healthcare-Associated Pathogens Due to the Contaminated Hospital Environment. Infect Control Hosp Epidemiol 2013;34:449–52.

7. Otter JA, Yezli S, Salkeld JA, et al. Evidence that contaminated surfaces contribute to the transmission of hospital pathogens and an overview of strategies to address contaminated surfaces in hospital settings. Am J Infect Control 2013;41(5 Suppl):S6–11.

8. Wu Y-L, Yang X-Y, Ding XX, et al. Exposure to infected/colonized roommates and prior room occupants increases the risks of healthcare-associated infections with the same organism. J Hosp Infect 2019;101(2):231–9.

9. National Academies of Sciences. Microbiomes of the built environment: a Research Agenda for indoor Microbiology, human health, and buildings. Washington, DC: The National Academies Press; 2017. https://doi.org/10.17226/23647.

10. Burmahl B, Morgan J. 2020 Hospital Construction Survey. Advanced planning, design and construction technology helps drive building project efficiency. Health Facilities Management, ASHE. 3/19/2020. Available at: https://www.hfmmagazine.com/articles/3859-hospital-construction-survey. Accessed February 22, 2021.

11. Centers for Disease Control and Prevention (CDC). The Role of Telehealth in Expanding Access to Healthcare During the COVID-19 Pandemic: Considerations for Vaccine Uptake and Monitoring for Adverse Events. 3/11/2021. Available at: https://emergency.cdc.gov/coca/calls/2021/callinfo_031121.asp. Accessed, March 15, 2021.

12. Centers for Medicare and Medicaid Services (CMS). CMS Announces Comprehensive Strategy to Enhance Hospital Capacity Amid COVID-19 Surge. 11/25/2020. Available at: https://www.cms.gov/newsroom/press-releases/cms-announces-comprehensive-strategy-enhance-hospital-capacity-amid-covid-19-surge. Accessed December 11, 2020.

13. Bartley JM. APIC State-of-the-Art Report: The role of infection control during construction in health care facilities. Am J Infect Control 2000;28:156–69.

14. American Society of Heating. Refrigerating and air-conditioning Engineers (ASHRAE), ventilation of health care facilities. ANSI/ASHRAE/ASHE standard 170-2021. Atlanta (GA): ASHRAE; 2021.

15. Facility Guidelines Institute (FGI). Guidelines for Design and Construction of Hospitals, 2018. FGI. Available at: https://fgiguidelines.org/guidelines/purchase-the-guidelines/. Accessed December 29, 2020.

16. American Hospital Association. Hospitals face continued financial challenges one year into the COVID-19 pandemic. Chicago, IL: AHA; 2021.

17. Rebmann T. Infectious Disease Disasters: Bioterrorism, Emerging Infections, and Pandemics. In: Boston KM, editor. APIC text online. Arlington, VA: APIC; 2020. p. 122–79. Chapter 122.

18. CDC. NIOSH. Hierarchy of controls. Available at: https://www.cdc.gov/niosh/topics/hierarchy/. Accessed January 15, 2021.

19. Morawska L, Milton DK. It is time to address airborne transmission of coronavirus disease 2019 (COVID-19). Clin Infect Dis 2020;71:2311–3.

20. Tang JW, Bahnfleth WP, Bluyssen PM, et al. Dismantling myths on the airborne transmission of severe acute respiratory syndrome coronavirus-2 (SARS-CoV-2). J Hosp Infect 2021;110:89–96.

21. Rasmussen AL, Popescu SV. SARS-CoV-2 transmission without symptoms. Symptomless transmission silently drives viral spread and is key to ending the pandemic. Science 2021;371:1206–7.

22. Weber DJ, Babcock H, Hayden MK, et al. Universal pandemic precautions—An idea ripe for the times. Infect Control Hosp Epidemiol 2020;41:1321–2.

23. CDC. Interim Infection Prevention and Control Recommendations for Healthcare Personnel During the Coronavirus Disease 2019 (COVID-19) Pandemic. 2/23/2021. Available at: https://www.cdc.gov/coronavirus/2019-ncov/hcp/infection-control-recommendations.html. Accessed, March 1, 2021.

24. ASHRAE. Core Recommendations for Reducing Airborne Infectious Aerosol Exposure. ASHRAE Epidemic Task Force. 1/6/2021. Available at: https://www.ashrae.org/file%20library/technical%20resources/covid-19/core-recommendations-for-reducing-airborne-infectious-aerosol-exposure.pdf. Accessed March 1, 2021.

25. ASHRAE. ASHRAE Position Document on Infectious Aerosols. Environmental Health Position Document Committee. 4/14/2020. Available at: https://www.ashrae.org/file%20library/about/position%20documents/pd_infectiousaerosols_2020.pdf. Accessed March 1, 2021.

26. Morgan J. Redesign increases isolation space UVA Medical Center implemented design changes mid-construction to increase airborne infectious isolation rooms. Healthcare Facilities Management. 3/8/2021. Available at: https://www.hfmmagazine.com/articles/4119-redesign-increases-isolation-space. Accessed March 15, 2021.

27. Booth RD, Ponce SJ, Corso GJ, et al. American society for health care engineering (ASHE) current/updated health care facilities ventilation controls and guidelines for management of patients with suspected or confirmed SARS-CoV-2 (COVID-19). Chicago, IL: ASHE; 2021.

28. CDC, National Institute for Occupational Safety and Health. Engineering Controls To Reduce Airborne, Droplet and Contact Exposures During Epidemic/Pandemic Response. Ventilated Headboard. 5/26/2020. Available at: https://www.cdc.gov/niosh/topics/healthcare/engcontrolsolutions/ventilated-headboard.html. Accessed February 18, 2021.

29. Yang J, Sekhar SC, Cheong KWD, et al. Performance evaluation of a novel personalized ventilation–personalized exhaust system for airborne infection control. Indoor Air 2015;25:176–87.

30. Kanamori H, Rutala WA, Sickbert-Bennett EE, et al. Review of Fungal Outbreaks and Infection Prevention in Healthcare Settings During Construction and Renovation. Clin Infect Dis 2015;61:433–44.

31. Kanamori H, Weber DJ, Rutala WA. Healthcare Outbreaks Associated With a Water Reservoir and Infection Prevention Strategies. Clin Infect Dis 2016;62(11):1423–35.

32. Perkins KM, Reddy SC, Fagan R, et al. Investigation of healthcare infection risks from water-related organisms: Summary of CDC consultations, 2014—2017. Infect Control Hosp Epidemiol 2019;40:621–6.

33. Parkes LO, Hota SS. Sink-Related Outbreaks and Mitigation Strategies in Healthcare Facilities. Curr Infect Dis Rep 2018;20:42–56.

34. Carling P. Wastewater drains: epidemiology and interventions in 23 carbapenem-resistant organism outbreaks. Infect Control Hosp Epidemiol 2018;39:972–9.

35. Garrison LE, Kunz JM, Cooley LA, et al. Vital signs: deficiencies in environmental control identified in outbreaks of legionnaires' disease — North America, 2000–2014. MMWR 2016;65:576–84.

36. CDC. Toolkit: Developing a Water Management Program to Reduce Legionella Growth and Spread in Buildings. 6/5/2017. Available at: https://www.cdc.gov/legionella/wmp/toolkit/index.html. Accessed February 10, 2021.

37. ASHRAE. ANSI/ASHRAE standard 188-2018, Legionellosis: risk management for building water systems. Atlanta (GA): ASHRAE; 2018.
38. Premier Inc. ICRA Definitions And Elements. Available at: https://www.premiersafetyinstitute.org/safety-topics-az/building-design/infection-control-risk-assessment-icra/. Accessed March 5, 2021.
39. CDC. Water Infection Control Risk Assessment (WICRA) for Healthcare Settings. Available at: https://www.cdc.gov/hai/pdfs/prevent/water-assessment-tool-508.pdf. Accessed March 29, 2021.
40. Scanlon MM, Gordon JL, McCoy WF, et al. Water management for construction: evidence for risk characterization in community and healthcare settings: a systematic review. Int J Environ Res Public Health 2020;17:2168.
41. Datta R, Platt R, Yokoe DS, et al. Environmental cleaning intervention and risk of acquiring multidrug-resistant organisms from prior room occupants. Arch Intern Med 2011;171:491–4.
42. Rupp ME, Fitzgerald T, Sholtz L, et al. Maintain the gain: program to sustain performance improvement in environmental cleaning. Infect Control Hosp Epidemiol 2014;35:866–8.
43. Chaudhury H, Mahmood A, Valente M. The use of single patient rooms versus multiple occupancy rooms in acute care environments. Coalition for Health Environments Research (CHER); 2005. Available at: https://www.healthdesign.org/sites/default/files/use_of_single_patient_rooms_v_multiple_occ._rooms-acute_care.pdf. Accessed February 4, 2021.
44. Root RD, Lindstrom M, Xie A, et al. Investigating the association of room features with healthcare-facility–onset Clostridioides difficile: An exploratory study. Infect Control Hosp Epidemiol 2020;1–6. https://doi.org/10.1017/ice.2020.1307.
45. Squire MM, Sessel GK, Lin G, et al. Optimal Design of Paired Built Environment Interventions for Control of MDROs in Acute Care and Community Hospitals. HERD 2021;14(2):109–29.
46. Thompson D, Hamilton K, Cadenhead CD, et al. Guidelines for intensive care unit design. Crit Care Med 2012;40:1586–600.
47. Buchanan MO, Thompson SC, DiBiase LM, et al. Does a mobile dust-containment cart reduce the risk of healthcare-associated fungal infections during above-ceiling work? Infect Control Hosp Epidemiol 2021;42(4):477–9.
48. Mousavi ES, Bausman D, Tafazzoli M. Renovation in hospitals: Training construction crews to work in health care facilities. Am J Infect Control 2020;48:403–9.

ADDITIONAL RESOURCES

ASHRAE. ASHRAE COVID-19 Response Resources. Available at: https://www.ashrae.org/technical-resources/resources. Accessed March 1, 2021.

Johnson L. Construction and Renovation, Chapter 118. In: Boston KM, editor. APIC Text Online. Arlington, VA: APIC; 2019. p. 118–24.

Michigan Regional Council of Carpenters and Millwrights. Construction Infection Control Risk Assessment (ICRA) Training. Available at: https://www.hammer9.com/icra. Accessed March 25, 2021.

Society of Critical Care Medicine, Halpern NA, Kaplan LJ, Rausen M, Yang JJ. Configuring ICUs in the COVID-19 Era 2020. Available at: https://www.sccm.org/getattachment/03130f42-5350-4456-be9f-b9407194938d/Configuring-ICUs-in-the-COVID-19-Era-A-Collection. Accessed March 9, 2021.

Occupational Health Update
Approach to Evaluation of Health Care Personnel and Preexposure Prophylaxis

Erica S. Shenoy, MD, PhD[a,b,c,*], David J. Weber, MD, MPH[d,e]

KEYWORDS

- Occupational health • Health care personnel • Vaccines • Immunization
- Preexposure prophylaxis

KEY POINTS

- Health care personnel (HCP) are at risk of exposure to infectious agents depending on their job duties and other factors.
- Effective occupational health services (OHS) programs are a key aspect of preventing exposure to infectious agents and subsequent infection.
- HCP must be educated on proper handling of sharps, early identification and isolation of potentially infectious patients, and implementation of standard and transmission-based precautions, including hand hygiene.
- OHS must ensure immunity to vaccine-preventable diseases.

RISKS TO HEALTH CARE PERSONNEL AND THE ROLE OF OCCUPATIONAL HEALTH SERVICES

Health care is one of the fastest-growing sectors of the US economy, employing more than 20 million persons.[1,2] Health care personnel (HCP) face a range of noninfectious hazards on the job, including back injuries, strains and sprains, latex allergy, violence, and stress.[3] HCP are at risk of exposure to infectious agents depending on their job duties and other factors. Risks include percutaneous exposure to blood-borne pathogens (BBP) via sharp injuries (eg, human immunodeficiency virus [HIV], hepatitis B virus [HBV], hepatitis C virus HCV]); exposure by direct contact, droplet, or

[a] Infection Control Unit, Massachusetts General Hospital, 55 Fruit Street, Bulfinch 334, Boston, MA 02114, USA; [b] Division of Infectious Diseases, Massachusetts General Hospital, 55 Fruit Street, Bulfinch 334, Boston, MA, USA; [c] Harvard Medical School, Boston, MA, USA; [d] Division of Infectious Disease, School of Medicine, University of North Carolina at Chapel Hill, Bioinformatics Building, Suite 2163, Campus Box 7030, 130 Mason Farm Road, Chapel Hill, NC 27599-7030, USA; [e] Department of Hospital Epidemiology, UNC Medical Center, Chapel Hill, NC, USA
* Corresponding author. Infection Control Unit, Massachusetts General Hospital, 55 Fruit Street, Bulfinch 334, Boston, MA 02114.
E-mail address: eshenoy@mgh.harvard.edu

Infect Dis Clin N Am 35 (2021) 717–734
https://doi.org/10.1016/j.idc.2021.04.008
0891-5520/21/© 2021 Elsevier Inc. All rights reserved.
id.theclinics.com

airborne-transmitted pathogens through direct patient care (eg, pertussis, meningo-coccal infections, tuberculosis); and indirect contact through transmission related to the contaminated health care environment (eg, *Clostridioides difficile*). Cases of nonfatal occupational injury and illness among HCP are among the highest of any industrial sector.[3] Approaches to preventing occupational acquisition of infection by HCP have been reviewed, and include implementation of the Hierarchy of Controls to assess implementation of feasible and effective control solutions.[4–7] The Hierarchy of Controls (**Fig. 1**), developed by the National Institute of Occupational Health and Safety (NIOSH), is a framework to assess the effectiveness of interventions to reduce hazards in the workplace and the risks of injury or illness.[8]

Minimizing the risk of communicable disease acquisition is based on 6 key recommended practices: (1) proper training of HCP at initiation of health care practice and annually (eg, infection prevention practices, sharp injury prevention, no eating or drinking in areas where care is delivered); (2) ensuring immunity to vaccine-preventable diseases[4,6,7,9–11]; (3) evaluation of HCP who were exposed to communicable diseases for receipt of postexposure prophylaxis (PEP)[6,7,12–14]; (4) adherence to standard precautions when providing patient care,[15] especially the performance of appropriate hand hygiene before and after patient care[16–18]; (5) rapid institution of appropriate transmission-based precautions for patients with a known or suspected communicable disease as part of the identify-isolate-inform framework[19–23]; and (6) proper use of personal protective equipment, such as surgical or procedural masks, N-95 respirators (including respiratory clearance and fit testing), eye protection, gloves,

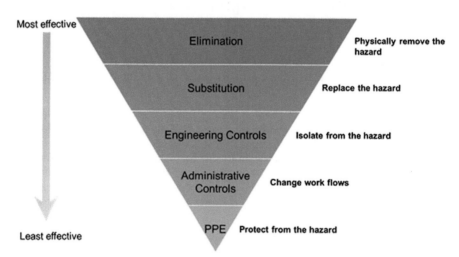

Fig. 1. The hierarchy of controls. Interventions at the top of the hierarchy can potentially be more effective than those at the bottom. Elimination and substitution strategies are highly effective but can be difficult to implement. An example of an effective elimination strategy is vaccination. Engineering controls are designed to remove a hazard before the hazard comes in contact with the worker. Use of airborne infection isolation rooms for airborne diseases such as measles is an example of engineering controls. Administrative controls, such as symptom screening of visitors, patients, and HCP, can be challenging to maintain over time. Use of personal protective equipment (PPE), although highly effective when used correctly and consistently, requires effort by HCP to achieve protection. (*Adapted from* The National Institute for Occupational Safety and Health (NIOSH). Hierarchy of Controls. Available at: https://www.cdc.gov/niosh/topics/hierarchy/default.html. 2015. Accessed November 20, 2020.)

and gowns when caring for patients with potentially communicable diseases, based on the mode of transmission (**Box 1**).[15] Prevention of clinical laboratory-acquired infection requires adherence to recommended administrative protocols (eg, no eating, drinking, or smoking in areas where microbiologic or pathologic samples are processed), engineering controls (eg, containment hoods), personal protective equipment (eg, N-95 respirators when culturing *Mycobacterium tuberculosis*), and appropriate immunizations.[24,25]

DEFINITIONS

The following definitions are from the Centers for Disease Control and Prevention (CDC).[7]

HCP refers to all paid and unpaid persons serving in health care settings who have the potential for direct or indirect exposure to patients or infectious materials, including body substances; contaminated medical supplies, devices, and equipment; contaminated environmental surfaces; or contaminated air. These HCP may include, but are not limited to, those listed in **Box 2**. In general, HCP who have regular or frequent contact with patients, body fluids, or specimens have a higher risk of acquiring or transmitting infections than do HCP who have only brief contact with patients and their environment (eg, beds, food trays, medical equipment). However, all HCP who work within the confines of a health care facility should be covered by the occupational health service (OHS) and receive appropriate screening and preexposure prophylaxis even if they do not provide direct patient care. Recommendations for HCP who work in dental health care settings, autopsy personnel, and clinical laboratory personnel are addressed elsewhere.[25–27]

Health care settings refer to locations where health care is delivered and includes, but is not limited to, acute care facilities, long-term acute care facilities, inpatient rehabilitation services, nursing homes and assisted living facilities, home health care, vehicles where care is delivered (eg, mobile clinics), and outpatient facilities such as dialysis centers and physician offices.

OHS refers to the group, department, or program that addresses many aspects of health and safety in the workplace for HCP, including the provision of clinical services for work-related injuries, exposures, and illnesses. In health care settings, OHS

Box 1
Modes of transmission of selected communicable diseases

Airborne	Bites	Blood Borne	Contact (Direct and Indirect)	Droplet
• Measles	• Rabies	• HBV	• Anthrax (cutaneous)	• Diphtheria
• Tuberculosis (pulmonary, laryngeal)	• Tetanus	• HCV	• *C difficile*	• Influenza
		• HIV	• Hepatitis A	• Invasive group A streptococcus
• Varicella zoster virus (primary varicella or disseminated herpes zoster)			• MRSA	• Invasive *Neisseria meningitidis*
			• SARS-CoV-2	
			• Varicella zoster virus (herpes zoster)	• Pertussis
			• Herpes simplex	• Plague
				• SARS-CoV-2

Abbreviations: MRSA, methicillin-resistant *Staphylococcus aureus*; SARS-CoV-2, severe acute respiratory syndrome coronavirus-2.

Box 2
Health care personnel whose care should be covered by an occupational health service

- Emergency medical service personnel
- Nurse and nursing assistants
- Physicians
- Technicians
- Therapists (eg, occupational health, physical, respiratory care)
- Phlebotomists
- Pharmacists
- Students and trainees
- Contractual staff not employed by the health care facility
- Persons not directly involved in patient care (for example, clerical, dietary, housekeeping, laundry, security, maintenance, engineering and facilities management, administrative, billing, volunteers, clinical laboratory personnel)

Note: HCP does not include dental health care personnel, autopsy personnel, and laboratory personnel, for whom recommendations are provided separately.[25–27]

---

addresses workplace hazards, including communicable diseases; slips, trips, and falls; patient handling injuries; chemical exposures; HCP burnout; and workplace violence. Most commonly, OHS are provided on site within the health care facility in which HCP are performing patient care but may also be provided off site. Occupational health programs should include a variety of activities designed to minimize the risk for HCP to acquire an infectious disease, to evaluate HCP with a potential exposure to a communicable disease, and to evaluate HCP with a communicable disease (**Box 3**).

Occupational health programs should be aware of appropriate guidelines from the CDC and professional organizations. They should adhere to appropriate state and federal laws and regulations. Specific regulations promulgated by the US Occupational Safety and Health Administration (OSHA) related to HCP include BBP (1910.1030)[28] and tuberculosis/respiratory protection (1910.134).[29] The Federal Needlestick Safety and Prevention Act (HR5178), which was enacted in 2000, requires the use of safety engineered devices whenever possible to reduce the likelihood of sharp injuries.[30] Commonly used references are provided in **Table 1**.

EVALUATION OF HEALTH CARE PERSONNEL AND PREEXPOSURE PROPHYLAXIS

OHS either provide or refer newly hired HCP for preplacement medical evaluations before initiation of employment, and periodically as needed during the course of employment.

Preexposure Screening

All HCP should undergo a new personnel orientation on hire. As part of the orientation process, HCP should undergo screening and education directed at reducing the risk of acquisition of infection diseases by health care providers (**Box 2**). All information obtained should be entered into an electronic database. Access to this database may be prescribed by state law because some states treat HCP occupational health records as personnel records. If OHS records are part of the organization's standard patient

Box 3
Components of an occupational health service for health care personnel at initial employment

At initial
employment

1. Evaluation for ability to perform job functions
2. Screen for illicit drugs
3. Medical evaluation of selected HCP
   a. Department of transportation (required for use of certain motor vehicles)
   b. Flight physical (required of pilots)
   c. Police/security for use of weapons
4. Review of immunity to vaccine-preventable diseases (**Tables 1** and **2**)
5. Evaluation for tuberculosis
   a. Symptom review for active tuberculosis
   b. Testing for latent tuberculosis (TST or IGRA; IGRA preferred)
6. Allergy screening for common health care–associated products
   a. Latex/natural rubber, germicides (antiseptics, disinfectants)
7. Counseling for pregnant or immunocompromised personnel (voluntary)
8. Education
   a. Fire and electrical safety
   b. Prevention of sharps injury
   c. Appropriate hand hygiene and proper use of personal protective equipment
   d. Workplace violence
   e. Disaster planning: weather, bomb threats, biothreats, chemical spills
   f. Reporting infectious disease exposures, injuries, illnesses
   g. OSHA required (if applicable): blood-borne pathogens, tuberculosis/respiratory protection

Annual

1. Symptom evaluation for tuberculosis
2. Review of immunity to vaccine-preventable diseases
   a. Influenza immunization

Miscellaneous

1. Hearing evaluation if part of OSHA-required hearing conservation program
2. Test for color blindness if performing high-level disinfection

Education

1. OSHA required (if applicable): blood-borne pathogens, tuberculosis/respiratory protection
2. Others as recommended/required by health care facility

When needed

1. Evaluation for possible communicable disease
   a. Consideration for treatment and job restriction/furlough if disease poses threat to patients or other HCP
2. Evaluation for postexposure prophylaxis
   a. Consideration for treatment and job restriction/furlough if disease poses threat to patients or other HCP
3. Evaluation of injured personnel (eg, strains, sprains, lacerations)
   a. Provide first aid
   b. Refer to emergency department or specialized clinic for severe injuries
   c. Provide long-term care
   d. Communicate with worker's compensation department
4. Return-to-work evaluation for non–work-related injuries/illnesses
5. Fit-for-duty examination (may include drug and alcohol testing)

Abbreviations: IGRA, interferon gamma release assay; OSHA, Occupational Safety and Health Administration; TST, tuberculin skin test.

electronic medical records, unauthorized access of provider's occupational health information by supervisors should be prohibited by the institutions privacy rules and periodically assessed.

Table 1
Commonly cited references related to health care personnel occupational exposure

Author	Title	Most Recently Updated	Link
CDC, National Center for Emerging and Zoonotic Infectious Diseases, Division of Healthcare Quality and Promotion	Infection Control in Healthcare Personnel: Infrastructure and Routine Practices for Occupational Infection Prevention and Control Services	2019	https://www.cdc.gov/infectioncontrol/guidelines/healthcare-personnel/index.html
CDC	Recommended Vaccines for Healthcare Workers	2020	https://www.cdc.gov/vaccines/adults/rec-vac/hcw.html
ACIP	ACIP Vaccine Recommendations and Guidelines	2020	https://www.cdc.gov/vaccines/hcp/acip-recs/index.html
Society for Healthcare Epidemiology of America	Management of Healthcare Personnel Living With Hepatitis B, Hepatitis C, or Human Immunodeficiency Virus in US Healthcare Institutions	2020	http://www.shea-online.org/index.php/practice-resources

Abbreviation: ACIP, Advisory Committee on Immunization Practices.

Immunizations

General recommendations regarding vaccination of HCP have been published by the CDC, the Advisory Committee on Immunization Practices (ACIP) for HCP[11,31] as well as the general public[32] and adults,[33] and the American Academy of Pediatrics (AAP) for children.[34] The most recent ACIP recommendations for adults, which are summarized yearly, should always be consulted. It is recommended that all HCP be immune to mumps, measles, rubella, varicella, influenza, and, in the context of the coronavirus disease 2019 (COVID-19) pandemic, severe acute respiratory syndrome coronavirus-2 (SARS-CoV-2).[35] Depending on the vaccine-preventable disease, immunity may be ensured by several different measures (**Table 2**). HCP who are not immune should receive appropriate immunizations (**Table 3**). However, even if HCP are considered immune to a vaccine-preventable disease transmitted by the droplet (ie, pertussis, invasive meningococcal infection, mumps, rubella, SARS-CoV-2) or airborne (ie, varicella, measles) route, they should wear appropriate respiratory protection as per transmission-based precautions while providing care to a patient with confirmed or suspected disease because immunization is not 100% effective in preventing infection. Further, failure of any provider to wear the appropriate respiratory protection may lead nonimmune providers (eg, persons with a contraindication to vaccination) to mistakenly believe that the transmission-based precautions have been discontinued.

HCP should be provided with all vaccines that are recommended for adults,[33] such as human papillomavirus, herpes zoster, Tdap (tetanus toxoid, diphtheria toxoid, acellular pertussis), and pneumococcal vaccines, or referred to their local medical providers for the same. In special circumstances, HCP should be offered immunization

Table 2
Methods of showing proof of immunity of health care personnel

Vaccine	Birth Before 1957	Physician Diagnosis	Positive Serology	Self-Report	Documented Appropriate Vaccine Series[a]
Mumps (MMR)	Yes[b]	Yes[d]	Yes	No	Yes
Measles (MMR)	Yes[b]	Yes[c]	Yes	No	Yes
Rubella (MMR)	Yes[b,c]	No	Yes	No	Yes
Varicella	No	Yes	Yes	Yes[e]	Yes
Hepatitis B	No	—	>10 mIU/mL[f]	No	Yes
Influenza	No	No	No	No	Yes
SARS-CoV-2	No	No	No	No	Yes

"Yes" in any column is acceptable evidence of immunity.
Greater than 96% of HCP born before 1957 were shown to be immune to measles, mumps, and/or rubella.[37]
Abbreviation: MMR, measles, mumps, rubella.
[a] Written documentation (ie, signed by a health care provider).
[b] Consider immunization of HCP born before 1957; recommend during an outbreak.
[c] All HCP of child-bearing potential should be immunized.
[d] Requires laboratory confirmation of infection.
[e] Based on published literature: greater than 97% of HCP born before 1980 were shown to be immune to varicella in 2014.[36]
[f] Obtain anti–hepatitis B surface antibody (anti-HBs) titer, 1 to 2 months after the last vaccine dose; if immunization is remote and anti-HBs titer not available, see text for management.

Table 3
Immunizations recommended for nonimmune health care personnel

Vaccine	Health Care Personnel	Comments
Mumps	All (2 doses)	Provide as MMR
Measles	All (2 doses)	Provide as MMR
Rubella	All (1 dose)	Provide as MMR
Varicella	All (2 doses)	—
Hepatitis B	HCP with potential exposure to blood or contaminated body fluids (2 or 3 doses depending on vaccine)	—
Meningococcal (serogroups A, C, Y, W)	Clinical microbiologists (1 dose; booster every 5 y)	All vaccines available are now conjugate products
Meningococcal (serogroup B)	Clinical microbiologists (2 or 3 doses, depending on manufacturer); booster every 2–3 y	MenB-FHbp and MenB-4C are not interchangeable
Influenza	All (1 dose each year)	HCP who care for severely immunocompromised persons who require care in a protected environment should receive IIV or RIV; HCP who receive LAIV should avoid providing care for severely immunocompromised persons (ie, persons receiving care in protected hospital unit such as BMTU) for 7 d after immunization
SARS-CoV-2	All (frequency of immunization not yet established)	

Abbreviations: BMTU, bone marrow transplant unit; IIV, inactivated influenza vaccine; LAIV, live, attenuated influenza vaccine; RIV, recombinant influenza vaccine.

Data from Refs[31,35] and ACIP.

with other vaccines, including polio, rabies, hepatitis A, vaccinia (smallpox),[38] Ebola virus, and anthrax (**Box 4**). HCP responding to an outbreak of Ebola virus disease (EVD), who work in one of the federally designated Ebola treatment centers in the United States, or work as laboratorians or other staff at biosafety level 4 facilities in the United States, are recommended for vaccination with EVD.[39] In addition, HCP who are traveling outside the United States for work-related activities should be evaluated and provided with CDC-recommended immunizations such as typhoid, cholera, and Japanese encephalitis.[40,41]

Vaccination for SARS-CoV-2 is recommended for HCP, including paid and unpaid personnel working in all health care settings. At this time, 2 vaccines, both messenger RNA (mRNA) vaccines, have been approved under Emergency Use Authorization: Pfizer-BioNTech's COVID-19 vaccine and Moderna's COVID-19 vaccine. Late-stage trials of additional vaccines are underway or planned (AstraZeneca, Janssen, and Novavax). There are few contraindications to vaccination. These contraindications include (1) severe allergic reaction (eg, anaphylaxis) after a previous dose of an mRNA COVID-19 vaccine or any of its components, (2) immediate allergic reaction of any severity to a previous dose of an mRNA COVID-19 vaccine or any of its components (including polyethylene glycol [PEG]), and (3) immediate allergic reaction of any severity to polysorbate (because of potential cross-reactive hypersensitivity with the vaccine ingredient PEG). Individuals in the last 2 categories should not receive mRNA COVID-19 vaccination unless they have been evaluated by an allergist-

---

Box 4
Special-use vaccines[a]

1. Anthrax: PEP, research, biothreat attack

2. Diphtheria (Tdap): outbreak

3. Ebola virus (Ervebo): adults who are responding, or may respond, to an outbreak of EVD, laboratorians or other staff working at biosafety level-4 facilities in the United States, or HCP working at federally designated Ebola treatment centers in the United States

4. Hepatitis A: PEP, outbreak, travel

5. Hepatitis B: PEP, travel

6. Measles (MMR): PEP, outbreak

7. Meningococcal serotypes A, C, W, Y: outbreak, travel

8. Meningococcal serotype B: outbreak

9. Mumps (MMR): outbreak

10. Pertussis (Tdap): outbreak

11. Poliomyelitis: research, outbreak

12. Rabies: PEP, research, travel

13. Rubella (MMR): outbreak

14. Smallpox (vaccinia): PEP, research, biothreat attack

15. Tetanus (Tdap or Td): PEP

16. Varicella: PEP, outbreak

Abbreviation: Td, tetanus toxoid, diphtheria toxoid. [a]Additional vaccines may be recommended for researchers or travel, such as yellow fever, Japanese encephalitis, and cholera.

immunologist who has determined that the vaccine can be safely administered with adequate observation and support. Detailed guidance is provided by the CDC. Individuals with a history of immediate allergic reaction to any other vaccine or injectable therapy can receive mRNA COVID-19 vaccines but must have received counseling in advance regarding potential risk of severe allergic reaction. If vaccination proceeds in these instances, the observation period should be extended from 15 minutes to 30 minutes for individuals with a history of immediate allergic reaction of any severity to a vaccine or injectable therapy and persons with a history of anaphylaxis of any cause.[42] Vaccination centers should have immediate availability of resuscitation equipment.

Immunocompromised Health Care Personnel

Immunocompromised HCP require special consideration in the provision of immunizations.[32] First, live, attenuated virus vaccines (eg, measles-mumps-rubella; varicella; live, attenuated influenza) may be contraindicated. Second, vaccines not routinely recommended may be indicated (eg, pneumococcal, meningococcal, *Haemophilus influenzae* type b). Third, higher antigen doses (eg, hepatitis B vaccine in people with end-stage renal disease), additional doses of vaccine (eg, rabies vaccine in immunocompromised persons), or postimmunization serologic evaluation may be indicated (eg, antibody response to rabies vaccine) because immunization of immunocompromised people may elicit a lower antibody response. In addition, such personnel should be individually evaluated for reassignment (with the consent of the employee) depending on their job duties. Of importance, caring for an immunocompromised patient is not a contraindication to receipt of a live, attenuated vaccine, although HCP receiving live, attenuated influenza vaccine (LAIV) should not work in a protected environment (ie, stem cell transplant unit) for 7 days postimmunization.[33,43]

Pregnant Health Care Personnel

Pregnant HCP also require special consideration in the provision of immunizations. The risks from immunization during pregnancy are largely theoretic.[32] The benefit of immunization among pregnant women usually outweighs the potential risks for adverse reactions, especially when the risk for disease exposure is high, infection would pose a special risk to the mother or fetus, and the vaccine is unlikely to cause harm.[44-47] Furthermore, newer information continues to confirm the safety of vaccines given inadvertently during pregnancy. Ideally, women of childbearing age, including HCP, should have been immunized against measles, mumps, rubella, varicella, tetanus, diphtheria, pertussis, meningococcus, polio, COVID-19, hepatitis A, and hepatitis B as children or adolescents before becoming pregnant. Nevertheless, live, attenuated vaccines should be provided only to nonpregnant HCP and deferred during pregnancy. The ACIP has recommended administration of Tdap during all pregnancies, preferably during weeks 27 to 36. If not administered during pregnancy, Tdap should be administered immediately postpartum before discharge from the hospital or birthing center for new mothers who have never received Tdap before or whose vaccination status is unknown. Women who are pregnant during respiratory virus season should receive inactivated influenza immunization. There is no convincing evidence of risk from immunizing pregnant women with other inactivated virus or bacterial vaccines, or toxoids. Susceptible pregnant women at high risk for specific infections should receive, as indicated, the following vaccines: hepatitis A, hepatitis B, pneumococcal polysaccharide, meningococcal, rabies, COVID-19, and poliovirus (inactivated) (see **Box 3**). Importantly, the indications for use of immunoglobulin preparations are the same in pregnant and nonpregnant women. Breastfeeding does not adversely affect the response to immunization and is not a contraindication for any of the currently routinely recommended routine vaccines.

Health Care Personnel with Contraindications or Precautions to Immunization

Before the administration of any vaccine, the HCP should be evaluated for the presence of conditions that are listed as a vaccine contraindication or precaution.[32] If such a condition is present, the risks and benefits of vaccination need to be carefully weighed by the health care provider and the patient. The most common contraindication is a history of an anaphylactic reaction to a previous dose of the vaccine or to a vaccine component. Factors that are not contraindications to immunization include the following: household contact with a pregnant woman; breastfeeding; reaction to a previous vaccination, consisting only of mild to moderate local tenderness, swelling, or both, or fever less than 40.5°C; mild acute illness with or without low-grade fever; current antimicrobial therapy (except for oral typhoid vaccine) or convalescence from a recent illness; personal history of allergies, except a history of an anaphylactic reaction to a vaccine component; and family history of allergies, serious adverse reactions to vaccination, or seizures.

Routine Immunization as a Condition of Employment

Despite the benefits of vaccination, challenges remain in ensuring a fully vaccinated health care workforce. In February 2012, the National Vaccine Advisory Committee issued a statement that provided recommendations on how to achieve the Healthy People 2020 annual influenza vaccine coverage goal (ie, 90%) for HCP; for facilities that have implemented the recommended initial strategies but have "not consistently achieved the Healthy People goal for vaccination coverage of HCP in an efficient and timely manner" it was recommended that they should "strongly consider an employer requirement for influenza immunization."[48] In the most recent season for which data are available, 80.6% of HCP reported receiving influenza vaccination during the 2019 to 2020 season. Among those who were required by their employer to receive the vaccination, compliance was higher at 94.4% compared with those without an employer mandate at 69.6%.[49] In 2020, the Society for Healthcare Epidemiology of America (SHEA) recommended that only medical contraindications should be accepted as a reason for not receiving all routine immunizations as recommended by the CDC.[50]

EVALUATION OF HEALTH CARE PERSONNEL WITH COMMUNICABLE DISEASES

HCP exposed to a communicable disease for which they are susceptible should be considered for work restrictions or furlough. Similarly, HCP ill with a communicable disease should be considered for work restrictions or furlough (**Table 4**). Importantly, infectious HCP have been the source for patient infection and the index case for outbreaks.[52,53] HCP-to-patient transmission has been well documented for HIV, HBV, and HCV, but has most commonly been reported with HBV. For this reason, infected HCP who perform invasive procedures should be evaluated by a special panel for the need for education, additional engineering controls, and/or work restrictions per current guidelines from the Society of Hospital Epidemiology of America[54] and CDC.[55]

SUMMARY

Although HCP are at risk of exposure to communicable diseases, effective occupational health programs can mitigate risk through thorough evaluation of HCP, ensuring appropriate preexposure prophylaxis, and management of HCP with communicable diseases.

Table 4
Recommended work restrictions for health care personnel colonized/exposed or infected with selected infectious agents

Infection or Infectious Agent	Exposed or Colonized	Infected (Duration of Restrictions)
Conjunctivitis (adenovirus)	Exposed; no restriction unless illness develops	Restrict from patient contact and contact with the patient's environment (until discharge ceases)
Cytomegalovirus	No restriction	No restriction
Diarrheal diseases	No restriction unless illness develops	Acute disease: exclude from duty (until >48–72 h after symptoms resolve) Convalescent stage (*Salmonella* spp): restrict from care of high-risk patients and food handling (until symptoms resolve; consult local and state authorities for HCP/food handlers with *Salmonella typhi*)
Diphtheria	Exposed: no restriction unless illness develops	Exclude from duty (until antimicrobial therapy completed and 2 cultures obtained ≥24 h apart are negative)
Hepatitis A	Exposed: no restriction unless illness develops	Restrict from patient contact, contact with patient's environment, and food handling (until 7 d after onset of jaundice)
Hepatitis B (chronic)	—	Restrictions based on review of only HCP who perform exposure-prone procedures by expert panel (see text)
Hepatitis C	—	Restrictions based on review of HCP who perform exposure-prone procedures by expert panel (see text)
Herpes simplex (genital)	—	No restriction
Herpes simplex (hands; herpetic whitlow)	—	Restrict from patient contact and contact with the patient's environment (until lesions heal)

Herpes simplex (orofacial)	—	Evaluate for need to restrict from care of high-risk patients
HIV	—	Restrictions based on review of HCP who perform exposure-prone procedures by expert panel (see text)
Measles	Exposed (susceptible HCP): exclude from duty (from the fifth day after first exposure through 21st day after last exposure and/or after rash appears)	Exclude from duty (until 4 d after the rash appears)
Meningococcal infections	Exposed: no restriction unless illness develops Colonized (unrelated to invasive case): no restriction	Exclude from duty (until 24 h after start of effective therapy)
Methicillin-resistant *Staphylococcus aureus*	Colonized: no restrictions unless or ill or epidemiologically/molecular test linked to patient infections	Allow to work provided lesions can be contained under a bandage and clothes; if lesions on exposed area (eg, hand/wrists, face/neck), exclude from duty (until lesions healed)
Mumps	Exposed (susceptible HCP): exclude from duty (from the 12th day after first exposure through 26th day after last exposure or after onset of parotitis)	Exclude from duty (until 9 d after onset of parotitis)
Pertussis	Exposure (asymptomatic): no restriction unless develops illness (PEP recommended) Exposed (symptomatic): per active disease	Exclude from duty (from beginning of catarrhal stage through third week after onset of paroxysms or until 5 d after start of effective antimicrobial therapy)
Rubella	Exposed (susceptible HCP): exclude from duty (from seventh day after first exposure through 21st day after last exposure)	Exclude from duty (until 5 d after rash appears)
Group A *Streptococcus*	Colonized: no restrictions unless or ill or epidemiologically/molecular test linked to patient infections	Restrict from patient care, contact with patient's environment, or food handling

(continued on next page)

Table 4
(continued)

Infection or Infectious Agent	Exposed or Colonized	Infected (Duration of Restrictions)
		(until 24 h after adequate treatment started)
Tuberculosis	Latent tuberculous infection: no restrictions	Active pulmonary tuberculosis; exclude from duty (until proved noninfectious)
Varicella	Exposed (susceptible): exclude from duty from 10th day after first exposure through 21st day (27th day if varicella immune globulin provided) after last exposure	Exclude from duty (until all lesions dried and crusted)
Zoster	Exposed (susceptible): same as varicella	Localized, in healthy HCP: allow to work provided lesions can be contained under a bandage and clothes; if lesions on exposed area (eg, hand/wrists, face/neck), exclude from duty (until lesions dried and crusted) Generalized or localized in immunosuppressed HCP: exclude from duty (until all lesions dried and crusted)
Viral respiratory tract infections (acute)	No restrictions unless illness develops[a]	Febrile: exclude from duty (until afebrile for >24 h) Afebrile: exclude from care of highly immunocompromised patients (ie, patients cared for in a protected environment) until afebrile for >24 h or 7 d since onset of symptoms, whichever is longer; HCP should wear a mask providing care until symptom free
SARS-CoV-2	Detailed recommendations related to HCP restrictions after exposure to SARS-CoV-2 are available

[a] Consider restrictions if HCP exposed to highly contagious disease transmitted by the respiratory route or close contact (eg, MERS-CoV [Middle East respiratory syndrome coronavirus], Ebola).[1]

Data from Refs.[6,7,51]

CLINICS CARE POINTS

- On hire, HCP should undergo screening and education directed at reducing the risk of acquisition of infection diseases by health care providers.
- Recommendations for immunization for HCP are provided by CDC and ACIP.
- Before the administration of any vaccine, the HCP should be evaluated for the presence of conditions that are listed as a vaccine contraindication or precaution.

DISCLOSURE

The authors have nothing to disclose.

REFERENCES

1. U.S. Bureau of Labor Statistics. BLS employment by major industry sector. Available at: https://www.bls.gov/emp/tables/employment-by-major-industry-sector. htm. Accessed January 7, 2021.
2. U.S. Bureau of Labor Statistics. Bls projections of industry employment 2016-2026. Available at: https://www.bls.gov/careeroutlook/2017/article/ projectionsindustry. htm#Fastest%20growing%20industries. Accessed 01/15/ 2021.
3. Centers for Disease Control and Prevention. Workplace safety & health topics. Healthcare workers. Available at: http://www.cdc.gov/niosh/topics/healthcare/. Accessed January 07, 2021.
4. Weber DJ, Rutala WA, Schaffner W. Lessons learned: protection of healthcare workers from infectious disease risks. Crit Care Med 2010;38(8):S306–14.
5. Sebazco S. APIC text of infection control and epidemiology. Section V. Occupational health. Washington, DC: APIC; 2005.
6. Bolyard EA, Tablan OC, Williams WW, et al. Guideline for infection control in health care personnel, 1998. Am J Infect Control 1998;26(3):289–354.
7. Centers for Disease Control and Prevention. Infection control in healthcare personnel: infrastructure and routine practices for occupational infection prevention and control services. Available at: https://www.cdc.gov/infectioncontrol/ guidelines/healthcare-personnel/index.html. Accessed 01/09/2021.
8. NIOSH. Hierarchy of controls. 2015. Available at: https://www.cdc.gov/niosh/ topics/hierarchy/default.html. Accessed 11/20/2020.
9. American Academy of Pediatrics. Red Book: 2015 report of communicable diseases. 30th edition. Elk Grove Village, IL: American Academy of Pediatrics; 2015. p. 95–8.
10. Talbot TR. Update on immunizations for healthcare personnel in the United States. Vaccine 2014;32(38):4869–75.
11. Shefer A, Atkinson W, Friedman C, et al. Immunization of health-care personnel recommendations of the advisory committee on immunization practices (ACIP). MMWR Recomm Rep 2011;60(7, Suppl. S):1–45.
12. Tolle MA, Schwarzwald HL. Postexposure prophylaxis against human immunodeficiency virus. Am Fam Physician 2010;82(2):161–6.
13. Grant RM. Antiretroviral agents used by HIV-uninfected persons for prevention: pre- and postexposure prophylaxis. Clin Infect Dis 2010;50:S96–101.
14. Bader MS, McKinsey DS. Postexposure prophylaxis for common infectious diseases. Am Fam Physician 2013;88(1):25–32.

15. Siegel JD, Rhinehart E, Jackson M, et al. 2007 guideline for isolation precautions: preventing transmission of infectious agents in health care settings. Am J Infect Control 2007;35(10 Suppl 2):S65–164.

16. Boyce JM, Pittet D. Guideline for hand hygiene in health-care settings - Recommendations of the Healthcare Infection Control Practices Advisory Committee and the HICPAC/SHEA/APIC/IDSA hand hygiene task force. Am J Infect Control 2002;30(8):S1–46.

17. World Health Organization. WHO guidelines on hand hygiene in health care. Available at: https://www.ncbi.nlm.nih.gov/books/NBK144013/. Accessed 01/15/2021.

18. Boyce JM. Update on hand hygiene. Am J Infect Control 2013;41(5):S94–6.

19. Siegel JD, Rhinehart E, Jackson M, et al, Committee HICPA. Management of multidrug-resistant organisms in health care settings, 2006. Am J Infect Control 2007;35(10 Suppl 2):S165–93.

20. Lledo W, Hernandez M, Lopez E, et al. Guidance for control of infections with carbapenem-resistant or carbapenemase-producing enterobacteriaceae in acute care facilities. MMWR Morb Mortal Wkly Rep 2009;58(10):256–60.

21. Koenig KL, Alassaf W, Burns MJ. Identify-isolate-inform: a tool for initial detection and management of measles patients in the emergency department. West J Emerg Med 2015;16(2):212.

22. Sánchez SM, Searle EF, Rubins D, et al. Travel-screening documentation to enable the "Identify-Isolate-Inform" framework for emerging infectious diseases: It's all in the details. Infect Control Hosp Epidemiol 2020;41(12):1449–51.

23. Centers for Disease Control and Prevention. Identify, isolate, inform: emergency department evaluation and management for patients under investigation (PUIs) for Ebola Virus Disease (EVD). In: Centers for Disease Control and Prevention.

24. Wagar E. Bioterrorism and the role of the clinical microbiology laboratory. Clin Microbiol Rev 2016;29(1):175–89.

25. Identify, isolate, inform: Emergency department evaluation and management for patients under investigation (puis) for ebola virus disease (evd). Centers for Disease Control and Prevention. Available at: https://www.cdc.gov/vhf/ebola/clinicians/emergency-services/emergencydepartments.html. Accessed 1/21/2021.

26. Miller JM, Astles R, Baszler T, et al. Guidelines for safe work practices in human and animal medical diagnostic laboratories. Recommendations of a CDC-convened, biosafety blue ribbon panel. MMWR Suppl 2012;61(1):1–102.

27. Kohn WG, Collins AS, Cleveland JL, et al. Guidelines for infection control in dental health-care settings–2003. MMWR Recommend Rep 2003;52(RR-17):1–61.

28. U.S. Occupational Safety and Health Administration. Bloodborne pathogens (1910.1030). Available at: https://www.osha.gov/pls/oshaweb/owadisp.show_document?p_table=STANDARDS&p_id=10051.

29. U.S. Occupational Safety and Health Administration. Respiratory Protection (1910.134). Available at: https://www.osha.gov/pls/oshaweb/owadisp.show_document?p_id=12716&p_table=standards. Accessed 01/15/2021.

30. Kanamori H, Weber DJ, DiBiase LM, et al. Impact of safety-engineered devices on the incidence of occupational blood and body fluid exposures among health-care personnel in an academic facility, 2000-2014. Infect Control Hosp Epidemiol 2016;37(5):497–504.

31. Centers for Disease Control and Prevention. Vaccine information for adults: recommended vaccines for healthcare workers. Available at: https://www.cdc.gov/vaccines/adults/rec-vac/hcw.html. Accessed 1/21/2021.

32. National Center for Immunization and Respiratory Diseases. General recommendations on immunization — recommendations of the Advisory Committee on Immunization Practices (ACIP). MMWR Recomm Rep 2011;60(2):1–64.

33. Kim DK, Bridges CB, Harriman KH. Advisory committee on immunization practices recommended immunization schedule for adults aged 19 years or older - United States, 2016. MMWR Morb Mortal Wkly Rep 2016;65(4):88–90.

34. Kimberlin DW. Red Book: 2018-2021 report of the committee on infectious diseases. Itasca, Illinois: American Academy of Pediatrics; 2018.

35. Dooling K, McClung N, Chamberland M, et al. The Advisory Committee on Immunization Practices' interim recommendation for allocating initial supplies of COVID-19 vaccine—United States, 2020. MMWR Morb Mortal Wkly Rep 2020; 69(49):1857.

36. Troiani L, Hill JJ III, Consoli S, et al. Varicella-zoster immunity in us healthcare personnel with self-reported history of disease. Infect Control Hosp Epidemiol 2015;36(12):1467–8.

37. Weber DJ, Consoli S, Sickbert-Bennett E, et al. Susceptibility to Measles, Mumps, and Rubella in Newly Hired (2006-2008) healthcare workers born before 1957. Infect Control Hosp Epidemiol 2010;31(6):655–7.

38. Centers for Disease Control and Prevention. Smallpox: for Clinicians. Available at: https://www.cdc.gov/smallpox/clinicians/index.html. Accessed January 09, 2021.

39. Choi MJ, Cossaboom CM, Whitesell AN, et al. Use of ebola vaccine: recommendations of the advisory committee on immunization practices, United States, 2020. MMWR Recomm Rep 2021;70(1):1–12.

40. Centers for Disease Control and Prevention. Yellow book. Available at: https://wwwnc.cdc.gov/travel/page/yellowbook-home. Accessed 1/14/2021.

41. Centers for Disease Control and Prevention. Epidemiology and prevention of vaccine-preventable diseases. Available at: http://www.cdc.gov/vaccines/pubs/pinkbook/index.html. Accessed 1/14/2021.

42. Centers for Disease Control and Prevention. Interim clinical considerations for use of mRNA COVID-19 vaccines currently authorized in the United States. Available at: https://www.cdc.gov/vaccines/covid-19/info-byproduct/clinical-considerations.html. Accessed 1/21/2021.

43. Pearson ML, Bridges CB, Harper SA. Influenza vaccination of health-care personnel; recommendations of the healthcare infection control practices advisory committee (HICPAC) and the advisory committee on immunization practices (ACIP) 2006.

44. Bazan JA, Mangino JE. Infection control and postexposure prophylaxis for the pregnant healthcare worker. Clin Obstet Gynecol 2012;55(2):571–88.

45. Rasmussen SA, Watson AK, Kennedy ED, et al. Vaccines and pregnancy: past, present, and future. Semin Fetal Neonatal Med 2014;19(3):161–9.

46. Chu HY, Englund JA. Maternal immunization. Clin Infect Dis 2014;59(4):560–8.

47. Swamy GK, Beigi RH. Maternal benefits of immunization during pregnancy. Vaccine 2015;33(47):6436–40.

48. National Vaccine Advisory Committee. Recommendations on strategies to achieve the healthy people 2020 annual vaccine coverage goal for health care personnel. Available at: http://nvac_adult_immunization_work_group.pdf. Accessed 01/15/2021..

49. Influenza vaccination coverage among health care personnel — united states, 2019–20 influenza season. Available at: https://www.cdc.gov/flu/fluvaxview/hcpcoverage_1920estimates.htm. Accessed 1/21/2021.

50. Weber DJ, Talbot TR, Weinmann A, et al. Policy statement from the Society for Healthcare Epidemiology of America (SHEA): only medical contraindications should be accepted as a reason for not receiving all routine immunizations as recommended by the Centers for Disease Control and Prevention. Infect Control Hosp Epidemiol 2021;42(1):1–5.
51. Centers for Disease Control and Prevention. Criteria for Return to work for health-care personnel with suspected or confirmed COVID-19 (interim guidance) 2020. Available at: https://www.cdc.gov/coronavirus/2019-ncov/hcp/return-to-work.html. Accessed January 07, 2021.
52. Sydnor E, Perl TM. Healthcare providers as sources of vaccine-preventable diseases. Vaccine 2014;32(38):4814–22.
53. Huttunen R, Syrjanen J. Healthcare workers as vectors of infectious diseases. Eur J Clin Microbiol Infect Dis 2014;33(9):1477–88.
54. Henderson DK, Dembry L-M, Sifri CD, et al. Management of healthcare personnel living with hepatitis B, hepatitis C, or human immunodeficiency virus in US health-care institutions. Infect Control Hosp Epidemiol 2020;1–9.
55. Holmberg SD, Suryaprasad A, Ward JW. Updated CDC recommendations for the management of hepatitis b virus-infected health-care providers and students. MMWR Recomm Rep 2012;61(3, Suppl. S):1–12.

Occupational Health Update

Evaluation and Management of Exposures and Postexposure Prophylaxis

Erica S. Shenoy, MD, PhD[a,b,c,*], David J. Weber, MD, MPH[d,e]

KEYWORDS

- Occupational health • Health care personnel • Postexposure prophylaxis
- Hepatitis B • Hepatitis C • Human immunodeficiency virus

KEY POINTS

- Health care personnel (HCP) are at risk of exposure to infectious agents depending on their job duties and other factors.
- Occupational health and safety must identify and manage exposures, and evaluate options for postexposure prophylaxis to HCP.

GENERAL APPROACH TO POSTEXPOSURE PROPHYLAXIS

Despite adherence to infection-control protocols and implementation of best practices with respect to preexposure prophylaxis, health care personnel (HCP) may be exposed to communicable diseases in the course of training or employment. General guidelines on postexposure prophylaxis (PEP) are available from the Centers for Disease Control and Prevention (CDC), Advisory Committee on Immunization Practices (ACIP),[1] American Academy of Pediatrics (AAP),[2] Association for Professionals in Infection Control and Epidemiology (APIC),[3] and the American Public Health Association (APHA).[4] All HCP should be educated at their initiation of employment or providing service when and how to report a potential infectious disease exposure.

Documentation of Potential Exposures and Occupational Health and Safety Evaluation

In general, HCP should complete an incident report (exposure report), which at most sites is now routinely submitted electronically to occupational health and safety (OHS).

[a] Infection Control Unit, Massachusetts General Hospital, 55 Fruit Street, Bulfinch 334, Boston, MA 02114, USA; [b] Division of Infectious Diseases, Massachusetts General Hospital, Boston, MA, USA; [c] Harvard Medical School, Boston, MA, USA; [d] Division of Infectious Disease, School of Medicine, University of North Carolina at Chapel Hill, Bioinformatics Building, Suite 2163, Campus Box 7030, 130 Mason Farm Road, Chapel Hill, NC 27599-7030, USA; [e] Department of Hospital Epidemiology, UNC Medical Center, Chapel Hill, NC, USA
* Corresponding author. Infection Control Unit, Massachusetts General Hospital, 55 Fruit Street, Bulfinch 334, Boston, MA 02114.
E-mail address: eshenoy@mgh.harvard.edu

Infect Dis Clin N Am 35 (2021) 735–754
https://doi.org/10.1016/j.idc.2021.04.009
id.theclinics.com

Occupational health evaluation should be available 24-7 for potentially exposed HCP. The exposure report should be reviewed by occupational health and communicated to the worker's compensation department. HCP with serious or life-threatening injuries or exposures should be referred to an emergency department or specialty clinic as appropriate. If patient or visitor exposures also occurred, the infection prevention and control department should be notified.

A well-defined protocol should be in place that details the steps in evaluation of any HCP potentially exposed to an infectious agent (**Box 1**). Proper counseling of the exposed HCP is critical (**Box 2**). Appropriate first aid should be provided, including proper care of any sharp injury or mucosal membrane exposure (eg, copious rinsing of eyes in the case of splash to eyes). A proper evaluation of the source case should also be conducted to confirm the report by the exposed HCP that the source patient does indeed have a communicable disease. Appropriate laboratory tests should be obtained from the source patient to determine whether the source patient can transmit human immunodeficiency virus (HIV), hepatitis B virus (HBV), or hepatitis C virus (HCV) as part of blood-borne pathogen (BBP) exposures.

Application of Exposure Definition: Did an Exposure Occur?

In all cases, if an infectious source is identified, OHS must then make a determination of whether an exposure has occurred to the HCP. Exposure definitions are widely used and generally include specifics regarding the source infection and infectious period, and the type and duration of the interaction, and may be mitigated through use of personal protective equipment (PPE). OHS has discretion to consider specific exposures on a case-by-case basis that may not meet standard exposure definitions. During the severe acute respiratory syndrome coronavirus-2 (SARS-CoV-2) pandemic, the CDC's exposure definitions have changed over time and include considerations for exclusion from work as well as recognition that, because of workforce shortages, exclusion from work after an exposure to SARS-CoV-2 may not be feasible.[5]

POSTEXPOSURE PROPHYLAXIS FOR SELECTED COMMUNICABLE DISEASES

PEP is available for many diseases, including, but not limited to, diphtheria, hepatitis A and B, HIV, influenza, measles, invasive meningococcal infection, pertussis, rabies,

---

Box 1
Management of an infectious disease exposure

1. Obtain name, medical record number, and location of source case

2. Determine whether source case has an infection and is infectious (ie, capable of transmitting infection)

3. Determine whether transmission is possible (ie, appropriate exposure without appropriate personal protection)

4. Determine whether HCP is susceptible (may require laboratory tests)

5. Determine whether PEP is available and indicated

6. Consider alternative prophylaxis (if available) if HCP has a contraindication to the prophylaxis of first choice

7. Administer prophylaxis with informed consent (HCP may choose not to accept prophylaxis)

8. Arrange follow-up

9. Document all of the above in the occupational health record

Box 2
Postexposure prophylaxis counseling of exposed health care providers

Information to be provided to HCP who are exposed to an infectious agent	1. Risk (if known) of acquiring the infectious disease 2. Risk (if known) of transmitting any infection that is acquired to patients, other HCP, and contacts (eg, household members) 3. Methods of preventing transmission of infection to other persons 4. Need for work restrictions (if any) 5. Recommended follow-up
Information to be provided to HCP who are offered prophylaxis	1. Recommendations for prophylaxis 2. Alternative methods of prophylaxis if the primary method is contraindicated 3. Degree of protection provided by the therapy 4. Potential side effects of the therapy 5. Safety laboratory tests (if recommended) 6. Risks (if known) of infection if PEP is refused

syphilis, tuberculosis, and varicella/zoster. PEP is also available for some exposures, including animal bites (eg, dogs, cats, rodents, primates) and human bites. However, PEP is not available for exposure to arboviruses, hepatitis C, mumps, parvovirus B19, rubella, SARS-CoV-2, and Middle East respiratory syndrome coronavirus (MERS-CoV). PEP may consist of antivirals, antibiotics, immunoglobulin preparations, and/or vaccines. Immunoglobulin (IG) preparations may be indicated as part of PEP for exposure to hepatitis A (IG), hepatitis B (hepatitis B IG [HBIG]), measles (IG), rabies (rabies IG), tetanus (tetanus IG [TIG]), varicella (varicella-zoster IG [VariZIG]), and vaccinia (vaccinia IG [VIG]). More than 1 modality may be recommended. Postexposure antimicrobial prophylaxis is still recommended for pertussis, invasive meningococcal infection, and diphtheria even when the HCP has received preexposure prophylaxis with recommended immunizations.

Exposures to Blood-Borne Pathogens

Occupational exposures to BBPs can occur by percutaneous injury with a sharps object or through mucocutaneous exposure with contact of a mucous membrane or nonintact skin with blood, tissue, or other potentially infectious bodily fluids. Occupational exposures to blood-borne pathogens remain a serious public health concern, with an estimated 385,000 needlesticks and other sharps-related injuries in hospital-based HCP, with similar injuries across other health care settings.[6] The CDC estimates that 5.6 million workers in the health care industry and related occupations are at risk of occupational exposure to BBPs. Dozens of different pathogens have caused documented occupational infection following exposure to blood or body fluids in HCP or hospital laboratory personnel,[7] but the most important BBPs are HIV, HBV, and HCV.[8,9] The key features for assessing the risk of transmission of HBV, HCV, and HIV are for each agent their seroprevalence in the general population, their environmental survival, and transmissibility via percutaneous, mucous membrane, or nonintact skin exposure. The seroprevalence of these viruses in the general population is HBV $\sim$0.3%,[10] HCV $\sim$3.4%,[11] and HIV $\sim$0.4%.[12,13] HBV has been shown to survive and remain infectious for 7 days or more on environmental surfaces.[14] The data on HCV environmental survival have varied with articles reporting survival of 16 hours,[15] 5 days,[16] and up to 6 weeks.[17] For HIV, the $t_{1/2}$ has been reported as 28 hours,[18] with a maximum of several days.[19] The risk of transmission of HBV depends on the route of exposure, whether the exposed person is immune (via immunization or natural infection), and serologic status of the source patient. Rates of clinical hepatitis or serologic evidence of HBV infection in susceptible exposed HCP following a percutaneous exposure have been reported as 22% to 31% and 37% to 62%, respectively. The risk of clinical hepatitis or serologic evidence of HBV infection if the source is hepatitis B surface antigen (HBsAg) positive and hepatitis B E antigen (HBeAg) positive has been reported as 1% to 6% and 23% to 37%, respectively.[20] The risk of transmission of HCV following percutaneous exposure has been reported as 1.8% to 1.9%, but more recently was reported as 0.2%.[13,21–23] The risk of transmission of HIV following percutaneous exposure has been reported as 0.23% (95% confidence intervals, 0.0%–0.46%).[13,24]

In addition to percutaneous transmission, the blood-borne viruses HBV, HCV, and HIV can be transmitted via blood or contaminated fluid exposure of mucous membranes, nonintact skin, or human bites. The risk of transmission by these routes has not been quantitated for HBV and HCV. The risk of transmission by the mucosal route for HIV has been reported to be 0.09% (95% confidence intervals, 0.01%–0.5%).[13] The risk of transmission of HIV via exposure of nonintact skin is likely less than 0.1% but has not been completely quantified. The risk from a human bite has also not been quantified. However, transmission of HBV,[25] HCV,[26] and HIV[27] by human bites has been reported. Importantly, human bites that penetrate the skin should be considered as possible 2-way exposure (ie, from patient to HCP and HCP to patient).

Although the incidence of needlestick injuries has been reduced by advances in education, needle disposal, engineering changes and personnel protection, institutions and HCP must continue to assume responsibility in further reducing the risk. Several methods of reducing exposure to blood and other potential infectious body fluids have been described (**Box 3**).

All occupational exposures to blood and other potentially infectious material place HCP at risk for infection with a BBP. The Occupational Safety and Health Administration (OSHA) defines blood to mean human blood, blood components, and products made from human blood.[25] Other potentially infectious material includes body fluids such as semen, vaginal secretions, cerebrospinal fluid, synovial fluid, pericardial fluid, pleural fluid, peritoneal fluid, human milk, amniotic fluid, saliva associated with dental procedures, and body fluid that is visibly contaminated with blood. All body fluids should be considered infectious in situations where it is difficult or impossible to differentiate between different types of bloody fluids. Any unfixed tissues or organs (other than intact skin) from a human (living or dead) are also considered potentially infectious material.

CLINICAL CARE AND EVALUATION AFTER POTENTIAL EXPOSURE TO BLOOD-BORNE PATHOGENS

Care for HCP who have been exposed to blood or potentially contaminated fluids has been reviewed.[13,20,21,28–32] Exposed HCP should immediately be provided with first aid. Exposed mucous membranes should be flushed with water. Wounds and skin sites that have been in contact with blood or body fluids should be washed with soap and water. Antiseptics, such as chlorhexidine, have not been shown to reduce the risk of HBV transmission. However, there is no contraindication to their use as long as they are not injected into the wound. It is not recommended to squeeze the wound to express fluid or use potentially harmful agents such as bleach. The following are not considered exposures and do not require PEP: (1) contact of intact skin with blood or body fluids; (2) skin was not breached by a sharp; (3) contact with saliva

---

Box 3
Methods of reducing percutaneous, mucous membrane, or nonintact skin exposure to blood or potentially infectious body fluids

1. Strict adherence to standard precautions, including appropriate hand hygiene and use of PPE as indicated by the task (eg, gloves, gowns, masks, eye protection)

2. Use of safety-engineered devices (eg, needles, syringes, scalpels)

3. Use of double gloves during surgical procedures with an increased risk of glove puncture

4. Use of blunted surgical needles, when possible

5. Work practice controls to reduce risk of injuries, such as elimination of capping needles, using tray to pass sharp devices, immediate and appropriately discarding used sharp instruments

6. Puncture-resistant sharp disposal units

7. Precautions should be taken to prevent sharps injuries during procedures and during cleaning and disinfection of instruments

8. Mouthpieces, resuscitation bags, or other ventilation devices should be available whenever their need can be anticipated

9. HCP who have exudative lesions or weeping dermatitis on exposed body areas (hands/ wrist, face/neck) must be excused from providing direct patient care or working patient equipment (Occupational Safety and Health Administration regulation)

10. HCP unable to perform hand hygiene (eg, cast or nonremovable splint) should be prohibited from providing patient care until able to perform hand hygiene

11. Enhanced education on the proper use of safety-engineered devices

---

(nondental), urine, sputum, vomit, or feces that was not visibly contaminated with blood; and (4) a sharp that was not used before the injury.

The source patient for blood and body fluid exposures should be tested for HIV using a fourth-generation test (ie, combined antibody and antigen test), HBsAg, hepatitis C RNA (preferred) or HCV antibody, and other tests as indicated by the source patient's medical history (eg, malaria, syphilis, human T-lymphotropic virus). If the source patient's HCV antibody test is positive, an HCV polymerase chain reaction test should be obtained from the source.

Potential Exposures to Hepatitis B

The risk of HBV acquisition by HCP has declined dramatically over the years. The number of HBV infections among HCP declined by approximately 98% from an estimated 17,000 infections in 1983 to 263 acute HBV infections in 2010. This decline was likely caused by decreased exposure from improved work practice controls (see **Box 3**) and HBV immunization of HCP. However, the risk of HBV transmission from patient to HCP provider remains because there are an estimated 800,000 to 1.4 million persons in the United States living with chronic HBV infection.[20]

The key method of preventing health care–associated HBV infection among HCP is HBV immunization before beginning direct patient care of all HCP with potential blood or body fluid exposure.[33] Further, all HCP should know their immune response to vaccination. For HCP immunized in training or at initiation of patient contact, an antibody to HBsAg (anti-HBs) quantitative titer should be drawn 1 to 2 months after the last dose of vaccine. HCP with greater than or equal to 10 mIU/mL anti-HBs are considered immune for life. HCP who do not respond adequately should be reimmunized with an additional course of HBV vaccine and tested for immunity 1 to 2 months after the last dose. HCP who have not responded adequately (ie, $\geq$10 mIU/mL anti-HBs) should be tested for HBsAg. Nonresponders to 2 appropriate courses of HBV vaccine should be counseled to report any exposures to blood or body fluids because they may be prophylaxed with HBIG (**Table 1**). HCP with a remote history of hepatitis B vaccine should have their immunity to HBV assessed using the algorithm recommended by the CDC.[20]

HCP exposed to an HBsAg-positive patient should be evaluated for prophylaxis per the recommended CDC algorithm (see **Table 1**). HCP known to have responded to vaccine (ie, $\geq$10 mIU/mL anti-HBs) do not need any prophylaxis; unimmunized HCP or HCP with an unknown response should be managed per the CDC algorithm, which may entail the use of hepatitis B vaccine and/or HBIG. PEP should be provided as soon as possible but always within 7 days of exposure. HBIG and hepatitis B vaccine can be administered simultaneously at separate injection sites.[20]

Potential Exposures to Hepatitis C

The incidence of HCV infection in the United States is increasing and thus HCP may be at increased risk of exposure to patients with HCV, including individuals early in disease without serologic evidence of infection. The CDC have updated their guidance on management of exposure of HCP to HCV.[34] Recommendations for source-patient testing include (1) testing with a nucleic acid test (NAT) for HCV RNA as the preferred option, particularly if the source patient is known or suspected to have recent behaviors that increase risk of HCV acquisition, such as injection drug use in the prior 4 months; or (2) testing for antibody to HCV with reflex to NAT if positive. Follow-up testing of HCP is recommended if the source patient is HCV RNA positive, anti-HCV positive with RNA status unknown, or cannot be tested. Recommendations for HCP testing include (1) baseline testing of HCP for antibody to HCV with reflex to NAT if positive within 48 hours after the exposure; (2) if follow-up testing of HCP is recommended based on the source-patient's status, test with an NAT at 3 to 6 weeks postexposure; (3) if the HCP is NAT negative at 3 to 6 weeks postexposure, conduct a final test for anti-HCV antibody at 4 to 6 months postexposure; (4) a source patient or HCP who is positive for HCV RNA should be referred to care.

Potential Exposures to Human Immunodeficiency Virus

The number of persons living with HIV infection has increased over the years in the United States because of the success of antiviral medications. The CDC has estimated that, at the end of 2018, an estimated 1.2 million people aged 13 years and older had HIV in the United States, including an estimated 161,800 (14%) people whose infections had not been diagnosed.[12,35] In the United States, 58 confirmed and 150 possible cases of occupationally acquired HIV infection were reported to the CDC between 1985 and 2013.[36] Since 1999, only 1 confirmed cases (a laboratory technician who sustained a needle puncture while working with a live HIV culture in 2008) has been reported.[36]

The management of HCP exposed to blood or body fluids from persons infected with HIV is well described in the literature.[9,13,29–31,37,38] OSHA requires that all US health care facilities provide postexposure management of HIV exposures consistent with the most recent US Public Health Service guidelines.[30] These guidelines delineate the situations for which expert consultation for HIV PEP is recommended as well as the recommended follow-up for HCP exposed to known or suspected HIV-positive sources. The preferred HIV PEP regimen is Truvada 1 tablet orally once daily (tenofovir disoproxil fumarate [Viread] 300 mg + emtricitabine [Emtriva; FTC] 300 mg) plus raltegravir (Isentress; RAL) 400 mg orally twice daily. The following antiretroviral agents

Table 1
Postexposure management to prevent hepatitis B infection of health care personnel after occupational percutaneous and mucosal exposure to blood and body fluids

HCP Status	Postexposure Testing		PEP		Postvaccination Serologic Testing[b]
	Source Patient (HBsAg)	HCP Testing (Anti-HBs)	HBIG[a]	Vaccination	
Documented responder[c] after complete series (≥3 doses)	No action needed				
Documented nonresponder[d] after 6 doses	Positive/unknown	—[e]	HBIG × 2 separated by 1 mo	—	No
	No action needed				
Response unknown after 3 doses	Positive/unknown	<10 mIU/mL[e]	HBIG × 1	Initial revaccination	Yes
	Negative	<10 mIU/mL	None	—	—
	Any	≥10 mIU/mL	No action needed		
Unvaccinated/incompletely vaccinated or vaccine refusers	Positive/unknown	—[e]	HBIG × 1	Complete vaccination	Yes
	Negative	—	None	Complete vaccination	Yes

[a] HBIG should be administered intramuscularly as soon as possible after exposure when indicated. The effectiveness of HBIG when administered greater than 7 days after percutaneous, mucosal, or nonintact skin exposures is unknown. HBIG dose is 0.06 mL/kg.

[b] Should be performed 1 to 2 months after the last dose of the hepatitis B vaccine series (and 4–6 months after administration of HBIG to avoid detection of passively administered anti-HBs) using a quantitative method that allows detection of the protective concentration of anti-HBs (≥10 mIU/mL).

[c] A responder is defined as a person with anti-HBs level greater than or equal to 10 mIU/mL after greater than or equal to 3 doses of hepatitis B vaccine.

[d] A nonresponder is defined as a person with anti-HBs level less than 10 mIU/mL after greater than or equal to 6 doses of hepatitis B vaccine.

[e] HCP who have anti-HBs level less than 10 mIU/mL, or who are unvaccinated or incompletely vaccinated, and sustain an exposure to a source patient who is HBsAg positive or has unknown HBsAg status, should undergo baseline testing for HBV infection as soon as possible after exposure, and follow-up testing approximately 6 months later. Initial baseline tests consist of total anti-hepatitis B core antibody (anti-HBc); testing at approximately 6 months consists of HBsAg and total anti-HBc.

From Schillie SF, Murphy TV, Sawyer M, et al. CDC guidance for evaluating health-care personnel for hepatitis B virus protection and for administering postexposure management. 2013. Available at: https://www.cdc.gov/mmwr/preview/mmwrhtml/rr6210a1.htm. Accessed.

should be used for PEP only with expert consultation: abacavir (Ziagen; ABC), efavirenz (Sustiva; EFV), enfuvirtide (Fuzeon; T20), fosamprenavir (Lexiva; FOSAPV), maraviroc (Selzentry; MVC), saquinavir (Invirase; SQV), and stavudine (Zerit; d4T). The following agents are generally not recommended for PEP: didanosine (Videx EC; ddl), nelfinavir (Viracept; NFV), and tipranavir (Aptivus; d4T). Nevirapine is contraindicated at PEP. In 2018, the CDC included an update to the existing guidelines to recommend avoidance of dolutegravir for nonpregnant women of childbearing potential who are sexually active or have been sexually assaulted and who are not using an effective birth control method and pregnant women early in pregnancy.[40]

POSTEXPOSURE PROPHYLAXIS FOR NON–BLOOD-BORNE PATHOGEN EXPOSURES
Neisseria meningitidis

Neisseria meningitidis, a gram-negative diplococcus and causative agent of invasive meningococcal disease, has at least 13 serogroups based on capsular typing. Five serogroups (ie, A, B, C, W, and Y) cause most disease worldwide; 3 of these serogroups (B, C, and Y) cause most of the illness in the United States.[41,42] The incidence of invasive meningococcal disease varies over time and by age and location.[43,44] In recent years, the incidence of invasive disease has declined in the United States, with a historic low in 2018. Based on reported cases in 2018, the CDC estimated that there were 330 cases (0.14 per 100,000) and 39 deaths in the United States.[45]

N meningitidis is transmitted person to person via respiratory and throat secretions (saliva or spit) during close (eg, coughing, kissing) or lengthy contact (eg, living in the same household). The carriage frequency of N meningitidis in children and young adults is ~10%.[46] Outbreaks most often occur in communities, schools, colleges, prisons, and other closed populations.[42] HCP have acquired invasive meningococcal infection as a result of providing direct care (eg, assisting in endotracheal intubation and airway suctioning) to infected patients.[47] It has been estimated that clinical microbiologists have an attack rate greater than 50 times high than the background rate of invasive meningococcal disease.[48] For this reasons, the CDC/ACIP recommend that clinical and research microbiologists who might be routinely exposed to isolates of N meningitidis receive both the quadrivalent meningococcal vaccine (Men4ACWY) and the meningococcal serogroup B vaccine (MenB) as preexposure prophylaxis. In addition, HCP at increased risk during an outbreak are recommended to receive both vaccines.[49] Recommendations for timing of booster doses are provided in the updated guidelines. In addition, if HCP have underlying medical conditions that place them at increased risk of invasive disease (ie, anatomic or functional asplenia; complement component deficiencies such as C3, C5–C9, properdin, factor H, or factor D; complement inhibitor such as eculizumab [Soliris] or ravulizumab [Ultomiris] use; or human immunodeficiency virus infection), vaccination is recommended with Men4ACWY and MenB, with the exception of individuals with HIV for the latter. Such HCP should receive a booster dose of MenACWY every 5 years if they remain at increased risk and a booster dose of serogroup B meningococcal vaccine at 1 year after completion of primary vaccination and every 2 to 3 years thereafter (MenB-FHbp and MenB-4C are not interchangeable).

Chemoprophylaxis of household members of an index case of invasive meningococcal disease is recommended.[43,44,50] Chemoprophylaxis of exposed HCP is advised for all persons who have had intensive, unprotected contact (ie, without wearing a mask) with infected patients (eg, via mouth-to-mouth resuscitation, endotracheal intubation, or endotracheal tube management) with invasive meningococcal disease.

Chemoprophylaxis for HCP should be recommended even if the HCP has been vaccinated with a meningococcal vaccine.[8] Because the rate of secondary disease for close contacts is highest immediately after onset of disease in the index patient, antimicrobial chemoprophylaxis should be administered as soon as possible (ideally <24 hours after identification of the index patient). In contrast, chemoprophylaxis administered more than 14 days after exposure to the index patient is probably of limited or no value. Oropharyngeal or nasopharyngeal cultures are not helpful in determining the need for chemoprophylaxis and might delay institution of this preventive measure unnecessarily. Chemoprophylaxis is not recommended for close contacts of patients with evidence of N meningitidis only in nonsterile sites (eg, oropharyngeal, endotracheal, or conjunctival); however, in some instances, meningococcal pneumonia may be managed as invasive disease. Asymptomatic nasopharyngeal carriers of N meningitidis without an exposure do not require treatment or chemoprophylaxis.

There is strong evidence that several antibiotics (ie, rifampin, ciprofloxacin, ceftriaxone) and moderate evidence that other antibiotics (ie, azithromycin, cefixime) are highly effective in eradication of meningococcal carriage (ie, 90%–95%).[51–53] The preferred drugs for exposed HCP are rifampin (600 mg orally every 12 hours for 2 days) or ciprofloxacin (500 mg orally for 1 dose). The preferred agent in pregnant women is ceftriaxone (250 mg intramuscularly for 1 dose, diluted with 1% lidocaine to decrease pain at the injection site).[53] Although sporadic resistance to rifampin and ciprofloxacin has been reported worldwide, meningococcal resistance to chemoprophylaxis antibiotics remains rare in the United States.[53] This finding was recently reaffirmed in a recent population-based surveillance of antimicrobial resistance in N meningitidis strains from the United States.[54] All strains tested were susceptible to ceftriaxone and azithromycin; 99% of strains were susceptible to ciprofloxacin and rifampin. In 2019 to 2020, 11 meningococcal isolates from US patients had isolates containing a β-lactamase gene associated with penicillin resistance and mutations associated with ciprofloxacin resistance. An additional 22 cases reported during 2013 to 2020 involved the same gene but did not have mutations associated with ciprofloxacin resistance. Based on these findings, in states that have experienced meningococcal disease cases caused by ciprofloxacin-resistant strains during the past 1 to 2 years, clinicians and public health staff members should consider antimicrobial susceptibility testing on meningococcal isolates to inform prophylaxis decisions.[55] Although azithromycin is not recommended for use as a first-line chemoprophylaxis agent, azithromycin has been recommended for chemoprophylaxis in the rare circumstance of sustained ciprofloxacin resistance in a community. Use of azithromycin as a single oral dose has been shown to be effective for eradication of nasopharyngeal carriage and can be used on a limited basis where ciprofloxacin resistance has been detected.[49]

Varicella

Before the introduction of the varicella vaccine in 1995, varicella was a common disease; an average of 4 million people got chickenpox, 10,500 to 13,000 were hospitalized (range, 8000–18,000), and 100 to 150 died each year.[56] Since the introduction of the varicella vaccine, there has been a dramatic decrease in the number of cases of varicella, hospitalizations, and deaths. However, because varicella may be acquired from exposure to varicella or zoster, exposure in health care settings will continue to occur. Multiple nosocomial outbreaks of varicella-zoster virus (VZV) have been reported.[1] Nosocomial transmission has been attributed to delays in the diagnosis or reporting of varicella or herpes zoster (HZ) and to failures to implement control measures promptly. In hospitals and other health care settings, airborne transmission of VZV from patients with either varicella or HZ has resulted in varicella in HCP and patients who had no direct contact with the index patient.[57] Although all susceptible patients in health care settings are at risk for severe varicella disease with complications, certain patients without evidence of immunity are at increased risk: pregnant women, premature infants born to susceptible mothers, infants born at less than 28 weeks' gestation or who weigh less than or equal to 1000 g regardless of maternal immune status, and immunocompromised persons of all ages (including persons who are undergoing immunosuppressive therapy, have malignant disease, or are immunodeficient).[56]

Guidelines for postexposure management of HCP exposed to varicella or zoster have been published by the CDC, AAP,[2] and APHA.[4] Exposure to VZV is defined as close contact with an infectious person, such as close indoor contact (eg, in the same room) or face-to-face contact. Experts differ regarding the duration of contact; some suggest 5 minutes, and others up to 1 hour; all agree that it does not include transitory contact.[2] PEP with vaccination or VariZIG (Cangene Corporation, Winnipeg, Canada)[58] depends on immune status of the exposed HCP. HCP who have history of natural infection to varicella (physician-diagnosed disease) or who received 2 doses of vaccine and who are exposed to VZV (varicella, disseminated HZ, and uncovered lesions of a localized HZ) should be monitored daily during days 8 to 21 after exposure for fever, skin lesions, and systemic symptoms suggestive of varicella. HCP can be monitored directly by occupational health program or infection-control practitioners or instructed to report fever, headache, or other constitutional symptoms and any atypical skin lesions immediately. HCP should be excluded from a work facility immediately if symptoms occur.[1] HCP who have received 1 dose of vaccine and who are exposed to VZV should receive the second dose within 3 to 5 days after exposure to rash (provided 4 weeks have elapsed after the first dose). After vaccination, management is similar to that of 2-dose vaccine recipients. Those who did not receive a second dose or who received the second dose more than 5 days after exposure should be excluded from work for 8 to 21 days after exposure.

For HCP at risk for severe disease for whom varicella vaccination is contraindicated (eg, pregnant or immunocompromised HCP without evidence of immunity), varicellazoster immune globulin after exposure is recommended. If indicated, VariZIG should be administered as soon as possible following VZV exposure, ideally within 96 hours for greatest effectiveness but always within 10 days.[58] VariZIG is supplied in 125-IU vials and should be administered intramuscularly; the recommended dose is 125 IU/10 kg of body weight, up to a maximum of 625 IU (5 vials). If VariZIG is indicated but not available or more than 10 days have elapsed since the exposure, PEP can be provided with oral acyclovir (20 mg/kg per dose administered 4 times per day; maximum daily dose, 3200 mg) or oral valacyclovir (20 mg/kg per dose administered 3 times per day; maximum daily dose, 3000 mg) beginning on day 8 postexposure and continuing for 7 to 14 days.

Pertussis

In the United States, the highest recorded annual incidence of pertussis occurred in 1934, when greater than 260,000 cases were reported.[23] After the introduction of diphtheria, tetanus, and whole-cell pertussis vaccine, the incidence dramatically declined. However, in recent years there has been a resurgence of pertussis. Possible explanations for this increase in disease include (1) genetic changes in *Bordetella pertussis*, making vaccine less effective; (2) waning immunity among children, adolescents, and adults vaccinated during childhood, especially those who received acellular pertussis vaccines; (3) lessened effectiveness of acellular pertussis vaccines compared with whole-cell vaccines; (4) greater awareness of pertussis and hence more diagnostic testing; and (5) the general availability of better laboratory tests.[59]

Multiple nosocomial outbreaks of pertussis have been reported, including outbreaks in which an infected HCP was the source.[60–62] Nosocomial outbreaks have occurred for several reasons: (1) failure of all HCP to have been immunized with Tdap; (2) failure to recognize and appropriately isolate infected patients, (3) failure to provide antibiotic prophylaxis to exposed staff, and (4) failure to furlough symptomatic staff.[39,63] Seroprevalence studies of HCP who did not receive pertussis vaccine since childhood have revealed that 6.4%[64] and 15%[65] had evidence of recent infection. At present, CDC guidelines permit the use of Tdap every 10 years instead of Td. Therefore, all HCP should be recommended to receive a Tdap every 10 years by their local medical provider as part of their standard immunizations.[66]

Prevention of pertussis transmission in health care settings involves diagnosis and early treatment of clinical cases, droplet isolation of infectious patients, exclusion from work of HCP who are infectious, and PEP.[1] Guidelines for postexposure management of HCP exposed to pertussis have been published by the CDC, AAP,[2] and APHA.[4] Data on the need for PEP in Tdap-vaccinated HCP are inconclusive, and prior immunization with Tdap may not preclude the need for PEP.[67] Postexposure antimicrobial prophylaxis is recommended for all HCP who have unprotected exposure to pertussis and, if infected during the exposure window, would be likely to subsequently expose a patient at risk for severe pertussis (eg, hospitalized neonates and pregnant women). Other HCP should either receive postexposure antimicrobial prophylaxis or be monitored daily for 21 days after pertussis exposure and treated at the onset of signs and symptoms of pertussis.

B pertussis is highly susceptible in vitro to erythromycin[68,69] and the newer macrolides, azithromycin and clarithromycin.[70] It is also susceptible to trimethoprim-sulfamethoxazole.[69–73] Azithromycin has been shown to be effective in the prophylaxis and treatment of pertussis.[74] It is now the preferred agent because, compared with erythromycin, it requires a short period of PEP or therapy (5 vs 7–14 days) and a reduced dosing frequency (1 vs 4 times per day), and is less likely to result in gastrointestinal distress.[74] Trimethoprim-sulfamethoxazole is the recommended alternative for treatment and for chemoprophylaxis of individuals intolerant to a macrolide, although its efficacy as a chemoprophylactic agent has not been evaluated.

POSTEXPOSURE PROPHYLAXIS: OTHERS
Tetanus

Tetanus is an uncommon disease in the United States, with approximately 30 reported cases per year.[47] Nearly all cases of tetanus are among people who have never received tetanus vaccine or adults who did not stay current with their 10-year booster shots. HCP are not at greater risk for tetanus than the general population but, like other adults, may acquire tetanus if they are insufficiently immunized and they have contaminated puncture wounds, open wounds, burns, or crush injuries. HCP with injuries that could lead to tetanus should be evaluated and provided appropriate PEP based on the nature of the wound (ie, clean, minor wound vs higher-risk wounds) and their history of receipt of tetanus toxoid per recommendations of the CDC[48,75] and AAP.[2] If a Td booster is indicated, Tdap can be substituted.

Diphtheria

Although diphtheria was a widespread disease in the United States before the use of vaccines, it is now a rare disease. Between 2004 and 2015, only 2 cases were reported in the United States, although the disease continues to cause illness globally.[50] Importantly, the case-fatality rate is still 5% to 10%. HCP are not at greater risk for diphtheria than the general population.[1] For HCP exposed to nasopharyngeal secretions of a patient known or suspected to have diphtheria, the following postexposure measures should be taken regardless of their immunization status: (1) surveillance for 7 days for evidence of disease, (2) culture for *Corynebacterium diphtheriae*, and (3) antimicrobial prophylaxis with erythromycin (up to 1 g orally for 7–10 days) or a single injection of penicillin G benzathine (1.2 million U intramuscularly × 1). Asymptomatic exposed HCP should also receive a booster dose of Td if they have not received a booster dose of a diphtheria toxoid–containing vaccine within 5 years.[43] Exposed HCP should not receive equine diphtheria antitoxin because there is no evidence that antitoxin provides additional benefits for contacts who have received antimicrobial prophylaxis.

Measles

The incidence of measles has decreased dramatically since the widespread use of MMR vaccine. Since 2000, when measles was declared eliminated from the United States, the annual number of cases has ranged from a low of 37 in 2004 to a high of 1282 in 2019.[76] Measles cases in the United States occur as a result of importations by people who were infected while in other countries and often further spread of measles in US communities with pockets of unvaccinated people. Nosocomial measles is well documented in the literature and may contribute to the propagation of community outbreaks.[54,62,77,78] Investigations of individual outbreaks have reported that 17% to 59% of infections were acquired in a medical setting. Measles represents an important health hazard for HCP because (1) it is highly infectious, (2) transmission occurs via the airborne route, (3) persons become infectious 4 days before the onset of the characteristic rash, and (4) transmission in the outpatient setting has occurred even though the index cases had left the waiting or examination room up to 75 minutes earlier. Because of the greater opportunity for exposure, HCP are at higher risk than the general population for becoming infected with measles.

If measles exposures occur in a health care facility, all nonprotected HCP should be evaluated immediately for presumptive evidence of measles immunity; HCP without evidence of immunity should be offered the first dose of MMR vaccine and excluded from work from day 5 to 21 following exposure.[1] Available data suggest that live virus measles vaccine, if administered within 72 hours of measles exposure, prevents or modifies disease. HCP without evidence of immunity who are not vaccinated after exposure should be removed from all patient contact and excluded from the facility from day 5 after their first exposure through day 21 after the last exposure, even if they have received postexposure intramuscular immune globulin of 0.25 mL/kg (40 mg of immunoglobulin G per kilogram). Daily monitoring should be implemented for HCP with evidence of immunity to measles who are exposed to measles for signs and symptoms of measles infection for 21 days from last exposure. Those with documentation of 1 vaccine dose may remain at work and should receive the second dose. Immunoglobulin PEP is especially recommended for serosusceptible pregnant women and immunocompromised persons (0.5 mL/kg; maximum dose 15 mL). If immune globulin is administered to an exposed person, observations should continue for signs and symptoms of measles for 28 days after exposure because immunoglobulin may prolong the incubation period. HCP with measles should be furloughed from work for 4 days after the rash appears. HCP with known or suspected measles should be excluded from work for 4 days after the rash seems. Consider excluding immunosuppressed HCP who acquire measles from work for the duration of their illness.

Hepatitis A

Occasional outbreaks of hepatitis A virus (HAV) have been reported in hospitals.[79] Risk factors for HAV transmission to personnel have included activities that increase the risk of fecal-oral contamination, including caring for a person with unrecognized hepatitis A infection; sharing food, beverages, or cigarettes with patients, their families, or the staff; nail biting; handling bile without proper precautions; and not washing hands or not wearing gloves when providing care to an infected patient.[79,80] However, routine immunization of HCP with hepatitis A vaccine is not recommended because seroprevalence studies have not shown that HCP are at increased risk for HAV infection because of occupational exposure.[1,79] Maintenance workers who may be exposed to sewage are also not at increased risk for acquisition of hepatitis A and do not need to be vaccinated.

Hepatitis A vaccine may be used for PEP and control of a nosocomial outbreak for persons more than 1 year of age.[81] In these cases, only monovalent hepatitis A vaccine should be used and should be administered within 14 days of exposure. Exposed immunocompetent HCP who have not completed a hepatitis A vaccine series should receive a single dose of hepatitis A vaccine, and, for those more than 40 years of age with additional risk factors as outlined in the CDC guidelines, hepatitis A immune globulin (0.1–0.2 mL/kg).[81] Exposed immunocompromised HCP who have not completed the 2-dose hepatitis A vaccine series should receive both hepatitis A vaccine and immune globulin simultaneously in a different anatomic site. HCP should complete the 2-dose series; however, the second dose is not necessary for PEP to be effective and the second dose should not be administered before 6 months after the first dose. The efficacy of hepatitis A vaccine and immune globulin for PEP when administered more than 2 weeks after exposure has not been established.

Human Bites

HCP occasionally receive a human bite, especially when caring for behavioral health patients. Following a human bite, a semicircular or oval area of erythema or bruising is usually visible; the skin itself may or may not be intact. Wound care of a human bite is similar to that of an animal bite.[82] The bite area should be managed as follows: (1) clean the wound with an antiseptic; (2) trim any superficial devitalized tissue; (3) remove any foreign bodies or gross wound contaminants; and (4) assess the injury for tendon damage, vascular damage, or penetration into bone or joint. Most human bites should be left open to heal by secondary intention. However, if the wound may lead to a poor cosmetic result (eg, facial bites), the clinician may choose to close the wound. Human bites frequently develop infection. In general, all HCP with a human bite should receive antimicrobial prophylaxis (eg, amoxicillin-clavulanate) with the first dose provided as soon as possible after the injury.[83] An initial parenteral dose of antibiotics is often provided to rapidly obtain an effective tissue level followed by 3 to 5 days of oral antibiotics.[83] Recommendations for specific antimicrobial therapy have been published.[2]

All HCP with a human bite should be assessed as to whether tetanus prophylaxis should be provided. As noted earlier, human bites may lead to patient-to-HCP and HCP-to-patient transmission of BBPs (ie, HIV, HBV, and HCV). Thus the HCP is both an exposed person as well as a potential source for transmission and, hence, the same blood work ordered on the source should be obtained regardless of whether the source was a patient or HCP.

Rabies

Rabies is primarily a disease of animals.[84] The epidemiology of human rabies is a reflection of both the distribution of the disease in animals and the degree of contact with these animals. Rabies is most commonly acquired via a bite or scratch from a rabid animal or from contact between nonintact skin and infective saliva. Saliva and nervous tissue are highly infectious. In general, contact with other body fluids does not constitute exposure. Uncommon routes of infection include contamination of mucous membranes, corneal transplant, exposure to aerosols from spelunking or laboratory activities, and iatrogenic infection through improperly inactivated vaccines. Human-to-human transmission has rarely been reported.[84] Human rabies cases in the United States are rare, with only 1 to 3 cases reported annually.[85]

Rabies prophylaxis occasionally needs to be provided to HCP who work out of doors (eg, maintenance workers, personnel who care for grounds) and receive a bite from a wild animal that could potentially transmit rabies (eg, fox, raccoon) or have bat exposure. Concern about rabies transmission is frequent among HCP who have cared for human patients with rabies, especially because fluids from the upper and lower respiratory tracts of humans frequently test positive for rabies virus. One review article reported that ~30% of HCP who provided direct care for a patient with rabies were provided PEP.[86] The CDC recommends that patients with possible or known rabies be cared for using standard precautions.[87] However, given HCP concerns and the rare possible risk of rabies transmission, the authors believe that HCP should use PPE to prevent contact with the patient's saliva and respiratory secretions (ie, gown, gloves, mask, eye protection). HCP with mucous membrane or percutaneous skin exposure to a potentially rabid animal or human should receive postexposure rabies vaccine and rabies immune globulin as recommended by the CDC.[88]

Ectoparasites

Exposure of HCP to ectoparasites (eg, scabies, pediculosis) is likely common. Such exposed personnel should be evaluated for signs and symptoms of an infestation and provided appropriate therapy for confirmed or suspected scabies.[89] For non-crusted scabies, consider prophylactic therapy for HCP who had prolonged skin-to-skin contact with suspected and confirmed cases. For crusted scabies, all HCP who may have been exposed to the patient, or to clothing, bedding, or furniture used by such a patient, should be identified and treated. Treatment should be strongly considered even in equivocal circumstances because of the complexity of controlling an institutional outbreak and the low risk associated with treatment.

Syphilis

HCP are at risk for acquired syphilis via unprotected contact with syphilitic skin lesions such as chancres (primary stage) and rashes or sores (secondary stage). It can also be acquired via contact with secretions of children with congenital syphilis.[90] Before the standard practice of using gloves by HCP to examine patients with nonintact skin, there were reports of extragenital syphilitic lesions on HCP. Therefore, HCP who have had unprotected direct contact with syphilitic skin lesions of early congenital syphilis before identification of the disease or during the first 24 hours of therapy should be examined clinically for the presence of lesions 2 to 3 weeks after contact.[2] Serologic testing should be performed and repeated 3 months after contact or sooner if symptoms occur. HCP with unprotected contact of skin lesions of a patient with primary or secondary disease should be similarly managed. If the degree of exposure is considered substantial, immediate treatment should be considered.[2] The most current CDC sexually transmitted disease treatment guideline should be used to guide postexposure therapy.[91]

Influenza

As noted earlier, all HCP should be immunized annually against influenza. However, CDC has provided detailed recommendations on PEP for HCP exposed to influenza as well as the use of antivirals in outbreak situations.[92,93] Unvaccinated HCP who have occupational exposures and who did not use adequate PPE at the time of exposure are potential candidates for chemoprophylaxis. Although postexposure use of influenza vaccine does not prevent infection, vaccine can be offered when exposed individuals are identified as not yet immunized. Decisions on whether to administer antivirals for chemoprophylaxis should take into account the exposed person's risk for influenza complications, the type and duration of contact, recommendations from local or public health authorities, and clinical judgment. Chemoprophylaxis with antiviral medications is not a substitute for influenza vaccination when influenza vaccine is available. HCP receiving PEP should be informed that chemoprophylaxis reduces but does not eliminate the risk for influenza, that susceptibility to influenza returns once the antiviral medication is stopped, and that influenza vaccination is recommended if available. Oral oseltamivir, inhaled zanamivir, or oral baloxavir are recommended for antiviral chemoprophylaxis of influenza virus infection. The emphasis is on early treatment as an alternative to chemoprophylaxis in managing HCP who have had a suspected exposure to influenza virus. Recommendations for dosing and duration of each agent are provided; however, PEP is typically administered for a total of 7 days (1 day for baloxavir).[92]

Chemoprophylaxis can also be used as a control measure in outbreaks in health care facilities, especially if they house patients at higher risk for influenza complications.[92] In addition to antiviral medications, other outbreak-control measures include instituting droplet and contact precautions and establishing cohorts of patients with confirmed or suspected influenza, reoffering influenza vaccination (if available) to unvaccinated staff and patients, restricting staff movement between wards or buildings, and restricting contact between ill staff or visitors and patients. For control of outbreaks in institutional settings (eg, long-term care facilities for elderly people and children) and hospitals, CDC recommends antiviral chemoprophylaxis with oral oseltamivir or inhaled zanamivir for a minimum of 2 weeks and continuing up to 1 week after the last known case was identified. Antiviral chemoprophylaxis is recommended for all residents, including those who have received influenza vaccination. Baloxavir is approved for PEP (single dose) of influenza in persons aged 12 years and older.

SUMMARY

Identification and confirmation of communicable diseases exposures, counseling and evaluation of exposed HCP, and provision of PEP is an essential function of occupational health programs.

CLINICS CARE POINTS

- All HCP should be educated at their initiation of employment or providing service when and how to report a potential infectious disease exposure.
- Postexposure evaluation and management for BBPs and non–blood-borne pathogens is pathogen specific

DISCLOSURE

The authors have nothing to disclose.

REFERENCES

1. Shefer A, Atkinson W, Friedman C, et al. Immunization of health-care personnel: recommendations of the Advisory Committee on Immunization Practices (ACIP). MMWR Recomm Rep 2011;60(7, Suppl. S):1–45.

2. Kimberlin DW. Red Book: 2018-2021 report of the committee on infectious diseases. Itasca, IL: American Academy of Pediatrics; 2018.

3. Sebazco S. APIC text of infection control and epidemiology. Section V. Occupational health. Washington, DC: APIC; 2005.

4. American Public Health Association, ed Control of Communicable Diseases Manual. 2020. Heymann D, ed.

5. Centers for Disease Control and Prevention. (2020b). Interim U.S. Guidance for Risk Assessment and Work Restrictions for Healthcare Personnel with Potential Exposure to COVID-19. Retrieved 1/16/2021 from https://www.cdc.gov/coronavirus/2019-ncov/hcp/guidance-risk-assesmenthcp.html.

6. Centers for Disease Control and Prevention. Sharps safety for healthcare settings. Available at: http://www.cdc.gov/sharpssafety/index.html. Accessed 1/21/2021.

7. Tarantola A, Abiteboul D, Rachline A. Infection risks following accidental exposure to blood or body fluids in health care workers: a review of pathogens transmitted in published cases. Am J Infect Control 2006;34(6):367–75.

8. Nelson CB, Birmingham M, Costa A, et al. Preparedness for infectious threats: public-private partnership to develop an affordable vaccine for an emergent threat: the trivalent Neisseria meningitidis ACW135 polysaccharide vaccine. Am J Public Health 2007;97(Suppl 1):S15–22.

9. Deuffic-Burban S, Delarocque-Astagneau E, Abiteboul D, et al. Blood-borne viruses in health care workers: prevention and management. J Clin Virol 2011; 52(1):4–10.

10. Centers for Disease Control and Prevention. Hepatitis B Questions and Answers for Health Professionals. Available at: https://www.cdc.gov/hepatitis/hbv/hbvfaq.htm#overview. Accessed 1/16/2021.

11. Centers for Disease Control and Prevention. Hepatitis C Questions and Answers for Health Professionals. Available at: https://www.cdc.gov/hepatitis/hcv/hcvfaq.htm#section1. Accessed 1/16/2021.

12. Centers for Disease Control and Prevention. HIV/AIDS. Basic statistics. Retrieved 1/21/2021 from http://www.cdc.gov/hiv/basics/statistics.html.

13. Chapman LE, Sullivent EE, Grohskopf LA, et al. Recommendations for postexposure interventions to prevent infection with hepatitis B virus, hepatitis C virus, or human immunodeficiency virus, and tetanus in persons wounded during bombings and other mass-casualty events–United States, 2008: recommendations of the Centers for Disease Control and Prevention (CDC). MMWR Recomm Rep 2008;57(RR-6):1–21 [quiz: CE21-24].

14. Bond WW, Favero MS, Petersen NJ, et al. Survival of hepatitis-B virus after drying and storage for one week. Lancet 1981;1(8219):550–1.

15. Kamili S, Krawczynski K, McCaustland K, et al. Infectivity of hepatitis C virus in plasma after drying and storing at room temperature. Infect Control Hosp Epidemiol 2007;28(5):519–24.

16. Doerrbecker J, Friesland M, Ciesek S, et al. Inactivation and survival of hepatitis C virus on inanimate surfaces. J Infect Dis 2011;204(12):1830–8.

17. Paintsil E, Binka M, Patel A, et al. Hepatitis C virus maintains infectivity for weeks after drying on inanimate surfaces at room temperature: implications for risks of transmission. J Infect Dis 2014;209(8):1205–11.

18. Tjotta E, Hungnes O, Grinde B. Survival of Hiv-1 activity after disinfection, temperature and Ph changes, or drying. J Med Virol 1991;35(4):223–7.

19. Vanbueren J, Simpson RA, Jacobs P, et al. Survival of human-immunodeficiency-virus in suspension and dried onto surfaces. J Clin Microbiol 1994;32(2):571–4.

20. Schillie SF, Murphy TV, Sawyer M, et al. CDC guidance for evaluating health-care personnel for hepatitis B virus protection and for administering postexposure management. MMWR Recomm Rep 2013;62(10):1-19.
21. Henderson DK. Managing occupational risks for hepatitis C transmission in the health care setting. Clin Microbiol Rev 2003;16(3):546–68.
22. Egro FM, Nwaiwu CA, Smith S, et al. Seroconversion rates among health care workers exposed to hepatitis C virus-contaminated body fluids: The University of Pittsburgh 13-year experience. Am J Infect Control 2017;45(9):1001–5.
23. Centers for Disease Control and Prevention. Pertussis: surveillance and reporting. Retrieved 1/15/2021 from http://www.cdc.gov/pertussis/surv-reporting.html.
24. Baggaley RF, Boily MC, White RG, et al. Risk of HIV-1 transmission for parenteral exposure and blood transfusion: a systematic review and meta-analysis. AIDS 2006;20(6):805–12.
25. Gane E, Calder L. Transmission of HBV from patient to healthcare worker. N Z Med J 2008;121(1269):87–8.
26. Akhtar S, Moatter T, Azam SI, et al. Prevalence and risk factors for intrafamilial transmission of hepatitis C virus in Karachi, Pakistan. J Viral Hepat 2002;9(4): 309–14.
27. Richman KM, Rickman LS. The Potential for Transmission of Human-Immunodeficiency-Virus through Human Bites. J Acquir Immune Defic Syndr (1988) 1993;6(4):402–6.
28. Michelin A, Henderson DK. Infection control guidelines for prevention of health care-associated transmission of hepatitis B and C viruses. Clin Liver Dis 2010; 14(1):119–36, ix-x.
29. Henderson DK. Management of needlestick injuries a house officer who has a needlestick. JAMA 2012;307(1):75–84.
30. Kuhar DT, Henderson DK, Struble KA, et al. Updated US Public Health Service Guidelines for the Management of occupational exposures to human immunodeficiency virus and recommendations for postexposure prophylaxis. Infect Control Hosp Epidemiol 2013;34(9):875–92.
31. Beekmann SE, Henderson DK. Prevention of Human Immunodeficiency Virus and AIDS: postexposure prophylaxis (including health care workers). Infect Dis Clin North Am 2014;28(4):601–13.
32. Riddell A, Kennedy I, Tong CYW. Management of sharps injuries in the healthcare setting. BMJ 2015;351:h3733.
33. Schillie S, Harris A, Link-Gelles R, et al. Recommendations of the Advisory Committee on Immunization Practices for use of a hepatitis B vaccine with a novel adjuvant. MMWR Morb Mortal Wkly Rep 2018;67(15):455.
34. Moorman AC. Testing and clinical management of health care personnel potentially exposed to hepatitis C virus—CDC guidance, United States, 2020. MMWR Recomm Rep 2020;69:1–8.
35. Centers for Disease Control and Prevention. HIV surveillance report, vol. 31, 2018. Available at: http://www.cdc.gov/hiv/library/reports/hiv-surveillance.html. Accessed 1/15/2021.
36. Joyce MP, Kuhar D, Brooks JT. Occupationally acquired HIV infection among health care workers - United States, 1985-2013. MMWR Morb Mortal Wkly Rep 2015;63(53):1245–6.
37. Grant RM, Smith DK. Integrating antiretroviral strategies for human immunodeficiency virus prevention: post- and pre-exposure prophylaxis and early treatment. Open Forum Infect Dis 2015;2(4):ofv126.

38. Ford N, Shubber Z, Calmy A, et al. Choice of antiretroviral drugs for postexposure prophylaxis for adults and adolescents: a systematic review. Clin Infect Dis 2015; 60:S170–6.

39. Weber DJ, Rutala WA. Pertussis: a continuing hazard for healthcare facilities. Infect Control Hosp Epidemiol 2001;22(12):736–40.

40. Centers for Disease Control and Prevention. (2018). Interim Statement Regarding Potential Fetal Harm from Exposure to Dolutegravir- Implications for HIV Post-exposure Prophylaxis (PEP). Retrieved 1/16/2021 from https://stacks.cdc.gov/view/cdc/20711.

41. Centers for Disease Control and Prevention. Meningococcal disease. Available at: http://www.cdc.gov/meningococcal/index.html. Accessed 1/21/2021.

42. Centers for Disease Control and Prevention. ABCs report: Neisseria Meningitidis, provisional-2014. Available at: http://www.cdc.gov/abcs/reports-findings/survreports/mening14.html. Accessed 1/22/2021.

43. Halperin SA, Bettinger JA, Greenwood B, et al. The changing and dynamic epidemiology of meningococcal disease. Vaccine 2012;30:B26–36.

44. Dwilow R, Fanella S. Invasive meningococcal disease in the 21st century-An update for the clinician. Curr Neurol Neurosci Rep 2015;15(3).

45. National Center for Immunization and Respiratory Diseases. Enhanced Meningococcal Disease Surveillance Report, 2018. Available at: https://www.cdc.gov/meningococcal/downloads/NCIRDEMS-Report-2018.pdf. Accessed 1/16/2021.

46. Abio A, Neal KR, Beck CR. An epidemiological review of changes in meningococcal biology during the last 100 years. Pathog Glob Health 2013;107(7): 373–80.

47. Centers for Disease Control and Prevention. About tetanus. Available at: http://www.cdc.gov/tetanus/about/index.html. Accessed 1/14/2021.

48. Centers for Disease Control and Prevention. (2015). Tetanus: epidemiology and prevention of vaccinepreventable disease. The pink book. Centers for Disease Control and Prevention. Retrieved 1/21/2021 from http://www.cdc.gov/vaccines/pubs/pinkbook/tetanus.html.

49. Mbaeyi SA, Bozio CH, Duffy J, et al. Meningococcal vaccination: recommendations of the advisory committee on immunization practices, United States, 2020. MMWR Recomm Rep 2020;69(9):1.

50. World Health Organization. Diphtheria reported cases. Available at: https://apps.who.int/immunization_monitoring/globalsummary/timeseries/tsincidencediphtheria.html. Accessed 1/15/2021.

51. Hanquet G, Stefanoff P, Hellenbrand W, et al. Strong public health recommendations from weak evidence? Lessons learned in developing guidance on the public health management of meningococcal disease. Biomed Res Int 2015;2015: 569235.

52. Trestioreanu AZ, Fraser A, Gafter-Gvili A, et al. Antibiotics for preventing meningococcal infections. Cochrane Database Syst Rev 2013;(10):CD004785.

53. Cohn AC, MacNeil JR, Clark TA, et al. Prevention and control of meningococcal disease: recommendations of the Advisory Committee on Immunization Practices (ACIP). MMWR Recomm Rep 2013;62(RR-2):1–28.

54. Botelho-Nevers E, Gautret P, Biellik R, et al. Nosocomial transmission of measles: an updated review. Vaccine 2012;30(27):3996–4001.

55. McNamara LA, Potts C, Blain AE, et al. Detection of ciprofloxacin-resistant, β-lactamase-producing Neisseria meningitidis Serogroup Y Isolates - United States, 2019-2020. MMWR Morb Mortal Wkly Rep 2020;69(24):735–9.

56. Centers for Disease Control and Prevention. Monitoring the impact of varicella immunization. Available at: http://www.cdc.gov/chickenpox/hcp/monitoring-varicella.html. Accessed 1/21/2021.

57. Josephson A, Gombert ME. Airborne transmission of nosocomial varicella from localized zoster. J Infect Dis 1988;158(1):238–41.

58. Marin M, Bialek SR, Seward JF. Updated recommendations for use of VariZIG - United States, 2013. MMWR Morb Mortal Wkly Rep 2013;62(28):574–6.

59. Cherry JD. Pertussis: challenges today and for the future. PLoS Pathog 2013; 9(7):e1003418.

60. Centers for Disease Control and Prevention (CDC). Outbreaks of pertussis associated with hospitals–Kentucky, Pennsylvania, and Oregon, 2003. MMWR Morb Mortal Wkly Rep 2005;54(3):67–71.

61. Baggett HC, Duchin JS, Shelton W, et al. Two nosocomial pertussis outbreaks and their associated costs - King County, Washington, 2004. Infect Control Hosp Epidemiol 2007;28(5):537–43.

62. Sydnor E, Perl TM. Healthcare providers as sources of vaccine-preventable diseases. Vaccine 2014;32(38):4814–22.

63. Weber DJ, Rutala WA. Pertussis: an underappreciated risk for nosocomial outbreaks. Infect Control Hosp Epidemiol 1998;19(11):825–8.

64. Cunegundes KSA, de Moraes-Pinto MI, Takahashi TN, et al. Bordetella pertussis infection in paediatric healthcare workers. J Hosp Infect 2015;90(2):163–6.

65. Urbiztondo L, Broner S, Costa J, et al. Seroprevalence study of B. pertussis infection in health care workers in Catalonia, Spain. Hum Vaccin Immunother 2015; 11(1):293–7.

66. Havers FP, Moro PL, Hunter P, et al. Use of tetanus toxoid, reduced diphtheria toxoid, and acellular pertussis vaccines: updated recommendations of the advisory committee on immunization practices - United States, 2019. MMWR Morb Mortal Wkly Rep 2020;69(3):77–83.

67. Goins WP, Edwards KM, Vnencak-Jones CL, et al. A comparison of 2 strategies to prevent infection following pertussis exposure in vaccinated healthcare personnel. Clin Infect Dis 2012;54(7):938–45.

68. Zackrisson G, Brorson JE, Krantz I, et al. Invitro sensitivity of Bordetella-Pertussis. J Antimicrob Chemother 1983;11(5):407–11.

69. Kurzynski TA, Boehm DM, Rottpetri JA, et al. Antimicrobial susceptibilities of Bordetella species isolated in a multicenter pertussis surveillance project. Antimicrob Agents Chemother 1988;32(1):137–40.

70. Hoppe JE, Eichhorn A. Activity of new macrolides against Bordetella-pertussis and Bordetella-parapertussis. Eur J Clin Microbiol Infect Dis 1989;8(7):653–4.

71. Granstrom G, Sterner G, Nord CE, et al. Use of erythromycin to prevent pertussis in newborns of mothers with pertussis. J Infect Dis 1987;155(6):1210–4.

72. Sprauer MA, Cochi SL, Zell ER, et al. Prevention of secondary transmission of pertussis in households with early use of erythromycin. Am J Dis Child 1992; 146(2):177–81.

73. Deserres G, Boulianne N, Duval B. Field effectiveness of erythromycin prophylaxis to prevent pertussis within families. Pediatr Infect Dis J 1995;14(11):969–75.

74. Altunaiji S, Kukuruzovic R, Curtis N, et al. Antibiotics for whooping cough (pertussis) (withdrawn paper. 2007, atr. no. CD004404). Cochrane Database Syst Rev 2007;(3):CD004404.

75. Liang JL, Tiwari T, Moro P, et al. Prevention of pertussis, tetanus, and diphtheria with vaccines in the United States: recommendations of the Advisory Committee on Immunization Practices (ACIP). MMWR Recomm Rep 2018;67(2):1.

76. Centers for Disease Control and Prevention. (2020c). Measles Cases and Outbreaks. Retrieved 1/21/2021 from https://www.cdc.gov/measles/cases-outbreaks.html.
77. Huttunen R, Syrjanen J. Healthcare workers as vectors of infectious diseases. Eur J Clin Microbiol Infect Dis 2014;33(9):1477–88.
78. Maltezou HC, Wicker S. Measles in health-care settings. Am J Infect Control 2013;41(7):661–3.
79. Weber DJ, Rutala WA, Weigle K. Selection and use of vaccines for healthcare workers. Infect Control Hosp Epidemiol 1997;18(10):682–7.
80. Nelson NP, Link-Gelles R, Hofmeister MG, et al. Update: recommendations of the Advisory Committee on Immunization Practices for use of hepatitis A vaccine for postexposure prophylaxis and for preexposure prophylaxis for international travel. MMWR Morb Mortal Wkly Rep 2018;67(43):1216.
81. Nelson NP, Weng MK, Hofmeister MG, et al. Prevention of hepatitis A virus infection in the United States: recommendations of the advisory committee on immunization practices, 2020 2020.
82. Weber DJ, Hansen AR. Infections resulting from animal bites. Infect Dis Clin North Am 1991;5(3):663–80.
83. Endom E. Initial management of animal and human bites. In: UpToDate. Waltham (MA): Wolters Kluwer; 2016.
84. Weber DJ, Rutala WA. Risks and prevention of nosocomial transmission of rare zoonotic diseases. Clin Infect Dis 2001;32(3):446–56.
85. Centers for Disease Control and Prevention. Rabies: human rabies. Retrieved 1/15/2021 from http://www.cdc.gov/rabies/location/usa/surveillance/human_rabies.html.
86. Helmick CG, Tauxe RV, Vernon AA. Is there a risk to contacts of patients with rabies. Rev Infect Dis 1987;9(3):511–8.
87. Siegel JD, Rhinehart E, Jackson M, et al, Committee HCICPA. 2007 guideline for isolation precautions: preventing transmission of infectious agents in health care settings. Am J Infect Control 2007;35(10 Suppl 2):S65–164.
88. Rupprecht CE, Briggs D, Brown CM, et al. Use of a reduced (4-dose) vaccine schedule for postexposure prophylaxis to prevent human rabies recommendations of the advisory committee on immunization practices. MMWR Recomm Rep 2010;59(RR2):1–9.
89. Centers for Disease Control and Prevention. (2010). Scabies: Resources for Health Professionals. Retrieved 1/17/2021 from https://www.cdc.gov/parasites/scabies/health_professionals/control.html.
90. Stoltey JE, Cohen SE. Syphilis transmission: a review of the current evidence. Sex Health 2015;12(2):103–9.
91. Workowski KA, Bolan GA. Sexually transmitted diseases treatment guidelines, 2015. MMWR Recomm Rep 2015;64(Rr-03):1–137.
92. Centers for Disease Control and Prevention. Influenza antiviral medications: summary for clinicians. Available at: https://www.cdc.gov/flu/professionals/antivirals/summary-clinicians.htm. Accessed 1/15/2021.
93. Fiore AE, Fry A, Shay D, et al. Antiviral agents for the treatment and chemoprophylaxis of influenza recommendations of the Advisory Committee on Immunization Practices (ACIP). MMWR Recomm Rep 2011;60(RR1):1–24.

Computer Informatics for Infection Control

Michael Y. Lin, MD, MPH[a],*, William E. Trick, MD[a,b]

KEYWORDS

- Infection control • Informatics • Surveillance • Prevention • Public health

KEY POINTS

- Computer informatics tools are integral to routine infection control activities.
- Computer software can partially or fully automate infection surveillance, improving efficiency and reliability.
- Informatics are used for infection prevention, often through improved situational awareness and clinical decision support.
- Computer networks enhance public health infection control activities such as electronic laboratory reporting, outbreak detection, and control of antibiotic resistance.

As medical information becomes digitized, computer applications become an increasingly essential part of everyday infection control practice. The term informatics describes the use of computer information systems to answer questions, solve problems, and make decisions.[1] Informatics have the potential to improve infection control outcomes in 3 major domains: surveillance, prevention, and public health (**Box 1**).

In a sense, informatics can connect individual facility infection control programs with each other in a way that is similar to what the Internet did for stand-alone desktop computers; such connectedness amplifies the ability to control infections by enhancing interfacility communication and facilitating outbreak detection across multiple facilities. As predicted by the Sun Microsystems tagline in the 1980s, "The network is the computer,"[2] the coordination of infection control activities through the larger interconnected computer network is a key to future infection control achievements. This article reviews the current and emerging use of informatics for infection control.

BACKGROUND

Electronic medical record systems in the United States are common in hospitals and increasingly so in postacute care facilities such as nursing homes.[3,4] Patient

---

[a] Department of Medicine, Rush University Medical Center, 600 S. Paulina St., Suite 143, Chicago, IL, USA; [b] Center for Health Equity & Innovation, Health Research & Solutions, Cook County Health, 1950 W. Polk St., Suite 5807, Chicago, Illinois, USA
* Corresponding author.
E-mail address: Michael_Lin@rush.edu

Infect Dis Clin N Am 35 (2021) 755–769
https://doi.org/10.1016/j.idc.2021.04.010
0891-5520/21/© 2021 Elsevier Inc. All rights reserved.

id.theclinics.com

Box 1
Uses of informatics in infection control

Surveillance
- Fully or semiautomated surveillance of infections
- Fully automated device counting (denominator)
- Outbreak detection, single facility or ward

Prevention
- Awareness of multidrug-resistant organism carriage on admission
- Enhanced interfacility communication
- Identifying inappropriate infection precautions
- Reducing device use
- Antimicrobial stewardship

Public health
- Electronic communicable disease reporting
- Syndromic surveillance
- Regional outbreak detection

From Lin MY, Trick WE. Informatics in Infection Control. Infect Dis Clin North Am. 2016 Sep;30(3):759-70; with permission.

---

information relevant to the infection control department (including microbiology and laboratory test results, patient location, presence of invasive devices, and infection precautions status) is often stored electronically in discrete, computable fields enabling computers to automate processes previously performed by hand.

The automation of infection control has improved efficiency, allowing a single infection preventionist to perform more surveillance than previously possible. Historically, surveillance of health care–acquired infections focused on the intensive care unit, in part because of feasibility; now, with the use of automated surveillance, infection surveillance is performed across the entire facility. The adoption of informatics likely results in improved efficiency for infection preventionists[5]; however, a trade-off is the generation of more data to review, which competes with time interacting with facility staff. Ultimately, the critical question is whether the implementation of informatics improves patient safety.

Although the benefits of introducing informatics tools into infection control processes to local institutions are well recognized and supported by market forces, the authors anticipate a future state in which there is better integration of data across systems. Interinstitutional data sharing is being realized by multi-institutional health systems but is also possible among institutions that share electronic health record vendor applications, and increasingly among participants who have structured their data in nonproprietary, shared, common data models.[6–8]

INFECTION SURVEILLANCE

Surveillance is a cornerstone of infection prevention. Health care facilities use surveillance data to identify trends within wards (eg, whether infection is increasing in a particular ward). Public health officials, payors, and consumers use surveillance data to compare performance between health care facilities (eg, whether facility A has a higher infection rate compared with similar facilities). The objectives of surveillance definitions explicitly differ from those of clinical diagnostic criteria, which are used to help providers treat patients. Thus, although clinical diagnostic criteria rely heavily on human judgment to determine whether or not a patient has a disease, surveillance definitions often work better when the definitions are as objective as possible, to reduce subjectivity and increase reliability between infection preventionists.[9]

An example of subjective versus objective surveillance definition is *Clostridium difficile* surveillance. The National Healthcare Safety Network (NHSN) endorses 2 options for tracking *C difficile* infection (CDI): the health care–associated infection (HAI) gastrointestinal CDI (GI-CDI), which is subjective, and the CDI laboratory-identified (LabID) event, which is objective.[10,11] Although both methods require a positive test for toxin-producing *C difficile* on an unformed stool specimen, the HAI GI-CDI surveillance definition requires infection preventionists to review the clinical presentation of the patient to determine whether diarrhea was present on admission. In contrast, CDI LabID event reporting is based strictly on the number of inpatient days between specimen collection date and date of patient admission; there is no consideration for clinical symptoms. Although some clinicians and reviewers are frustrated with not being able to interpret nuanced information, laboratory-based surveillance events are computable and theoretically do not need human effort for each determination, improving reliability and reducing burden on infection preventionists.

Surveillance metrics typically comprise both numerator counts (how many events occurred?) and denominator counts (how many patient days at risk?). Ideally, infection control software assists infection preventionists with determining both types of counts.

FULLY AUTOMATED VERSUS SEMIAUTOMATED SURVEILLANCE

In general, computer surveillance of HAIs can be fully automated or semiautomated.[12,13] Fully automated surveillance is possible when the surveillance definition is completely computable (eg, *C difficile* LabID event). Alternatively, semiautomated surveillance occurs when the computer performs part of the surveillance (for example, case finding using specified criteria) and serves up putative infection episodes for human confirmation. For example, a computer may identify a candidate central line–associated bloodstream infection (CLABSI), based on a positive blood culture and the presence of a central line; the infection preventionist then reviews the chart to judge whether the bloodstream pathogen originated from a central line versus an alternative source (such as a pneumonia).

COMMON DATA SOURCES NEEDED FOR SURVEILLANCE INFORMATICS

All computer software for infection control require access to specific types of data. For most infection surveillance, software systems need microbiology and laboratory results to determine positive cultures and diagnostic tests. To determine where the patient is at the time of infection, software also need access to the admission/discharge/transfer (ADT) dataset. Other metric-specific data requirements are outlined later and in **Table 1**. Historically, microbiology data have been challenging to represent in discrete fields because of the dynamic nature of laboratory testing and the desire and necessity of personnel to add structured or unstructured textual annotations to results.

EXAMPLES OF SURVEILLANCE METRICS ENHANCED BY INFORMATICS
Central Line–Associated Bloodstream Infection

The NHSN definition of CLABSI requires judgment on the part of infection preventionists, who must decide whether a positive blood culture originated from a central line

Table 1
Key data elements necessary for electronic surveillance of health care–associated infections

NHSN Surveillance Metric	Key Electronic Data Elements	Barriers to Fully Automated Electronic Surveillance
Central line–associated line infection	Microbiology cultures (blood and nonblood sites), ADT, central venous catheter presence	Current definition requires judgment regarding the origin of the blood pathogen
Catheter-associated urinary tract infection	Microbiology cultures (urine only), ADT, vital signs (fever), urinary catheter presence	Current definition requires assessment of patient symptoms
Surgical site infection	Microbiology cultures (superficial or deep wound cultures), procedure billing codes (eg, CPT codes), billing codes (eg, ICD-10), ADT (to detect readmissions), antibiotic administration (optional)	Current definition requires judgment as to whether infection occurred, because not all infections have a positive culture; depth of infection requires assessment
Ventilator-associated event	Ventilator settings (PEEP, Fio_2), presence of endotracheal intubation device, ADT, antimicrobial use, vital signs (temperature), laboratory (white blood cell count), microbiology culture results	None
MDRO module (LabID)	Microbiology cultures, ADT	None
C difficile module (LabID)	Microbiology (C difficile), ADT	None

Abbreviations: CPT, current procedural therapy; Fio_2, fraction inspired oxygen; ICD-10, International Classification of Diseases, 10th Revision; MDRO, multidrug-resistant organism; PEEP, positive end-expiratory pressure.

Adapted from Woeltje, K. F., Lin, M. Y., Klompas, M., Wright, M. O., Zuccotti, G., & Trick, W. E. 2014. Data requirements for electronic surveillance of healthcare-associated infections. Infection Control & Hospital Epidemiology, 35(09), 1083-1091; with permission.

versus a nonblood source. Thus, agreement between infection preventionists is imperfect, even when reviewing an identical case,[14] hampering the ability to compare hospitals based on CLABSI rates.[15] In response, NHSN has made the CLABSI definition more objective over time (for example, making the definition of a secondary bacteremia more strict). Because some elements of CLABSI case finding require human judgment, most surveillance software programs offer a semiautomated approach to bloodstream infection surveillance: candidate positive blood cultures that occur in the presence of a central line are presented by the software to the infection preventionist for review. Semiautomated approaches work best when the computer algorithm has a high negative predictive value for infection,[16] thereby sparing the infection preventionist from having to review positive blood cultures that are unlikely to be true CLABSIs. To perform CLABSI surveillance, basic database sources are needed; microbiology, ADT, and ideally patient-specific central line data.

Some health care facilities have implemented fully automated CLABSI surveillance, as an alternative to traditional semiautomated surveillance.[15–17] Such approaches are useful in performing surveillance in units where there may not be enough resources to perform traditional surveillance (eg, non–intensive care unit areas of the hospital).[18] In addition, completely automated approaches are likely more reliable when performing interfacility comparisons, compared with traditional surveillance.[19] However, because fully automated CLABSI measurements produce infection rates that are higher than those derived from traditional methods, health care facilities reporting automated CLABSI rates would need to be compared with other facilities using the same automated surveillance definition.

Surgical Site Infection

Surgical site infection (SSI) surveillance requires some human judgment, because the depth of infection (superficial vs deep vs organ/space) must be determined, and not all SSIs involve a positive microbiologic culture. Thus, SSI surveillance is typically semi-automated, with software used to identify candidate surgical cases (eg, triggered by antimicrobial prescribing) and to count the denominator of qualified procedures in a given time. SSI rates are typically risk adjusted by the American Society of Anesthesiologists score, wound class, and duration of surgery; these elements are usually available electronically through the surgical information system, but the accuracy of these data sources must be validated at each facility before use.

Case finding of SSIs is extremely valuable, reducing the amount of chart review needed. Because not all SSIs result in a positive culture, surveillance systems that rely solely on positive cultures are likely to undercount infections. Ideally, case-finding algorithms would use a combination of culture results, diagnosis codes, facility readmission, and antibiotic use; different algorithms have been developed for a variety of SSIs.[20–26] For example, a multicenter study of SSI surveillance focusing on coronary artery bypass graft, caesarian section, and breast surgeries showed that enhanced surveillance (that identified postoperative patients with inpatient antimicrobial exposure of various thresholds of duration) had sensitivity of 88% to 91% sensitivity, compared with 38% to 64% for routine surveillance, and surveillance for caesarian section infection was further enhanced with the addition of infection diagnosis codes.[20] Enhanced case-finding strategies ideally should be adopted uniformly across health systems to make interfacility comparisons equitable.

Ventilator-Associated Pneumonia/Ventilator-Associated Event

In 2013, NHSN released a new surveillance metric called ventilator-associated event (VAE); these definitions were designed to rely only on objective criteria (such as changes in ventilator settings).[27] The VAE definition marked a departure from older definitions of ventilator-associated pneumonia that relied heavily on subjective criteria (such as interpretation of clinical signs/symptoms and radiographic signs). In the process, the VAE definition shifted the focus of prevention from pneumonia alone to general complications of mechanical ventilation.

VAE surveillance starts by identifying patients with ventilator-associated conditions (VACs), defined as a sustained increase in ventilator settings after a period of stable or improving ventilator settings.[28] Among VAC cases, additional criteria (white count, temperature, antibiotic receipt) define a subgroup of VAC called infection-related ventilator-associated complication (IVAC)." Among IVAC cases, a subgroup of possible ventilator-associated pneumonia is defined by sputum purulence and respiratory microbiologic test results. VAE surveillance can be fully automated in hospitals that can electronically access all required data elements: daily minimum positive end-expiratory pressure (PEEP), daily minimum fraction of inspired oxygen (Fio_2), daily minimum and maximum temperature, daily minimum and maximum white blood cell count, and antibiotic start/stop dates. To assess possible ventilator-associated pneumonia, Gram stain, culture, neutrophil counts, and epithelial cell counts from respiratory specimens are needed. Facilities that cannot access all required data elements electronically may perform the surveillance in a semiautomated manner, which may include review of some data elements by infection preventionists.

Catheter-Associated Urinary Tract Infection

The NHSN definition for catheter-associated urinary tract infection (CAUTI) relies on determining whether bacteria in the urine are associated with symptoms of infection (eg, fever, urgency, frequency, dysuria, suprapubic tenderness, and costovertebral angle pain or tenderness) and whether a urinary catheter is present.[29] Symptoms, as documented in clinical notes, are difficult for software to extract from the medical record; thus, CAUTI surveillance usually is semiautomated with a human making a final determination based on chart review. The presence or absence of an indwelling urinary catheter is the starting point for determining whether a CAUTI has occurred and also for counting denominator data (urinary catheter days). Furthermore, surveillance software must be able to interpret a urine culture result based on NHSN criteria, by counting the number of species in the urine culture (no more than 2 species allowed, with at least 1 species at a concentration of $\geq 10^5$ colony-forming units).

Multidrug-Resistant Organism Module

The NHSN multidrug-resistant organism (MDRO) module contains the LabID surveillance option, which relies on completely objective and computable metrics (microbiology culture results and patient location data). Candidate bacterial pathogens include methicillin-resistant *Staphylococcus aureus* (MRSA), methicillin-susceptible *S aureus*, vancomycin-resistant *Enterococcus* (VRE), cephalosporin-resistant *Klebsiella*, carbapenem-resistant Enterobacterales (CRE), multidrug-resistant *Acinetobacter* spp, and *C difficile*. These surveillance metrics allow determination of community-onset versus facility-onset infection, and unit-specific surveillance. The LabID surveillance definitions are good examples of infection metrics that can be calculated completely by computers without human effort.

OUTBREAK DETECTION

Infection preventionists typically perform outbreak detection of health care facility–acquired infections using simple rules, such as 3 or more new cases of a single pathogen within 2 weeks in a single ward. Such approaches do not account for the natural variation of pathogen prevalence over time and can miss outbreaks spanning multiple facility units. Surveillance software offer the opportunity to perform automated cluster detection using statistical principles. For example, in 1 study, investigators used a space-time permutation scan statistic (WHONET-SaTScan) approach to identify clusters of pathogens that were of same species and antibiotic susceptibility profiles.[30] Over 5 years, such an approach identified 59 clusters, 95% of which were deemed by the hospital epidemiologists to merit consideration or warrant active investigation/intervention; importantly, 72 out of 73 previously designated MRSA clusters and 87 out of 87 VRE clusters were found to have likely occurred by chance alone (ie, not significant), potentially saving infection preventionist resources. Statistical surveillance systems use baseline prevalence data to automate evaluation of whether a statistically significant increase in infections or organisms has occurred. Such automated outbreak detection systems can be applied at a facility level[31] or across a region.[32,33]

INFECTION PREVENTION

Although infection control software is used predominantly to improve data collection and surveillance, there are many opportunities for software to actively prevent infections and improve patient care. Such approaches often use clinical decision support tools that present information to the end user (infection preventionist or health care facility staff) to prompt immediate action.[34]

Identifying Multidrug-Resistant Organism Colonization at Time of Admission

Health care facilities may want to identify MDRO-colonized patients in order to place them in appropriate infection control precautions.[35] Infection control software, or the health system's electronic medical record, can flag patients with a history of MDRO carriage.[36] For example, a computer alerting system allowed a hospital to increase staff awareness of patient MRSA colonization from 15% at baseline to 90%, with a similar increase in appropriate contact precautions.[37] Other investigational systems allow health care facilities to identify those patients who are at higher risk of MDRO carriage, to then prompt further culture testing at the time of admission (ie, active surveillance).[38]

Health care facilities find it difficult to ascertain patients' MDRO status at the time of admission if the MDRO test information resides at another health care facility. Such awareness requires a regional health informatics system (sometimes called a health information exchange) to share MDRO information between facilities. MDRO information sharing is being developed in certain regions of the United States.[39] One example is the Illinois Extensively Drug Resistant Organism (XDRO) registry, which facilitates sharing of targeted pathogens such as carbapenem-resistant organisms and *Candida auris* among all facilities in Illinois (**Fig. 1**).[32,40] Infection preventionists are mandated to report patients colonized by targeted MDROs to the Illinois Department of Public Health, and thereafter, any health care facility can query the registry to determine whether a given patient has ever been reported to the registry. Such alerts can be automated, which is important for large health care facilities with high admission rates. A potential evolution of the system will be to identify individuals at high probability of colonization by MDROs on admission to a health care facility using regional data sources and use active surveillance methods for these patients.[41]

Identifying Inappropriate Infection Precautions

During a patient's health care facility stay, infection preventionists spend considerable time ensuring that appropriate isolation precautions are placed for patients with relevant

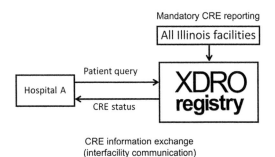

Fig. 1. Conceptual framework of the XDRO registry, Illinois. (*From* Trick WE, Lin MY, Cheng-Leidig R, et al. Electronic Public Health Registry of Extensively Drug-Resistant Organisms, Illinois, USA. *Emerging Infectious Diseases.* 2015;21(10):1725-1732. https://doi.org/10.3201/eid2110.150538.)

pathogens. For example, a patient with a positive AFB (acid-fast bacilli) smear may need to be placed in airborne precautions because of tuberculosis transmission risk. If a given patient's infection control precautions can be captured electronically in real time, then infection control software can identify patients with specific pathogens (eg, MDROs, C difficile, varicella zoster virus, Mycobacterium tuberculosis) and identify patients with inappropriate isolation precautions for further infection preventionist review.[42,43]

Reducing Device Use

Clinical decision support can reduce device use, leading to fewer device-related infections. For example, a multihospital academic system instituted measures to reduce the use of indwelling urinary catheters, including alerts to providers to reassess the need for the urinary catheter if not removed within the recommended time. Urinary catheter use declined during the study period, as well as CAUTIs.[44] Similar interventions for urinary catheters have been described elsewhere.[45,46]

Antibiotic Stewardship

Antimicrobial stewardship is a complementary component of infection control, because antimicrobial use affects C difficile infection rates and increases risk for antimicrobial resistance. Many software programs are available to augment stewardship strategies in health care facilities.[47] Prospective audit and feedback strategy is enhanced by electronically identifying patients on target antimicrobials for review (eg, all patients on broad-spectrum antimicrobials) or for patients treated with antimicrobials that have redundant spectra.[48] Formulary restriction and preauthorization uses clinical decision support at the time of antimicrobial prescribing to alter prescribing behavior (eg, avoiding certain antimicrobial drug classes, or prompting the ordering provider to obtain approval from the infectious diseases department). Guideline-based treatment recommendations can be provided to physicians by the computer software at the time of antibiotic decision making. In addition, software can encourage appropriate antimicrobial use by identifying new clinical information (eg, a positive blood culture result) that should prompt modification of antimicrobial therapy.

Numerous examples of computer-assisted antimicrobial stewardship are available,[49–52] including a randomized control trial that showed that a clinical decision support system could increase appropriate antimicrobial therapy and decrease antimicrobial expenditures[53] (this topic is discussed in further detail in the Shiwei Zhou and colleagues' article, "Antimicrobial Stewardship and the Infection Control Practitioner: A Natural Alliance," in this issue).

INFORMATICS AND PUBLIC HEALTH

Informatics systems have strengthened and expanded the interface between infection preventionists and public health agencies. Incentives such as the Centers for Medicare and Medicaid Services' Meaningful Use Program have encouraged hospitals to adopt technologies such as electronic laboratory reporting and syndromic surveillance, although uptake has been inconsistent and hampered by the complexity of microbiology data.[54] Such connections facilitate opportunities for infection prevention activities to be integrated across regions, which has been shown to be pivotal for control of MDROs.[55]

Electronic Communicable Disease Reporting

Most public health reporting of communicable diseases has now moved to the Internet, with users reporting via a computer interface. A computer interface allows the infection preventionist to input complete report information, including microbiology results and patient demographic/epidemiologic information. Electronic laboratory reporting (ELR) facilitates some of the reporting, allowing the microbiology laboratory information to be automatically sent to the public health department using reporting rules. ELR has been shown to increase the completeness and timeliness of communicable disease reporting,[56] although a major limitation is that certain patient data, such as demographic and epidemiologic data, still require manual infection preventionist entry.[57,58]

Syndromic Surveillance and Outbreak Detection

Syndromic surveillance is preferred to traditional case reporting for monitoring common conditions such as influenza or for rapid identification of outbreaks and bioterrorism events.[54] To track influenza, public health officials monitor for influenzalike illness by categorizing chief complaints from emergency department assessments and some ambulatory care settings. Reports typically contain basic demographic information, but lack detailed clinical, vaccination, or laboratory information.

Inclusion of patient identifiers in syndromic surveillance feeds allows public health agencies to join syndromic surveillance data to other public health data. In Illinois, health systems have been instructed to indicate whether an individual was admitted to a health care facility in the syndromic surveillance messages, which, when joined to the XDRO registry database, enables rapid alerting of facilities that admit patients known to harbor target MDROs such as carbapenem-resistant organisms and *C auris*.

GENERAL CONSIDERATIONS FOR IMPLEMENTING INFORMATICS SOFTWARE

Infection control staff need to work closely with their information technology and laboratory specialists to implement and maintain informatics software. Some of the general considerations in working with informatics software and strategies to maintain quality of data through internal/external validation are discussed next.

Challenges of Microbiology Data

Microbiology data are inherently complex. Although some tests have a single dichotomous result value (eg, *C difficile* assay is positive/negative), culture results can include multiple organisms, each with its own antibiotic susceptibility profile. Furthermore, the bacterial taxonomy can change based on genetic analysis; for example, in 2017, *Enterobacter aerogenes* was renamed *Klebsiella aerogenes*.[59] Thus, informatics software must map each organism to standardized terminology (eg, SNOMED [Systemized Nomenclature of Medicine], College of American Pathologists), and determine when new data are coming from the microbiology laboratory that are unrecognized because of naming or format changes. Furthermore, any changes in the underlying information systems that supply data to infection control software require a complete reassessment of data integrity at the time of transition.

Challenges of Device Data

Information from routine nurse charting can allow software to detect the presence of invasive devices such as central lines, indwelling urinary catheters, and mechanical ventilation.[60] Based on our experience, start/stop orders for devices are less reliable than continuous (eg, per shift) nursing documentation for determining whether a device is present in a patient on a given day. For example, a patient can be discharged from a health care facility without a device discontinuation order, and then it is unclear on readmission whether the device is still present.

When enumerating device days electronically, infection control personnel are responsible for mapping local device names to device types. For example, the NHSN CAUTI definition measures infection complications of indwelling urethral catheters, so suprapubic catheters (which are outside the urethra) should not count as qualifying catheters. If local device names cannot discriminate between qualifying versus nonqualifying devices, infection control personnel need to work with the informatics team to modify the device name list. Similar distinctions need to be made for central venous catheters, because some devices, such as midline catheters, are not considered central lines.

Validation of Data

Surveillance of HAIs has high-stakes implications; besides the direct role of surveillance in monitoring patient safety, health care facility infections rates are publicly reported and affect reimbursement in pay-for-performance models.[61,62] Validation is the process that ensures high quality of infection control data. In the context of informatics, it means that the products of electronic surveillance are compared with a reference standard (usually manual review). Validation can be divided into 2 activities: internal validation, which refers to self-assessment by the reporting facility, and external validation, which is performed by an agency outside the reporting facility (usually the health department). Validation is an iterative process that should be performed periodically, particularly when there are changes to the process, such as a new electronic system, and any subsequent validation should still be compared with a manually collected reference standard.[63] Both numerator and denominator data need periodic validation, because poor quality in either domain can adversely affect infection rates.

NHSN recommends each facility's infection control program use the following steps for internal validation. (1) Ensure and document current training in NHSN surveillance competency. (2) Ensure that risk-adjustment variables are accurate and reliable (eg, for CLABSI/CAUTI, this involves verifying location mapping, bed size, and facility teaching status). (3) Ensure numerator quality by maintaining a decision record of all positive culture investigation results (blood cultures and urine cultures for CLABSI and CAUTI, respectively), and request a summary line listing of all positive cultures from the laboratory to compare with the list of previously investigated cultures. (4) Verify that denominator collection is accurate; if performed electronically, facilities are required to document that electronic data counts are within 5% of manual data counts for 3 months. Validation steps specific for infection type can be found on NHSN's data validation Web site (http://www.cdc.gov/nhsn/validation/).

Impact of COVID-19 Pandemic

The COVID-19 (coronavirus disease 2019) pandemic will likely accelerate interconnectedness between public health agencies and clinical databases. The urgency for public health agencies to monitor and respond to the COVID-19 pandemic created demands for data relevant to health care facility infection control departments, such as bed occupancy, personal protective equipment supplies, rapid reporting of COVID-19 cases, and questions about the effectiveness of various protective measures both for staff and patients. Some of these metrics were accommodated by existing data streams: for example, COVID-19 infections could be reported to public health departments through electronic laboratory interfaces. However, other critical information did not have reliable systems for making real-time decisions. Notably, real-time capacity monitoring of hospitals, nursing homes, intensive care units, and mechanical ventilators required creation of systems that sometimes relied on manual counting and centralized reporting through newly developed processes.

In the wake of COVID-19, there will be calls to action on how to upgrade public reporting systems. The authors expect that the Centers for Disease Control and Prevention and the infection control community will work together to identify critical enhancements. Based on our local experience, a few key modifications are needed. For example, electronic health record vendors should capture bed and ventilator use daily in a standardized format for reporting to a national agency. Furthermore, mandated reporting of medical conditions will be accompanied by more rigorous attention to patient address data to facilitate geocoding and linkage to metadata such as the social vulnerability index, which can graphically identify hotspots and recognize health disparities.

An additional area of promise for connectivity between public health agencies and clinical systems is for health care facilities to connect through health information exchanges with vendor-agnostic national common data models developed primarily for clinical research activities but that can be leveraged for public health activities.[64] Two such existing data models are the PCORnet and Observational Medical Outcomes Partnership (OMOP) structures.[65,66] The PCORnet regional networks provide a common data model structure with terms mapped to nationally endorsed vocabularies and routinely scheduled data curation queries. In addition, there are existing agreements and governance structures to protect patient privacy and to build trust among participants. OMOP is a foundational data structure for contributions to the National COVID Cohort Collaborative (N3C) data enclave.

As common data models and networks mature, there will be future opportunities for clinical and public health partnerships, not just for COVID-19 but for additional infection control and antimicrobial stewardship initiatives.

SUMMARY

The use of computer informatics is now a routine part of infection control practice. Such computer systems still require effort from infection preventionists to establish and maintain because of the complexity and changing nature of electronic data. As with any tool, it is important to understand situations where computers can benefit infection prevention (eg, automated surveillance, decision support, connecting to networks) and situations where computers can cause pitfalls (eg, inaccurate device denominator data because of lack of validation). The authors believe that the ability of computer networks to coordinate infection control activities beyond the walls of the health care facility (eg, regional network surveillance of outbreaks) represents the next major leap for infection control.

CLINICS CARE POINTS

- Information generated from electronic data are only as accurate as the data inputs going into the software.
- When using electronic software for surveillance of infections, ensure that the data sources for both the numerator (eg, organism names) and denominator (eg, device days) remain valid over time.
- When performing surveillance using partial computer assistance, look for computerized screening approaches that are highly accurate in ruling out cases (ie, have a high negative predictive value).
- Like surveillance definitions designed for infection control, electronic surveillance definitions are not intended to be used for clinical decision making.

DISCLOSURE

The authors have nothing to disclose.

REFERENCES

1. Kulikowski CA, Shortliffe EH, Currie LM, et al. AMIA Board white paper: definition of biomedical informatics and specification of core competencies for graduate education in the discipline. J Am Med Inform Assoc 2012;19:931–8.
2. The Network Is the Computer, Again. Networkcomputing.com. 2014. Available at: https://www.networkcomputing.com/cloud-infrastructure/network-computer-again. Accessed February 4, 2021.
3. Gold M, McLaughlin C. Assessing HITECH implementation and lessons: 5 years later. Milbank Q 2016;94:654–87.
4. Henry J, Pylypchuk Y, Patel V. ONC Data Brief: Electronic Health Record Adoption and Interoperability among U.S. Skilled Nursing Facilities and Home Health Agencies in 2017. In: The Office of the National Coordinator for Health Information Technology, ed.2018:1-13.
5. Russo PL, Shaban RZ, Macbeth D, et al. Impact of electronic healthcare-associated infection surveillance software on infection prevention resources: a systematic review of the literature. J Hosp Infect 2018;99:1–7.
6. Hripcsak G, Duke JD, Shah NH, et al. Observational Health Data Sciences and Informatics (OHDSI): opportunities for observational researchers. Stud Health Technol Inform 2015;216:574.
7. Observational Medical Outcomes Partnership (OMOP). Available at: https://fnih. org/what-we-do/major-completed-programs/omop. Accessed January 29, 2021.
8. Collins FS, Hudson KL, Briggs JP, et al. PCORnet: turning a dream into reality. London: BMJ Publishing Group; 2014.
9. Rubin MA, Mayer J, Greene T, et al. An agent-based model for evaluating surveillance methods for catheter-related bloodstream infection. AMIA Annu Symp Proc. 2008 Nov 6;2008:631-5.
10. Surveillance for C. difficile, MRSA, and other Drug-resistant Infections. Available at: https://www.cdc.gov/nhsn/acute-care-hospital/cdiff-mrsa/index.html. Accessed February 1, 2021.
11. Distinguishing healthcare-associated infection (HAI) and LabID events. Available at: https://www.cdc.gov/nhsn/faqs/faq-mdro-cdi.html#q12. Accessed February 1, 2021.
12. Woeltje KF, Lin MY, Klompas M, et al. Data requirements for electronic surveillance of healthcare-associated infections. Infect Control Hosp Epidemiol 2014; 35:1083–91.
13. Klompas M, Yokoe DS, Weinstein RA. Automated surveillance of health care–associated infections. Clin Infect Dis 2009;48:1268–75.
14. Mayer J, Greene T, Howell J, et al. Agreement in classifying bloodstream infections among multiple reviewers conducting surveillance. Clin Infect Dis 2012; 55:364–70.
15. Lin MY, Hota B, Khan YM, et al. Quality of traditional surveillance for public reporting of nosocomial bloodstream infection rates. JAMA 2010;304:2035–41.
16. Woeltje KF, Butler AM, Goris AJ, et al. Automated surveillance for central line–associated bloodstream infection in intensive care units. Infect Control Hosp Epidemiol 2008;29:842–6.
17. Trick WE, Zagorski BM, Tokars JI, et al. Computer algorithms to detect bloodstream infections. Emerg Infect Dis 2004;10:1612–20.

18. Woeltje KF, McMullen KM, Butler AM, et al. Electronic surveillance for healthcare-associated central line—associated bloodstream infections outside the intensive care unit. Infect Control Hosp Epidemiol 2011;32:1086–90.

19. Lin MY, Woeltje KF, Khan YM, et al. Multicenter evaluation of computer automated versus traditional surveillance of hospital-acquired bloodstream infections. Infect Control Hosp Epidemiol 2014;35:1483–90.

20. Yokoe DS, Noskin GA, Cunnigham SM, et al. Enhanced identification of postoperative infections among inpatients. Emerg Infect Dis 2004;10:1924–30.

21. Yokoe DS, Khan Y, Olsen MA, et al. Enhanced surgical site infection surveillance following hysterectomy, vascular, and colorectal surgery. Infect Control Hosp Epidemiol 2012;33:768–73.

22. Calderwood MS, Ma A, Khan YM, et al. Use of Medicare diagnosis and procedure codes to improve detection of surgical site infections following hip arthroplasty, knee arthroplasty, and vascular surgery. Infect Control Hosp Epidemiol 2012;33:40–9.

23. Olsen MA, Fraser VJ. Use of diagnosis codes and/or wound culture results for surveillance of surgical site infection after mastectomy and breast reconstruction. Infect Control Hosp Epidemiol 2010;31:544–7.

24. Bolon MK, Hooper D, Stevenson KB, et al. Improved surveillance for surgical site infections after orthopedic implantation procedures: extending applications for automated data. Clin Infect Dis 2009;48:1223–9.

25. Cho SY, Chung DR, Choi JR, et al. Validation of semiautomated surgical site infection surveillance using electronic screening algorithms in 38 surgery categories. Infect Control Hosp Epidemiol 2018;39:931–5.

26. Sips ME, Bonten MJ, van Mourik MS. Semiautomated surveillance of deep surgical site infections after primary total hip or knee arthroplasty. Infect Control Hosp Epidemiol 2017;38:732–5.

27. Magill SS, Klompas M, Balk R, et al. Developing a New, National Approach to Surveillance for Ventilator-Associated Events: Executive Summary. Clin Infect Dis 2013;57:1742–6.

28. Ventilator-Associated Event (VAE). 2021. Available at: https://www.cdc.gov/nhsn/pdfs/pscmanual/10-vae_final.pdf. Accessed February 2, 2021.

29. Urinary Tract Infection (Catheter-Associated Urinary Tract Infection [CAUTI] and Non-Catheter-Associated Urinary Tract Infection [UTI]) Events 2021. Available at: https://www.cdc.gov/nhsn/pdfs/pscManual/7pscCAUTIcurrent.pdf. Accessed February 2, 2021.

30. Huang SS, Yokoe DS, Stelling J, et al. Automated detection of infectious disease outbreaks in hospitals: a retrospective cohort study. PLoS Med 2010;7:e1000238.

31. Stachel A, Pinto G, Stelling J, et al. Implementation and evaluation of an automated surveillance system to detect hospital outbreak. Am J Infect Control 2017;45:1372–7.

32. Trick WE, Lin MY, Cheng-Leidig R, et al. Electronic public health registry of extensively drug-resistant organisms, Illinois, USA. Emerg Infect Dis 2015;21:1725–32.

33. Octaria R, Griffith H, Estes M, et al. Comparing Automated Cluster Detection Methods for Carbapenem-Resistant Enterobacteriaceae (CRE): Rule-Based Versus Statistical. Infect Control Hosp Epidemiol 2020;41:s27–.

34. Wright M-O, Robicsek A. Clinical decision support systems and infection prevention: To know is not enough. Am J Infect Control 2015;43:554–8.

35. Facility Guidance for Control of Carbapenem-resistant Enterobacteriaceae (CRE) The Centers for Disease Control and Prevention. 2015. Available at: http://www.cdc.gov/hai/pdfs/cre/CRE-guidance-508.pdf. Accessed February 12, 2021.

36. Kho AN, Dexter PR, Warvel JS, et al. An Effective Computerized Reminder for Contact Isolation of Patients Colonized or Infected with Resistant Organisms. Int J Med Inf 2008;77:194–8.

37. Kac G, Grohs P, Durieux P, et al. Impact of Electronic Alerts on Isolation Precautions for Patients with Multidrug-Resistant Bacteria. Arch Intern Med 2007;167: 2086–90.

38. Robicsek A, Beaumont JL, Wright M-O, et al. Electronic prediction rules for methicillin-resistant *Staphylococcus aureus* colonization. Infect Control Hosp Epidemiol 2011;32:9–19.

39. Kho AN, Lemmon L, Commiskey M, et al. Use of a regional health information exchange to detect crossover of patients with MRSA between urban hospitals. J Am Med Inform Assoc 2008;15:212–6.

40. XDRO registry. Available at: at.xdro.org. Accessed February 3, 2021.

41. Lin MY, Rezny S, Ray MJ, Jovanov D, Weinstein RA, Trick WE. Predicting carbapenem-resistant Enterobacteriaceae (CRE) carriage at the time of admission using a state-wide hospital discharge database. Open Forum Infectious Diseases 2019; 6(12). https://doi.org/10.1093/ofid/ofz483.

42. Ross B, Marine M, Chou M, et al. Measuring compliance with transmission-based isolation precautions: Comparison of paper-based and electronic data collection. Am J Infect Control 2011;39:839–43.

43. Chen ES, Wajngurt D, Qureshi K, et al. Automated real-time detection and notification of positive infection cases. AMIA Annu Symp Proc; 2006. 2006:883.

44. Baillie CA, Epps M, Hanish A, et al. Usability and Impact of a Computerized Clinical Decision Support Intervention Designed to Reduce Urinary Catheter Utilization and Catheter-Associated Urinary Tract Infections. Infect Control Hosp Epidemiol 2014;35:1147–55.

45. Meddings J, Rogers MA, Macy M, et al. Systematic review and meta-analysis: reminder systems to reduce catheter-associated urinary tract infections and urinary catheter use in hospitalized patients. Clin Infect Dis 2010;51:550–60.

46. Youngerman BE, Salmasian H, Carter EJ, et al. Reducing indwelling urinary catheter use through staged introduction of electronic clinical decision support in a multicenter hospital system. Infect Control Hosp Epidemiol 2018;39:902–8.

47. Forrest GN, Van Schooneveld TC, Kullar R, et al. Use of electronic health records and clinical decision support systems for antimicrobial stewardship. Clin Infect Dis 2014;59:S122–33.

48. Glowacki RC, Schwartz DN, Itokazu GS, et al. Antibiotic combinations with redundant antimicrobial spectra: clinical epidemiology and pilot intervention of computer-assisted surveillance. Clin Infect Dis 2003;37:59–64.

49. Pestotnik SL, Classen DC, Evans RS, et al. Implementing antibiotic practice guidelines through computer-assisted decision support: clinical and financial outcomes. Ann Intern Med 1996;124:884–90.

50. Evans RS, Pestotnik SL, Classen DC, et al. A computer-assisted management program for antibiotics and other antiinfective agents. N Engl J Med 1998;338: 232–8.

51. Samore MH, Bateman K, Alder SC, et al. Clinical decision support and appropriateness of antimicrobial prescribing: a randomized trial. JAMA 2005;294: 2305–14.

52. Curtis CE, Al Bahar F, Marriott JF. The effectiveness of computerised decision support on antibiotic use in hospitals: a systematic review. PLoS One 2017;12: e0183062.

53. McGregor JC, Weekes E, Forrest GN, et al. Impact of a computerized clinical decision support system on reducing inappropriate antimicrobial use: a randomized controlled trial. J Am Med Inform Assoc 2006;13:378–84.

54. Birkhead GS, Klompas M, Shah NR. Uses of electronic health records for public health surveillance to advance public health. Annu Rev Public Health 2015;36: 345–59.

55. Slayton RB, Toth D, Lee BY, et al. Vital signs: estimated effects of a coordinated approach for action to reduce antibiotic-resistant infections in health care facilities—United States. MMWR Morb Mortal Wkly Rep 2015;64:826.

56. Effler P, Ching-Lee M, Bogard A, et al. Statewide system of electronic notifiable disease reporting from clinical laboratories: comparing automated reporting with conventional methods. JAMA 1999;282:1845–50.

57. Dixon BE, Siegel JA, Oemige TV, et al. Electronic health information quality challenges and interventions to improve public health surveillance data and practice. Public Health Rep 2013;546–53.

58. Willis SJ, Cocoros NM, Randall LM, et al. Electronic Health Record Use in Public Health Infectious Disease Surveillance, USA, 2018–2019. Curr Infect Dis Rep 2019;21:1–9.

59. Tindall B, Sutton G, Garrity G. Enterobacter aerogenes Hormaeche and Edwards 1960 (Approved Lists 1980) and Klebsiella mobilis Bascomb et al. 1971 (Approved Lists 1980) share the same nomenclatural type (ATCC 13048) on the Approved Lists and are homotypic synonyms, with consequences for the name Klebsiella mobilis Bascomb et al. 1971 (Approved Lists 1980). Int J Syst Evol Microbiol 2017;67:502–4.

60. Wright M-O, Fisher A, John M, et al. The electronic medical record as a tool for infection surveillance: Successful automation of device-days. Am J Infect Control 2009;37:364–70.

61. Totten AM, Wagner J, Tiwari A, et al. Closing the quality gap: revisiting the state of the science (vol. 5: public reporting as a quality improvement strategy). 2012.

62. Kahn CN, Ault T, Potetz L, et al. Assessing Medicare's Hospital Pay-For-Performance Programs And Whether They Are Achieving Their Goals. Health Aff 2015;34:1281–8.

63. National Healthcare Safety Network (NHSN). Patient safety component manual 2021. Available at: https://www.cdc.gov/nhsn/pdfs/pscmanual/pcsmanual_current.pdf. Accessed February 3, 2021.

64. Dixon BE, Grannis SJ, McAndrews C, et al. Leveraging Data Visualization and a Statewide Health Information Exchange to Support COVID-19 Surveillance and Response: Application of Public Health Informatics. J Am Med Inform Assoc 2021. https://doi.org/10.1093/jamia/ocab004.

65. The National Patient-Centered Clinical Research Network (PCORnet). Available at: https://pcornet.org/. Accessed February 3, 2021.

66. OMOP Common Data Model. Available at: https://www.ohdsi.org/data-standardization/the-common-data-model/. Accessed February 3, 2021.

Antimicrobial Stewardship and the Infection Control Practitioner: A Natural Alliance

Shiwei Zhou, MD[a], Jerod L. Nagel, PharmD[b],
Keith S. Kaye, MD, MPH[c], Kerry L. LaPlante, PharmD[d,e,f,g,h],
Owen R. Albin, MD[i], Jason M. Pogue, PharmD[j],*

KEYWORDS

- Antimicrobial stewardship • Infection control and prevention
- Multidrug resistant organisms • *Clostridioides difficile* colitis
- Asymptomatic bacteriuria

KEY POINTS

- Antibiotic misuse is a serious patient safety concern and a national public health priority.
- Years of indiscriminate antibiotic use have led to selection of antibiotic-resistant bacteria and *Clostridioides difficile* infection, which ultimately lead to poor patient outcomes.
- Antimicrobial stewardship programs are designed to promote judicious use of antimicrobials by optimizing antimicrobial selection, dose, route, and duration.
- Infection preventionists can enhance stewardship efforts through policy and guideline development, collaboration on diagnostic stewardship interventions, and by working together to decrease the incidence and improve outcomes of infections owing to drug-resistant organisms.

Continued

[a] Division of Infectious Diseases, Department of Internal Medicine, Michigan Medicine, F4171A University Hospital South, 1500 East Medical Center Drive, Ann Arbor, MI 48109, USA; [b] Department of Pharmacy, Michigan Medicine, University of Michigan College of Pharmacy, 428 Church Street, Ann Arbor, MI 48109, USA; [c] Division of Infectious Diseases, Department of Internal Medicine, Michigan Medicine, 5510A MSRB 1, SPC 5680, 1150 West Medical Center Drive, Ann Arbor, MI 48109-5680, USA; [d] Infectious Diseases Research Program, Providence Veterans Affairs Medical Center, Providence, RI, USA; [e] Center of Innovation in Long-Term Support Services, Providence Veterans Affairs Medical Center, Veterans Affairs Medical Center (151), Building 7, 830 Chalkstone Avenue, Providence, RI 02908, USA; [f] College of Pharmacy, University of Rhode Island, University of Rhode Island College of Pharmacy, Suite 255A-C, 7 Greenhouse Road Suite, Kingston, RI 02881, USA; [g] Department of Health Services Policy & Practice, Center for Gerontology & Health Care Research, Brown University School of Public Health, Providence, RI, USA; [h] Division of Infectious Diseases, Warren Alpert Medical School of Brown University, Providence, RI, USA; [i] Division of Infectious Diseases, Department of Internal Medicine, Michigan Medicine, University Hospital South F4009, 1500 East Medical Center Drive, Ann Arbor, MI 48109, USA; [j] Department of Clinical Pharmacy, University of Michigan College of Pharmacy, 428 Church Street, Ann Arbor, MI 48109, USA
* Corresponding author.
E-mail address: jmpogue@med.umich.edu

Infect Dis Clin N Am 35 (2021) 771–787
https://doi.org/10.1016/j.idc.2021.04.011
0891-5520/21/© 2021 Elsevier Inc. All rights reserved.

id.theclinics.com

Continued

- These common goals lead to a natural alliance between antimicrobial stewardship clinicians and infection control practitioners.

CONSEQUENCES OF ANTIMICROBIAL RESISTANCE: IMPACT ON PUBLIC HEALTH AND SAFETY

One of the greatest achievements in science and medicine of the last century was the discovery and the subsequent development of antibiotics for human use. Antibiotics have enabled many of the achievements in modern medicine, including transplantation, invasive forms of surgery, chemotherapy, and successful management of critically ill patients.[1] Unfortunately, antibiotic efficacy has been compromised by the development and vast expansion of antimicrobial resistance. The impact that antimicrobial resistance has on the international community is well-recognized by governing bodies. The World Health Organization has identified antimicrobial resistance as 1 of the 3 greatest threats to human health,[2] placing it in the same category as climate change and widespread poverty. In 2004, the Infectious Diseases Society of America raised the alert level in the United States with their Bad Bugs, No Drugs campaign introducing the cleverly titled ESKAPE pathogens,[3] which can escape the effects of the antimicrobial armamentarium and endanger susceptible patients. The ESKAPE pathogens include the gram-positive pathogens methicillin-resistant *Staphylococcus aureus* (MRSA) and vancomycin-resistant enterococcus (VRE), as well as the gram-negative pathogens *Klebsiella pneumoniae*, *Pseudomonas aeruginosa*, *Acinetobacter baumannii*, and Enterobacter species.[3] The Centers for Disease Control and Prevention (CDC) built on this awareness and call for action in their 2013 Antibiotic Resistance Threats Report, in which they detailed the drastic impact that resistant organisms have on patient outcomes. In this report, the CDC estimated that annually in the United States at least 2 million people become infected with bacteria that are resistant to antibiotics and at least 23,000 people die each year as a direct result of these infections, with even more perishing from conditions that were complicated by these infections.[4] In 2019, the CDC built on this report, revising their estimates to 2.8 million infections and more than 35,000 deaths annually from antimicrobial resistant organisms.[5] A report from the UK in 2014 highlighted the impact of this increasing trend throughout the globe. In this report, it was projected that unless action was taken to reverse the trend of increasing antimicrobial resistance, infections owing to resistant pathogens will become the largest cause of attributable deaths annually throughout the globe by 2050, accounting for 10 million deaths each year, more than cancer and diabetes combined.[6]

THE IMPACT OF ANTIMICROBIAL USE, MISUSE, AND OVERUSE

The overuse and misuse of antimicrobial agents have detrimental effects to the individual patient, the health care system, and society as a whole. Among other negative consequences, inappropriate antimicrobial use has contributed to the rising costs of health care, the emergence of multidrug-resistant organisms (MDROs) and superinfections (most notably *Clostridioides difficile* infections), as well as unnecessary adverse drug reactions. It is estimated that up to 50% of antimicrobial use is inappropriate in acute care settings[7] and up to 75% of antibiotic use in inappropriate in long-term care facilities.[8] These staggering numbers add considerable costs to patient care. According to the Office of Technology Assessment, antibiotics are the second most commonly prescribed class of drugs in the United States.[9] Upwards of 40% of all hospitalized patients receive at least 1 antibiotic during admission.

Although it is intuitive that use of a particular antimicrobial, through the process of selective pressure, will lead to the development of resistance to that agent or class of agents in an organism present in a patient, it is actually a much more complex process. Cross-resistance to structurally unrelated antimicrobials can also occur with alarming frequency, by 1 of 2 main methods. First is the presence of shared resistance pathways. An example of this is multidrug-resistant efflux pumps that have the capability to remove structurally unrelated drugs out of the bacterial cell. Second is the presence of resistance islands within the genetic material of certain pathogens that carry diverse resistance mechanisms to structurally different antimicrobials. In this scenario, receipt of antibiotic A can select for the strain of bacteria with resistance to that antibiotic. However, because that resistance determinant coexists on the genetic material of the organism with resistance determinants for other antimicrobials, the strain selected displays multidrug resistance. Because of this, scrutiny of every antimicrobial exposure is warranted to prevent the emergence of MDROs. For example, the impact of each antimicrobial exposure on the development and subsequent isolation of carbapenem-resistant Enterobacteriaceae (CRE), an organism to which the CDC has given the highest threat level, is well-described. In addition to data showing carbapenem exposure as a risk factor for isolation of CRE,[10] there are equally compelling data showing that any antimicrobial exposure,[11] each additional antimicrobial exposure,[12] and each additional day of antimicrobial exposure[13] are all associated with an increased risk of CRE isolation.

In addition to antimicrobial-resistant organisms, published data have demonstrated an independent association with virtually every class of antimicrobial agent and the development of C difficile infection.[14] Encouragingly, however, a meta-analysis investigating the impact stewardship programs can have on C difficile rates reported that a variety of stewardship strategies can be used to decrease rates by more than 50%.[15] In addition to the association between antibiotic use and antibiotic resistance and C difficile, data also show that a prolonged duration of antimicrobial exposure will also increase the likelihood of potentially serious adverse events. For these reasons, it is essential that health care professionals are continually assessing all patients on antimicrobials to determine whether or not there is a continued need for antimicrobial therapy.

NATIONAL INITIATIVES CALLING FOR IMPROVED ANTIMICROBIAL USE

Owing to the high degree of inappropriate antimicrobial use, the impact that all use has on resistance, superinfections, and safety, and the negative impact of infections owing to resistant pathogens and C difficile on patient outcomes, national initiatives have been implemented to improve antimicrobial use. In September of 2014, President Barack Obama signed an executive order titled Combating Antibiotic-Resistant Bacteria, furthering the previous efforts of the CDC and continuing to move forward the call for enhanced antimicrobial stewardship to combat this natural security priority. This executive order led to the establishment of a task force that developed a national action plan recommending enhanced antimicrobial stewardship to decrease inappropriate antimicrobial use by at least 20%.[16] This action plan covered inpatient settings as well as antimicrobial stewardship efforts across the continuum of care, including the community, as well as long-term care facilities, where up to 75% of antimicrobial use is inappropriate.[6] This call for enhanced stewardship was subsequently embraced by regulatory agencies including The Joint Commission (TJC) and the Centers for Medicare and Medicaid Services (CMS). In 2017, TJC enacted minimum antimicrobial stewardship standards that were required for accreditation of hospitals and critical access hospitals. These standards were expanded in 2020 to ambulatory health care organizations that routinely prescribe antimicrobial medications, including organizations providing medical or dental services, episodic care, occupational and worksite health, and urgent and immediate care. The CMS first required antimicrobial stewardship programs as a condition of participation for long-term care facilities in 2017 and expanded this to include hospitals and critical access hospitals in 2020. Although these efforts have enhanced activities and awareness around appropriate antimicrobial use, stewardship remains a national priority and the presidential advisory council recently laid out their second national action plan for 2020 to 2025 to continue to build on this momentum.

WHAT IS ANTIMICROBIAL STEWARDSHIP AND WHAT ARE THE GOALS?

Antimicrobial stewardship is globally defined as any activity to optimize the drug selection, dose, route, or duration of an antimicrobial.[17,18] Antimicrobial stewardship programs implement, direct, and monitor appropriate antimicrobial use at a health care institution. Antimicrobial stewardship programs provide a standard, evidence-based approach to judicious antimicrobial use. The most effective antimicrobial stewardship programs that incorporate multiple strategies and collaborate with various specialties within a given health care facility, although interventions on a smaller scale to improve antimicrobial use are also valuable in some settings.

Although there are multiple goals of antimicrobial stewardship programs, such as curbing the alarming increase in antimicrobial resistance, the primary function of stewardship programs is to optimize the outcome of a given patient with an infectious disease.[18] This process is done in part by optimizing the 4 components of antimicrobial therapy for a patient: agent selection, dose, route, and duration. Appropriate antimicrobial selection encompasses the narrowest spectrum of therapy to treat the suspected organism that also penetrates the site of infection. Appropriate selection for empiric therapy takes into account likely pathogens, local susceptibility data, and patient-specific factors, such as allergies, severity of illness, and comorbidities. Once a causative pathogen is identified, empiric therapy should be de-escalated or streamlined to the narrowest spectrum therapy that covers that pathogen. Dose optimization includes strategies for optimizing the likelihood of achieving pharmacokinetic or pharmacodynamic targets (eg, extended infusion of beta-lactams) or dose reduction in the presence of renal insufficiency to ensure that patients do not have unnecessarily high concentrations of the antimicrobial, which can be associated with toxicity. Appropriate route includes transitioning patients to oral therapy once indicated, and the optimal duration of therapy is based on the clinical course of the infection, in combination with evidence-based guidelines.

In optimizing these 4 facets of antimicrobial exposures, clinicians can minimize the unintended consequences of antimicrobial use. Most notably, from a public health standpoint, a decrease in the emergence of antimicrobial resistance and preservation of existing and future antimicrobial agents are priorities. Although there are numerous examples of stewardship approaches in the literature that have led to decreases in unnecessary antimicrobial use, there are few that have demonstrated clearly correlated decreases in antimicrobial resistance. The lack of evidence is likely related to difficulties in measuring these outcomes rather than an inability for stewardship programs to achieve this goal. In fact, the 2019 updated CDC threat report demonstrated 20% to

40% decreases in infections owing to MRSA, VRE, carbapenem-resistant *A baumannii*, and multidrug-resistant *P aeruginosa* when compared with the data from the 2013 report, suggesting a benefit of contemporaneous stewardship interventions in curbing antimicrobial resistance.[6] Furthermore, as described previously, there are clear data describing the impact of stewardship programs on the reduction of *C difficile*.[15]

It is also important to consider benefits other than reduction in resistance when justifying the existence of an antimicrobial stewardship program. Improvements in patient outcomes and safety as well as decreasing inappropriate antibiotic exposure are easier to demonstrate and may be more palatable for individual providers as reasons to endorse stewardship. An additional goal of antimicrobial stewardship, of particular interest to administrators, is to decrease health care costs without compromising the quality of medical care. Antimicrobials account for up to 20% of hospital pharmacy budgets.[18] It is estimated that up to 50% of antimicrobial use is inappropriate,[5] adding considerable costs to patient care. As discussed elsewhere in this article, antibiotics are the second most commonly prescribed class of drugs in the United States and upwards of 40% of all hospitalized patients receive antibiotics in the United States annually.[9] Antimicrobial stewardship programs have demonstrated significant annual savings in both large academic hospitals as well as smaller community hospitals in the range of $200,000 to $900,000, without sacrificing the quality of clinical care.[19-25] However, cost reductions may not be sustainable, especially as inappropriate antibiotic use decreases, and should not be the primary metric by which stewardship programs are judged.

KEY MEMBERS AND DEPARTMENTS REPRESENTED ON THE ANTIMICROBIAL STEWARDSHIP TEAM

Antimicrobial stewardship programs must harness the talents of all members of the health care team to effectively develop and maintain a program with optimal patient outcomes. This section discusses the members of the antimicrobial stewardship team and provides a brief overview of their roles.[18]

Infectious Diseases Physician

Essential to a successful antimicrobial stewardship program is the presence of at least 1 infectious disease-trained physician who dedicates a portion of their time to the design, implementation, and/or evaluation of the program. Having a stewardship team led by an infectious diseases physician may increase the acceptance of and compliance with the program by other physicians. This factor may also reduce the perception that a stewardship program is a pharmacy-driven cost-savings scheme. Even if the infectious diseases physician does not perform many of the daily activities of the program, it is essential to have someone trained in infectious diseases available to provide clinical guidance and support to those administering the program.

Clinical Pharmacist

One or more clinical pharmacists with specialized training in infectious diseases is highly recommended for establishing and maintaining a stewardship program. Infectious diseases pharmacists can perform most of the day-to-day activities of a stewardship program, including antimicrobial education, before and after prescription review, and guideline development. Because many institutions do not currently have access to infectious diseases-trained clinical pharmacists, it is important to note that pharmacists without training in infectious diseases can play an important part in antimicrobial stewardship, and the CDC Core Elements of Antimicrobial

Stewardship highlight the importance of pharmacy expertise as a co-leader of the stewardship program. The roles of pharmacists should be tailored based on the structure of the stewardship program. Multiple stewardship training programs are available in the United States to further their development of clinical pharmacists with regard to stewardship activities.

Infection Preventionist and Health Care Epidemiologist

Expertise in infection control and prevention (ICP), and health care epidemiology plays a pivotal role in the development, justification, and impact measurement of an antimicrobial stewardship program.[26] Health care professionals with this expertise can assist with the early identification of organisms and infected patients to further the mission of stewardship programs (see the discussion of opportunities for collaboration elsewhere in this article). Additionally, these individuals are a standing presence within the health care institution and can promote compliance with standard and transmission-based precautions, bundle care practices, vaccination efforts, and hand hygiene to help limit the development and spread of MDROs and C difficile. They also provide experience in educating staff, patients, and visitors.

Microbiology Laboratory

The clinical microbiology laboratory plays a critical role in antimicrobial stewardship by providing patient-specific culture and susceptibility data to optimize individual therapy. A stewardship program and the microbiology laboratory should work collaboratively on the institution's antibiogram as well as in selecting which antimicrobials are on the susceptibility panels. Local antibiograms with microbe-specific susceptibility data updated at least annually can assist with developing treatment guidelines for certain infections within an institution. In addition, because the stewardship program directly observes how providers use microbiology data, it can provide important feedback to the laboratory regarding optimal mechanisms for communication of laboratory tests as well as new testing modalities (including rapid diagnostics) that should be considered to enhance patient care. Furthermore, stewardship programs can work with the microbiology laboratory on reporting practices to facilitate rational antibiotic use. Selective reporting of antimicrobial susceptibilities can help to improve compliance with institutional recommendations for pathogen specific therapy (eg, if a program wants to limit fluoroquinolone use, they can work with the microbiology laboratory to suppress susceptibility information for fluoroquinolones).

Information Technology

Access to experts in information technology is critical in the development and management of a stewardship program. These individuals can capture data on microbiology and antimicrobial use from existing electronic sources, facilitate the detection of patients warranting daily intervention by stewardship personnel, and assist with measuring the impact of the stewardship program.

Hospital Administration

It is unlikely that an antimicrobial stewardship program will be successfully implemented without endorsement by the hospital administration. A commitment to the implementation of antimicrobial stewardship programs must come from upper levels of the hospital administration that are willing to invest resources in program development; otherwise, funding for initiating and sustaining a stewardship program may be inadequate. If support from hospital leadership is lacking, some physicians may be less likely to comply with antimicrobial recommendations.

Pharmacy and Therapeutics Committee

The pharmacy and therapeutics committee determines which drugs, including antibiotics, should be placed on an institution's formulary. Antimicrobials are chosen based on efficacy, costs, safety profiles, and pathogen resistance profiles. An effective committee limits the number of agents that have a similar antimicrobial spectrum to simplify therapeutic options, decrease the impact of pharmaceutical detailing on antimicrobial selection by physicians, and decrease antimicrobial costs through contract negotiation. Members of the stewardship team should be involved in the pharmacy and therapeutics committee to assist in antimicrobial formulary selection.

INFECTION CONTROL AND ANTIMICROBIAL STEWARDSHIP

Both ICP and antimicrobial stewardship programs have become mandatory in health care facilities. Of the two, ICPs are better established in hospital systems and have long been subject to regulatory and federal mandates, whereas the mandate for Antimicrobial stewardship programs (ASPs) in hospitals and nursing homes in the United states by TJC and CMS has been more recent. The CDC Core Elements of Antimicrobial Stewardship provides guidance to ASPs, and the World Health Organization has published core components of infection prevention and control as shown in **Table 1**.

The day-to-day responsibilities of antimicrobial stewardship programs and ICP departments can be very different. Infection prevention is tasked with health care–associated infection (HAI) process measures, outcomes reporting, outbreak investigations, and feedback to specific hospital units. Stewardship is involved in the approval of restricted antimicrobials, formulary review, and daily patient care interventions related to drug- and disease-based antimicrobial stewardship.[18,27] Because of different institutional needs, stewardship and infection prevention can become compartmentalized and even isolated from one another owing to the differences in their quotidian duties.

Collaboration between ASPs and ICPs is increasingly common. In the United States, the CMS and TJC have required hospitals to submit data on HAIs including MDRO-related infections, catheter-associated urinary tract infections, surgical site infections, catheter-related blood stream infections and to make these data publicly available. In 2008, the CMS started implementing reimbursement penalties for institutions that are underperforming compared with peer institutions with regard to the management of a variety of disease states.[28] This change in reimbursement, as well as an overall focus toward transparency and quality improvement, has led ICP to renew their focus on monitoring and prevention of HAIs.[29] ASPs have become a part of that work, particularly with regards to decreasing antibiotic use, preventing MDRO emergence, and decreasing rates of *C difficile* infection.

In addition to the shared goals mentioned above, ICPs and ASPs often have overlapping membership, complementary skill sets, and are critical to helping each other accomplish their specific goals. Both groups are tasked with providing educational programs and training for hospital staff and are involved in quality improvement projects that impact patient care. In addition, ASPs and ICPs share technology infrastructure, data, and metrics.[30] Close collaboration between ICPs and ASPs is essential for policy and guideline development, for implementation of diagnostic stewardship interventions, and to decrease the incidence of and improve outcomes from infections owing to drug-resistant organisms (see **Table 1**).

Synergy and collaboration between ASPs and ICPs is essential in improving patient outcomes, providing cost-effective care, decreasing the development of resistance, and preventing the spread of infection. The section on Diagnostic Stewardship Initiatives provides specific examples of how infection control practitioners can collaborate

Table 1
Antimicrobial stewardship and infection prevention: core elements and commonalities

CDC Core Elements of Hospital Antimicrobial Stewardship Programs (ASPs)	WHO Components of ICP Programs
Leadership commitment: Human, financial, information technology to ASPs	*Organization of IP program*: designate leadership and authority, establish preparedness responses
Accountability: Single leader appointed to lead ASPs, ideally an infectious disease physician	*Human resources:* training for health-care workers and IP professionals
Pharmacy expertise: pharmacist ideally co-lead of ASP to lead implementation efforts	*Microbiology laboratory:* establish liaison and communicate with microbiology laboratory
Action: implement interventions to improve antibiotic use	*Technical guidelines*: adapt/implement evidence based infection prevention guidelines at local level
Tracking: monitor antibiotic prescribing, impact of interventions, and outcomes like *C difficile*, MDRO	*Surveillance and assessment IP practices:* define local objectives and surveillance methods, conduct appropriate surveillance, monitor compliance
Reporting: regularly report information on antibiotic use and resistance	*Clean/safe environment*: identify infection risks in the environment and intervene
Education: educate prescribers, pharmacist, nurses and patients	*Link with public health and other services*

Commonalities Between ASPs and ICPs
Education programs for hospital staff
Reporting outcomes for benchmarking to the CDC's National Healthcare Safety Network
Development of hospital policy and guidelines
Multidisciplinary approach – infectious disease, pharmacy, microbiology lab, information technology, etc
Quality improvement and research activities
Outbreak response (ie, coronavirus disease 2019)

with antimicrobial stewardship programs to improve patient care while also helping to meet important targets for each group.

DIAGNOSTIC STEWARDSHIP INITIATIVES

In recent years, diagnostic stewardship has come into wider practice as an intervention to improve antibiotic use and decrease HAIs. Interventions in diagnostic stewardship target the different phases of the diagnostic testing pathway, including ordering, collection, and reporting of tests, processes that occur before any antibiotics are prescribed. The goal is to avoid unnecessary testing and the subsequent overtreatment of asymptomatic patients—those who are colonized, but not infected. Diagnostic stewardship interventions involve both ASPs and ICP practitioners, because changes in diagnosis can significantly impact both the HAI standardized infection ratios (SIR) (in particular for *C difficile* and catheter-associated urinary tract infections) and antibiotic prescribing.[31]

Clostridioides difficile Infections

C difficile is a common cause of antibiotic-associated diarrhea and a leading HAI. Notably, health care facility onset *C difficile* rates are one of the SIRs monitored by the National Healthcare Safety Network (NHSN). From a stewardship perspective, *C difficile* infections are a consequence of antimicrobial use and therefore decreasing rates of *C difficile* infection is a shared goal of ICP and ASPs. One key consideration when addressing *C difficile* infection rates from both a stewardship and infection prevention standpoint is ensuring that infection, and not colonization, is being detected.

Rates of asymptomatic colonization of *C difficile* in the population vary widely, but is not an uncommon occurrence, with estimates ranging between 0% and 18% in healthy adults to as high as 51% in residents of long-term care facilities.[32,33] In hospitalized patients, the use of nucleic acid amplification tests, which only detect the presence of the organism from stool samples, can lead to overdiagnosis in up to one-half of the patients who are simply colonized without being infected.[34] The treatment of *C difficile* in colonized patients has been shown to increase the risk of subsequent colonization of VRE, and leads to increased costs overall without improving outcomes.[34] To limit the overdiagnosis and overtreatment of suspected *C difficile* infection, more recent guidelines recommend that testing be done only in patients with clinical signs and symptoms of infection using a 2-step diagnostic algorithm that includes the detection of stool toxin to improve performance, rather than the nucleic acid amplification tests alone.[35]

To address these issues, ASPs and ICPs have implemented diagnostic stewardship initiatives at different phases of the diagnostic pathway. To decrease inappropriate testing, hospitals have implemented computerized clinical decision support tools for patients with diarrhea who recently started laxatives or tube feeds, to prompt the clinician to reconsider ordering *C difficile* testing when there is an alternate cause for diarrhea.[36] In another example of a diagnostic stewardship collaboration between ICPs and ASPs, providers at 1 institution were asked to page ASP pharmacists to discuss the rationale for *C difficile* testing when the tests were ordered outside of institutional guidelines.[37] This intervention led to a significant decrease in testing and a 32% decrease in the health care onset *C difficile* rate. Similarly, Yen and colleagues[38] found that 43% fewer tests were processed and a 63% decrease in false-positive hospital-onset *C difficile* infection events were demonstrated after mandating that stool samples be canceled if they were not received within 24 hours and samples rejected if their characteristics were not in accordance with the standardized criteria.[38]

In addition to diagnostic interventions to decrease the incidence of *C difficile* infection, collaborations between ICPs and ASPs are also well-documented for the prevention of *C difficile* disease.[15,39] As mentioned elsewhere in this article, a meta-analysis of 16 studies demonstrated that focused stewardship interventions targeting reductions in antimicrobial prescribing decreased the incidence of *C difficile* infection by 52% (pooled risk ratio, 0.48; 95% confidence interval, 0.38–0.62).[15]

Asymptomatic Bacteriuria

The diagnosis of urinary tract infections requires a combination of clinical signs and symptoms as well as a positive urine culture. Growth of bacteria in a urine culture from an asymptomatic patient is known as asymptomatic bacteriuria (ASB). The diagnosis of ASB impacts ICP by spuriously increasing rates of catheter-associated urinary tract infection, another NHSN benchmarked SIR. Because treatment for ASB treatment is not recommended except in patients who are pregnant or requiring invasive urologic procedures,[40] limiting both the incidence and treatment of ASB is a significant target for stewardship programs as well. The treatment of ASB in hospitalized patients has been associated with increases in antimicrobial exposures, selection of resistant organisms, antimicrobial adverse events, future symptomatic urinary tract infections,[41] and longer lengths of hospital stay,[42] without improvement in outcomes.

This factor has spurred collaborations between ICPs and ASPs for diagnostic stewardship interventions targeting more appropriate ordering, collection, and reporting of urine cultures. Tratner and colleagues[43] reported on a multifaceted guideline intervention to decrease urine culture ordering and antimicrobial prescribing for catheter-associated ASB at 2 Department of Veterans Affairs hospitals in patients with urinary catheters. The authors were able to demonstrate a 43% decrease in urine culture ordering and a 65% decrease in ASB treatment with the intervention. In another example, Lee and colleagues[44] made an educational intervention in the long-term care setting, which led to a significant decrease in ASB antibiotic prescribing from 90% to 63% (P = .003) at their institution. More recently, Luu and colleagues[45] implemented an education, audit, and feedback program at an academic center that led to significantly decreased inpatient urine culture ordering and subsequently a decreased catheter-associated urinary tract infection SIR.

These examples demonstrate how collaborations between ICPs and ASPs targeting ASB can improve patient care while allowing both programs to meet their targets in reducing HAIs and inappropriate antimicrobial use, respectively.

MULTIDRUG-RESISTANT ORGANISM COLLABORATIONS

Antibiotic exposure is a main driver for the development or acquisition of infection owing to an MDRO. This finding is consistent among most publications evaluating the risk factors for the development of bacterial resistance, regardless of the organisms or infection analyzed.[46] Thus, infection control departments must rely on stewardship programs to help minimize excessive antibiotic exposure, which ultimately decreases the level of risk that patients face with regard to acquiring infections owing to MDROs. Antimicrobial stewardship programs rely on good infection control practices, in a complementary fashion, to minimize the patient-to-patient spread of multidrug resistant bacteria. Poor infection control practices can lead to an increasing number of patients with multidrug-resistant infections, leading to more broad spectrum antibiotic use and the further development of resistance in a downward spiral.

The development of local antibiograms is a critical collaboration of microbiology, ICPs, ASPs, and information technology, and can be used to inform changes in empiric treatment as well as surgical prophylaxis guidelines. The antibiograms can be categorized for different patient locations—inpatient, outpatient, and specific hospital units such as the intensive care unit. These measures may improve health care system-wide empiric antibiotic use.[47] The importance of improving empiric therapy appropriateness cannot be overstated as inappropriate empiric therapy is the most important modifiable risk factor for mortality in patients with sepsis.

In addition to antibiogram development, which reflects the resistance rates in clinical cultures at the hospital level, infection control screening of individuals for colonization by target organisms, such as VRE, CRE, MRSA, or extended spectrum beta-lactamase–producing Enterobacteriaceae, can be extremely valuable for providing antimicrobial stewardship programs information that can refine empiric antimicrobial recommendations on a patient level. Two examples that follow are with VRE and MRSA; however, these types of data can help to improve empiric therapy for infection owing to a pathogen resistant to standard empiric antimicrobial therapy.

VRE colonization in high-risk populations is a risk factor for the development of VRE bacteremia.[48,49] Active surveillance for infection control purposes, followed by communication between infection control and stewardship team members regarding which patients are colonized with VRE can lead to the timely initiation of anti-VRE therapy. In patients with enterococcal bloodstream infections, delay of effective therapy for more than 48 hours was associated with a 3-fold increase in 30-day mortality.[50] If stewardship personnel know that a patient is colonized with VRE, they can adjust empiric therapy accordingly and improve outcomes. Additionally, the lack of colonization with VRE is associated with a strong negative predictive value for the development of VRE infection.[48,49] Therefore, informing stewardship personnel about which patients screen negative for VRE could help antimicrobial stewardship programs to avoid or de-escalate unnecessary empiric anti-VRE therapy.

The prevention and management of MRSA infection and bacteremia is another important area of collaboration between ICPs and ASPs. ICP activities and interventions include routine screening and isolation of patients who are MRSA positive. In patients who screen negative, ASPs can recommend prompt de-escalation of MRSA-active antibiotics, which has been efficacious in decreasing the duration of antibiotic exposure, adverse events, and costs.[51,52] The use of MRSA nares screening in particular has shown promise in facilitating de-escalation of antibiotic therapy in nosocomial pneumonia.[51,52]

Barriers to the Implementation and Maintenance of Stewardship Programs

Implementing a successful stewardship program is challenging and faces numerous potential barriers. A recent survey suggested that only 18% of infectious diseases physicians participating in antimicrobial stewardship programs are reimbursed for their services, despite guideline recommendations recommending compensation.[18,53]

Developing appropriate goals is another common barrier in defining the success of a stewardship program, particularly because there is not a consistent definition of what appropriate antimicrobial prescribing entails.[54] Although most physicians recognize antimicrobial resistance as an important public health issue, they are primarily concerned with the acute needs of the individual patient for whom they are caring.[55] Therefore, it is essential that stewardship personnel work closely with key stakeholders at an institution (eg, front-line providers, hospital administrators) to determine institution specific targets for the ASP that meet the needs of all members of the team.

Practicing antimicrobial stewardship on a day-to-day basis with a properly established antimicrobial stewardship team also faces several barriers. One barrier relates to infectious diseases physicians sometimes accommodating antimicrobial requests to make their daily interactions with the requesting physicians more collegial. Forty-five percent of infectious diseases physicians believe that participation in antimicrobial stewardship programs leads to a loss of consultation requests.[53] Stewardship programs should facilitate educational sessions that promote communication and include infectious diseases physicians in the development of guidelines, restriction criteria, and pathways. Antimicrobial stewardship programs should augment the activities of infectious diseases departments by encouraging primary physicians to request formal infectious diseases consultation in medically complex cases. Other barriers to the implementation of stewardship programs include developing a process to handle situations in which stewardship recommendations are not accepted, the need to continually educate incoming residents and interns, and targeting areas of inappropriate prescribing in the face of ever-changing rates of antimicrobial resistance and publication of new literature.

Making a Business Case for Antimicrobial Stewardship

Antimicrobial stewardship activities currently do not directly impact hospital reimbursement or generate revenue, although having a program that meets the CDC core elements for antimicrobial stewardship is a requirement for TJC accreditation and a condition of participation for CMS. Similar to most infection control undertakings, stewardship activities are mostly cost avoiding in nature. Stewardship teams have consistently and successfully demonstrated a decrease in the costs associated with decreased antimicrobial use. Additionally, some disease-based stewardship activities have demonstrated a decrease in the length of stay and hospital readmissions, which improve profit margins in a fixed reimbursement system. Finally, stewardship teams that decrease unnecessary antimicrobial use will likely decrease the risk for *C difficile* infection and the risk for development of multidrug-resistant pathogen colonization or infection, which impacts the cost of health care.

Building a business case for stewardship depends on the activities of the stewardship program and the current state of health care–associated infections, as well as the levels of antimicrobial resistance at the institution. Hospitals with very high rates of hospital-acquired *C difficile* infection or high rates of multidrug-resistant infections could have an increased perceived value of their stewardship programs.

Measuring the Impact of the Program

There are no current standardized metrics to evaluate the performance of stewardship programs, and measuring the impact of a program remains a primary challenge. Measuring the success of an antimicrobial stewardship program depends on the predefined goals for that program. Although programs should be encouraged to evaluate antibiotic use and costs, the impact of interventions on the quality of care and patient outcomes are likely more important. The 3 most common metrics for antibiotic use include days of therapy, defined daily dose, and mean duration of antimicrobial therapy. Evaluating use trends over time within the hospital can help to identify areas of potential inappropriate antimicrobial overutilization. Furthermore, antimicrobial stewardship programs can compare use across similar hospitals. The NHSN offers benchmarking of days of therapy per 1000 patient-days stratified by location type, using identical location codes to those used by infection control when reporting health care–associated infections.[56] The NHSN has implemented the standardized antimicrobial administration ratio, which is the stewardship analogue to the SIR in infection control. The reporting of antimicrobial use is relatively nascent compared with the current reporting performed by infection control programs and is currently not required. However, as antimicrobial use benchmarking improves and becomes more commonly performed, facilities will have the capability to better understand the relationship between antimicrobial use, health care–associated infections, and patient outcomes. Additionally, improvements in specificity are needed to compare antibiotic use among patient populations that are not be linked to an NHSN unit classification, such as solid organ transplant recipients, neurosurgery patients, or patients with diabetic foot infections. Polk and colleagues[57] evaluated use stratified by these types of patient populations using International Classification of Diseases-9 codes; however, current benchmarking at this level is not available to most hospitals.

Although antimicrobial stewardship programs have consistently documented a decrease in antimicrobial costs after implementation, there is a plateau effect that is reached over time and it is important that this fact is established as an expectation among hospital administrators. The focus of antimicrobial stewardship should not be continual reduction of costs year over year; however, evaluating costs can help programs to identify areas for cost improvement. Antimicrobial stewardship programs can adjust formulary, guidelines, and antimicrobial restriction criteria to decrease the antimicrobial budget, without influencing overall use rates.

The primary goal of antimicrobial stewardship programs is to improve patient outcomes. The ideal way to improve and measure outcomes is through disease-based stewardship and/or multidisciplinary bundles. Individual hospitals will need to decide on which diseases to focus efforts, evaluate outcomes, and measure costs. One common area of focus is among patients with positive blood culture results (with or without implementation of rapid diagnostic testing) and often involves real-time stewardship team review and intervention. Numerous studies have demonstrated that stewardship review for patients with bloodstream infection improves timeliness of appropriate antibiotic therapy, decreases antimicrobial costs, and improves clinical outcomes, including both mortality and length of hospitalization.[58–63] Multiple studies have also evaluated the impact of total hospital costs, rather than only antimicrobial costs, and demonstrated a total cost savings ranging from $19,583 to $26,298 per blood stream infection.[64–66] This practice can lead to millions in cost savings over the course of a year. Stewardship programs that implement blood culture review should clearly communicate their impact on outcomes and costs to hospital administration. In many situations, microbiology cost is increased with the implementation of new technology or modification of technician workflow to alert the stewardship program to positive results. There might not be major changes in antimicrobial expenses because, in response to results provided by new technology, antimicrobials are often started or modified, rather than being completely discontinued. Therefore, a silo cost structure might not demonstrate any significant decrease in costs for the microbiology or pharmacy departments, despite there being a decrease in the overall hospital costs owing to the collaborative efforts of microbiology and pharmacy. Thus, it is important to communicate expectations and outcomes to administration so as to garner the necessary resources to implement and maintain effective disease-based stewardship and quality improvement efforts.

SUMMARY

The continued increase in the rates of antimicrobial-resistant organisms, the devastating impact of infections that these pathogens have on patient outcomes, and the leanness of the antibiotic pipeline have created a health care industry in desperate need of enhanced antimicrobial stewardship strategies to optimize outcomes in patients infected with these types of pathogens and to decrease the development and spread of MDROs. Common goals of improved patient outcomes and MDRO reduction lead to a natural alliance between antimicrobial stewardship clinicians and infection control practitioners.

Antimicrobial stewardship and infection control within an institution should develop collaborative goals and strategies for decreasing the development and spread of problematic pathogens, as well as defining optimal evidence-based strategies for management of patients infected with these pathogens. These strategies could include joint efforts to decrease C difficile infections, including decreasing the inappropriate use of high-risk antimicrobials and improving hand hygiene and contact precaution compliance, as well as the development of diagnostic stewardship interventions surrounding C difficile. Other opportunities for collaboration include diagnostic stewardship interventions pertaining to ASB, and screening for problematic MDROs within an institution to ensure both rapid isolation of colonized patients as well as communication to stewardship personnel so that future empiric therapies can be tailored accordingly. Furthermore, infection control and stewardship teams can work together to tailor educational strategies to ensure that the message of each discipline reaches the widest possible audience.

Finally, stewardship and infection control personnel should determine the best metrics for measuring the success (or failures) of their combined efforts. These measures could include outcomes in patients infected with target pathogens (including time to appropriate or optimal antimicrobial therapy and time until a patient is placed in contact isolation), trends in C difficile rates within hospitalized patients, and/or antimicrobial use metrics. Ideally, institutions will develop a multifaceted dashboard including several of these types of metrics that most appropriately measure the success of these complementary programs.

DISCLOSURE

The authors have nothing to disclose.

REFERENCES

1. Laxminarayan R, Duse A, Wattal C, et al. Antibiotic resistance-the need for global solutions. Lancet Infect Dis 2013;13(12):1057–98.
2. Infectious Diseases Society of America. The 10 × '20 Initiative: pursuing a global commitment to develop 10 new antibacterial drugs by 2020. Clin Infect Dis 2010; 50(8):1081–3.
3. Boucher HW, Talbot GH, Bradley JS, et al. Bad bugs, no drugs: no ESKAPE! An update from the Infectious Diseases Society of America. Clin Infect Dis 2009; 48(1):1–12.
4. Centers for Disease Control and Prevention. Antibiotic resistance threats in the United States, 2013. Atlanta (GA): US Department of Health and Human Services. Available at: http://www.cdc.gov/drugresistance/threat-report-2013/. Accessed April 6, 2016.
5. Centers for Disease Control and Prevention. Antibiotic resistance threats in the United States, 2013. Atlanta (GA): US Department of Health and Human Services. Available at: www.cdc.gov/DrugResistance/Biggest-Threats.html. Accessed February 28, 2021.
6. Review on Antimicrobial Resistance. Antimicrobial resistance: tackling a crisis for the health and wealth of nations. 2014. Available at: https://amr-review.org/ Publications.html. Accessed February 28, 2021.
7. Reimann HA, D'Ambola J. The use and cost of antimicrobials in hospitals. Arch Environ Health 1966;13:631–6.
8. Morrill HJ, Caffrey AR, Jump RL, et al. Antimicrobial stewardship in long-term care facilities: a call to action. J Am Med Dir Assoc 2016;17(2). 183.e1–16.
9. Office of Technology Assessment USC. Impacts of antibiotic-resistant bacteria. OTA-H-629. Washington, DC: Government Printing Office; 1995.
10. McLaughlin M, Advincula MR, Malczynski M, et al. Correlations of antibiotic use and carbapenem resistance in Enterobacteriaceae. Antimicrob Agents Chemother 2013;57(10):5131–3.
11. Marchaim D, Chopra T, Bhargava A, et al. Recent exposure to antimicrobials and carbapenem-resistant Enterobacteriaceae: the role of antimicrobial stewardship. Infect Control Hosp Epidemiol 2012;33(8):817–30.
12. Patel N, Harrington S, Dihmess A, et al. Clinical epidemiology of carbapenem intermediate or -resistant Enterobacteriaceae. J Antimicrob Chemother 2011;66(7): 1600–8.
13. Swaminathan M, Sharma S, Poliansky Blash S, et al. Prevalence and risk factors for acquisition of carbapenem-resistant Enterobacteriaceae in the setting of endemicity. Infect Control Hosp Epidemiol 2013;34(8):809–17.
14. Slimings C, Riley TV. Antibiotics and hospital-acquired Clostridium difficile infection: update of systematic review and meta-analysis. J Antimicrob Chemother 2014;69(4):881–91.

15. Feazel LM, Malhotra A, Perencevich EN, et al. Effect of antibiotic stewardship programmes on Clostridium difficile incidence: a systematic review and metaa-nalysis. J Antimicrob Chemother 2014;69(7):1748–54.
16. Morton JB, LaPlante KL. Impact of the presidential executive order on decreasing antimicrobial resistance. Am J Health Syst Pharm 2015;72(14):1171–2.
17. Centers for Disease Control and Prevention. The core elements of antibiotic stewardship for nursing homes. Atlanta (GA): US Department of Health and Human Services; CDC; 2015. Available at: http://www.cdc.gov/longtermcare/index.html. Accessed April 6, 2016.
18. Dellit TH, Owens RC, McGowan JE Jr, et al. Infectious Diseases Society of America and the Society for Healthcare Epidemiology of America guidelines for developing an institutional program to enhance antimicrobial stewardship. Clin Infect Dis 2007;44:159–77.
19. Schentag JJ, Ballow CH, Fritz AL, et al. Changes in antimicrobial agent usage resulting from interactions among clinical pharmacy, the infectious disease division, and the microbiology laboratory. Diagn Microbiol Infect Dis 1993;16:255–64.
20. Carling P, Fung T, Killion A, et al. Favorable impact of a multidisciplinary antibiotic management program conducted during 7 years. Infect Control Hosp Epidemiol 2003;24:699–706.
21. LaRocco A Jr. Concurrent antibiotic review programs- a role for infectious diseases specialists at small community hospitals. Clin Infect Dis 2003;37:742–3.
22. Ansari F, Gray K, Nathwani D, et al. Outcomes of an intervention to improve hospital antibiotic prescribing: interrupted time series with segmented regression analysis. J Antimicrob Chemother 2003;52:842–8.
23. Ruttimann S, Keck B, Hartmeier C, et al. Long-term antibiotic cost savings from a comprehensive intervention program in a medical department of a university affiliated hospital. Clin Infect Dis 2004;38:348–56.
24. Lutters M, Harbarth S, Janssens J-P, et al. Effect of a comprehensive, multidisciplinary, educational program on the use of antibiotics in a geriatric university hospital. J Am Geriatr Soc 2004;52:112–6.
25. Scheckler WE, Bennett JV. Antibiotic usage in seven community hospitals. JAMA 1970;213(2):264–7.
26. Moody J, Cosgrove SE, Olmsted R, et al. Antimicrobial stewardship: a collaborative partnership between infection preventionists and healthcare epidemiologists. Infect Control Hosp Epidemiol 2012;33(4):328–30.
27. Wagner B, Filice GA, Drekonja D, et al. Antimicrobial stewardship programs in inpatient hospital settings: a systematic review. Infect Control Hosp Epidemiol 2014;35(10):1209–28.
28. CMS. Available at: https://www.cms.gov/Medicare/Medicare.html8. Accessed December 14, 2015.
29. Nagel JL, Stevenson JG, Eiland EH III, et al. Demonstrating the value of antimicrobial stewardship programs to hospital administrators. Clin Infect Dis 2014; 59(Suppl 3):S146–53.
30. Abbas S, Stevens MP. The role of the hospital epidemiologist in antibiotic stewardship. Med Clin North Am 2018;102(5):873–82.
31. Madden GR, Poulter MD, Sifri CD. Diagnostic stewardship and the 2017 update of the IDSA-SHEA clinical practice guidelines for clostridium difficile infection. Diagnosis (Berl) 2018;5(3):119–25.
32. Riggs MM, Sethi AK, Zabarsky TF, et al. Asymptomatic carriers are a potential source for transmission of epidemic and nonepidemic Clostridium difficile strains among long-term care facility residents. Clin Infect Dis 2007;45(8):992–8.

33. Schaffler H, Breitruck A. *Clostridium difficile* – from colonization to infections. Front Microbiol 2018;9:646.

34. Polage CR, Gyorke CE, Kennedy MA, et al. Overdiagnosis of clostridium difficile infection in the molecular test era. JAMA Intern Med 2015;175(11):1792–801.

35. McDonald LC, Gerding DN, Johnson S, et al. Clinical practice guidelines for clostridium difficile infection in adults and children: 2017 update by the Infectious Diseases Society of America (IDSA) and Society for Healthcare Epidemiology of America (SHEA). Clin Infect Dis 2018;66(7):e1–48.

36. White DR, Hamilton KW, Pegues DA, et al. The impact of a computerized clinical decision support tool on inappropriate clostridium difficile testing. Infect Control Hosp Epidemiol 2017;38(10):1204–8.

37. Tran NT, Mills JP, Zimmerman C, et al. Incorporating preauthorization into antimicrobial stewardship pharmacist workflow reduces Clostridioides difficile and gastrointestinal panel testing. Infect Control Hosp Epidemiol 2020;41(10): 1136–41.

38. Yen C, Holtom P, Butler-Wu SM, et al. Reducing clostridium difficile colitis rates via cost-saving diagnostic stewardship. Infect Control Hosp Epidemiol 2018;39(6): 734–6.

39. Yeung SS, Yeung JK, Lau TT, et al. Evaluation of a clostridium difficile infection management policy with clinical pharmacy and medical microbiology involvement at a major Canadian teaching hospital. J Clin Pharm Ther 2015;40(6): 655–60.

40. Nicolle LE, Gupta K, Bradley SF, et al. Clinical practice guideline for the management of asymptomatic bacteriuria: 2019 update by the Infectious Diseases Society of America. Clin Infect Dis 2019;68(10):1611–5.

41. Cai T, Mazzoli S, Mondaini N, et al. The role of asymptomatic bacteriuria in young women with recurrent urinary tract infections: to treat or not to treat. Clin Infect Dis 2012;55(6):771–7.

42. Petty LA, Vaughn VM, Flanders SA, et al. Risk factors and outcomes associated with treatment of asymptomatic bacteriuria in hospitalized patients. JAMA Intern Med 2019;179(11):1519–27.

43. Tratner BW, Grigoryan L, Petersen NJ, et al. Effectiveness of an antimicrobial stewardship approach for urinary catheter-associated asymptomatic bacteriuria. JAMA Intern Med 2015;175(7):1120–7.

44. Lee C, Phillips C, Vanstone JR. Educational intervention to reduce treatment of asymptomatic bacteriuria in long-term care. BMJ Open Qual 2018;7(4):e000483.

45. Luu A, Dominguez F, Yeshoua B, et al. Reducing catheter associated urinary tract infections via cost-saving diagnostic stewardship. Clin Infect Dis 2021;72(11): e883–6.

46. Andersson DI. Improving predictions of the risk of resistance development against new and old antibiotics. Clin Microbiol Infect 2015;21(10):894–8.

47. Furuno JP, Comer AC, Johnson JK, et al. Using antibiograms to improve antibiotic prescribing in skilled nursing facilities. Infect Control Hosp Epidemiol 2014; 35(Suppl 3):S56–61.

48. Ziakas PD, Thapa R, Rice LB, et al. Trends and significance of VRE colonization in the ICU: a meta-analysis of published studies. PLoS One 2013;8(9):e75658.

49. Weinstock DM, Conlon M, Iovino C. Colonization, bloodstream infection, and mortality caused by vancomycin-resistant enterococcus early after allogeneic hematopoietic stem cell transplant. Biol Blood Marrow Transplant 2007;13:615–21.

50. Zasowski EJ, Claeys KC, Lagnf AM, et al. Time is of the essence: the impact of delayed antibiotic therapy on patient outcomes in hospital-onset enterococcal bloodstream infections. Clin Infect Dis 2016;62(10):1242–50.
51. Smith MN, Erdman MJ, Ferreira JA, et al. Clinical utility of methicillin-resistant Staphylococcus aureus nasal polymerase chain reaction assay in critically ill patients with nosocomial pneumonia. J Crit Care 2017;38:168–71.
52. Baby N, Faust AC, Smith T, et al. Nasal methicillin-resistant staphylococcus aureus (MRSA) PCR testing reduces the duration of MRSA-targeted therapy in patients with suspected MRSA pneumonia. Antimicrob Agents Chemother 2017;61(4):e02432-16.
53. Sunenshine RH, Kiedkte LA, Jernigan DB, et al. Role of infectious diseases consultants in management of antimicrobial use in hospitals. Clin Infect Dis 2004;38: 934–8.
54. DePestel DD, Eiland EH 3rd, Lusardi K. Assessing appropriateness of antimicrobial therapy: in the eye of the interpreter. Clin Infect Dis 2014;59(Suppl 3): S154–61.
55. Metlay JP, Shea JA, Crossette LB, et al. Tensions in antibiotic prescribing: pitting social concerns against interests of individual patients. J Gen Intern Med 2002; 17:87–94.
56. National Healthcare Safety Network. Antimicrobial use and resistance options website. Available at: http://www.cdc.gov/nhsn/acute-care-hospital/aur/. Accessed December 15, 2015.
57. Polk RE, Hohmann SF, Medvedev S, et al. Benchmarking risk-adjusted adult antibacterial drug use in 70 US academic medical center hospitals. Clin Infect Dis 2011;53(11):1100–10.
58. Bauer KA, Perez KK, Forrest GN, et al. Review of rapid diagnostic tests used by antimicrobial stewardship programs. Clin Infect Dis 2014;59(Suppl 3):S134–45.
59. Loeb M, Brazil K, Lohfeld L, et al. Effect of a multifaceted intervention on number of antimicrobial prescriptions for suspected urinary tract infections in residents of nursing homes: cluster randomised controlled trial. BMJ 2005;331(7518):669.
60. Skarda DE, Schall K, Rollins M, et al. Response-based therapy for ruptured appendicitis reduces resource utilization. J Pediatr Surg 2014;49(12):1726–9.
61. Antworth A, Collins CD, Kunapuli A, et al. Impact of an antimicrobial stewardship program comprehensive care bundle on management of candidemia. Pharmacotherapy 2013;33(2):137–43.
62. Pogue JM, Mynatt RP, Marchaim D, et al. Automated alerts coupled with antimicrobial stewardship intervention lead to decreases in length of stay in patients with gram-negative bacteremia. Infect Control Hosp Epidemiol 2014;35(2):132–8.
63. Nguyen CT, Gandhi T, Chenoweth C, et al. Impact of an antimicrobial stewardship-led intervention for Staphylococcus aureus bacteraemia: a quasiexperimental study. J Antimicrob Chemother 2015;70(12):3390–6.
64. Perez KK, Olsen RJ, Musick WL, et al. Integrating rapid diagnostics and antimicrobial stewardship improves outcomes in patients with antibiotic-resistant Gram-negative bacteremia. J Infect 2014;69(3):216–25.
65. Perez KK, Olsen RJ, Musick WL, et al. Integrating rapid pathogen identification and antimicrobial stewardship significantly decreases hospital costs. Arch Pathol Lab Med 2013;137(9):1247–54.
66. Wong JR, Bauer KA, Mangino JE, et al. Antimicrobial stewardship pharmacist interventions for coagulase-negative staphylococci positive blood cultures using rapid polymerase chain reaction. Ann Pharmacother 2012;46(11):1484–90.

Behind Every Great Infection Prevention Program is a Great Microbiology Laboratory

Key Components and Strategies for an Effective Partnership

Paul Lephart, PhD, D(ABMM)[a],*, William LeBar, MS[a], Duane Newton, PhD, D(ABMM), FIDSA[b]

KEYWORDS

- Infection prevention • Infection control • Clinical microbiology
- Health care–associated infection • Hospital-acquired infection

KEY POINTS

- A successful infection prevention program depends on an integrated, resourced, and enabled clinical microbiology laboratory.
- The advance of technology and automation in the clinical microbiology laboratory now allows more rapid and effective infection control and prevention strategies.
- The clinical microbiology laboratory must work closely with the infection prevention program to construct financial models to promote advancement in health care–associated infection diagnostic testing.
- Collaboration between clinical microbiology, antibiotic stewardship, and infectious diseases in the context of the infection prevention program is essential to develop effective screening programs for specific pathogens and diseases.

INTRODUCTION

In the decade since Diekema and Saubolle[1] authored their comprehensive review of the role of the clinical microbiology laboratory (CML) in an infection prevention program (IPP), much has changed in the capabilities that the CML can provide in support of an IPP. This period has shown a prolific expansion of testing platforms with

[a] Clinical Microbiology Laboratory, Department of Pathology, University of Michigan Medical School, 2800 Plymouth Road Building 36-1221-52, Ann Arbor, MI 48109-2800, USA; [b] NaviDx Consulting, Department of Pathology, University of Michigan Medical School, 2800 Plymouth Road Building 36-1221-52, Ann Arbor, MI 48109-2800, USA
* Corresponding author.
E-mail address: plephart@umich.edu

Infect Dis Clin N Am 35 (2021) 789–802
https://doi.org/10.1016/j.idc.2021.04.012
id.theclinics.com

excellent performance characteristics, an impressive decrease in the time to actionable results, and a concomitant substantial increase in the breadth of pathogens and antimicrobial resistance markers that can be detected rapidly and concurrently. Although the global coronavirus disease 2019 (COVID-19) pandemic has shone a bright light on the importance of testing provided by clinical microbiology laboratories, members of the IPP team have long recognized and relied on these valuable resources provided by the laboratory.

Effective partnerships between the CML and IPP have depended on well-coordinated and well-communicated decisions on the use of the valuable, but often limited, resources available to the CML. Although the novel technologies and diagnostic approaches discussed in this article have substantially improved the quality and efficiency with which the CML has been able to function, well-trained and experienced clinical laboratory scientists still provide the foundation for the clinical services provided by CMLs. As the existing laboratory workforce has aged, and the prospects for replacement of retirees has been limited by administrative restrictions and/or a lack of qualified applicants,[2] it is increasingly important for decisions on resource use in the CML to be managed to maximize the clinical benefit. These decisions cannot be made in a silo, and require close collaboration between the CML and IPP, as well as the antimicrobial stewardship team, infectious diseases services, and other clinical partners when appropriate.

The authors have used the PDCA (plan-do-check-adjust) quality systems tool as a model for implementing and managing alterations in laboratory practice. When clinical needs change or new technologies are identified and thought to be useful, the CML, IPP, and appropriate clinical stakeholders convene to discuss the benefits and limitations of the prospective changes and develop a strategy for implementation (plan). Once the laboratory completes the process of test performance verification/validation, and/or incorporates operational changes to respond to the clinical needs, messaging is developed as a team, and communication of the new process occurs through clinical networks (do). Once implemented, continuous analysis of the new process occurs to ensure that the test performance, clinical use, and patient impact occur as expected or desired (check). Frequently, modifications to the process are required; these often involve revisions to reporting language to improve clarity for clinical users, or changes to production schedule to optimize the clinical impact (adjust). This quality systems process is used not only for each new initiative but also throughout the life of existing processes to monitor and confirm that clinical needs continue to be met. Through this dynamic and iterative process, the CML can contribute its expertise in clinical decision making and optimize its partnership with IPP to protect the health and safety of patients.

BACKGROUND

Although the CML has specific roles in facilitating the execution of the IPP's core missions, implementation of novel technologies to enhance clinical care are critical to ensure success in this partnership. The CML at its foundation serves as the source of microbial culture and eventual organism identification and antimicrobial susceptibility testing information as a component of diagnostic testing for infectious diseases. Although traditional methods remain the gold standard for many aspects of this testing, they can suffer from long turnaround times and suboptimal performance, both of which can prevent results from having more immediate and relevant clinical impact. In recent years, multiple technologies have been developed or enhanced that have mitigated many of the shortcomings associated with conventional methods.

As a result, speed and accuracy of laboratory results have improved substantially, which has been key to optimizing IPP initiatives and improving impact on patient care. The application of matrix-assisted laser desorption ionization–time of flight (MALDI-TOF) mass spectrometry (MS) technology in the identification of cultured organisms has been arguably the most transformative advance in the CML in the past decade. MALDI-TOF MS enables identification of multiple organisms in a matter of minutes compared with traditional biochemical methods of identification that require hours to days. Organism identification using MALDI-TOF MS identification is rooted in the gold standard of organism identification (nucleic acid sequence analysis of 16S ribosomal RNA genes) allowing an unparalleled improvement in specificity compared with traditional biochemical identification.[3–6]

Organism detection and characterization by molecular techniques have grown substantially, particularly with the availability of multiplex microarrayed nucleic acid probe and amplification panels for nearly every specimen type possible, providing results in hours directly from the specimen. Although these panels offer rapid clinical and IPP-relevant insight into the infection and/or colonization status of a patient, they are limited to a dozen or two target organisms and resistance gene markers compared with traditional culture, and results often require confirmation with traditional culture and susceptibility testing.[7–10] Technological advances have also been applied more directly to traditional microbiologic processing and culture techniques, resulting in improvements in efficiency and time to identification pertinent to the standard, essential components of the CML. Implementation of total laboratory automation systems that are designed to automate much of the processing, incubation, and culture monitoring inherent to the most basic functions of the CML has resulted in more efficient and rapid growth of organisms on routine culture media, leading to a faster time to identification and susceptibility reporting.[11–15] Although data showing the clinical value of these systems are limited, they provide antimicrobial stewardship program (ASP) and IPPs with the opportunity to initiate appropriate interventions in a more timely manner than was historically possible.

An integral part of any IPP is surveillance for health care–associated infections (HAIs) and working to prevent HAIs, as indicated by the Centers for Disease Control and Prevention (CDC) National Healthcare Safety Network (NHSN) and required by the Centers for Medicare and Medicaid Services (CMS). CMLs serving acute care hospitals need robust protocols and methodologies to ensure rapid and reliable detection of central line–associated bloodstream infections (CLABSIs), pneumonia (ventilator-associated pneumonia [VAP] and non–ventilator-associated pneumonia), catheter-associated urinary tract infections (CAUTIs), surgical site infections (SSIs), nosocomial *Clostridioides difficile* infections (CDIs), and nosocomial methicillin-resistant *Staphylococcus aureus* (MRSA) bacteremia.

BACTEREMIA

The standard of care for the detection of microorganisms from blood culture uses continuously monitored automated detection systems designed to optimize time to detection in all blood cultures, including in cases of CLABSI and MRSA bacteremia. After detection of culture growth, it is equally important to have efficient methodologies in place to identify organisms as specifically as possible and detect resistance mechanisms in an expedient fashion to allow timely administration of targeted therapies and appropriate risk management. Advances in technology over the last decade have seen the application of molecular probe microarray and multiplexed nucleic acid amplification tests (NAATs) applied toward the identification of the primary causative pathogens in bloodstream infections, as well as the most common blood culture contaminants. In addition, these panels allow detection of notable resistance genes, such as mecA (MRSA), vanA/B (vancomycin-resistant *Enterococcus* [VRE]), ctxM (extended spectrum beta-lactamase-producing Enterobacteriaceae [ESBL]), as well as K. pneumoniae carbapenemase (KPC) New Delhi Metallo-beta-lactamase (NDM) Verona Integron-Encomded Metallo-beta-lactamase (VIM) Imipenemase (IMP) Oxacillinase (OXA) genes associated with carbapenem resistance. Application of this technology is integral in supporting optimal IPP surveillance and control of CLABSIs and MRSA bacteremia.[16–18]

HOSPITAL-ACQUIRED PNEUMONIA

Hospital-acquired pneumonia, including both VAP and non–ventilator associated pneumonia, is one of the, if not the, most common HAIs in acute care hospitals in the United States.[19] Of key importance in cultures of respiratory specimens from patients suspected of pneumonia is the rapid and sensitive identification of S aureus (SA) and *Pseudomonas aeruginosa* (PSAE), because this is critically important to limiting the spread of these pathogens in the hospital, optimizing patient care, and limiting of the morbidity and mortality associated with them. Although SA and PSAE are key pathogens to recognize in any respiratory culture, some IPPs (such as our own) find it important for the CML to have protocols in place for hospitalized patients to explicitly note the presence of any amount of SA and PSAE in respiratory cultures. This practice is supported by recent American Thoracic Society (ATS)/Infectious Diseases Society of America (IDSA) guidelines that recommend performing sputum culture in hospitalized patients when risk factors for MRSA and PSAE are present.[20] Although recognition of these organisms on culture media is not difficult, many laboratories have different methods of reporting these organisms. In our laboratory, historically, respiratory cultures with no predominant organisms, and no PSAE and no SA isolated, were reported as oral flora present, with predominance of an organism defined as significantly more colonies than any other organism. The *Clinical Microbiology Procedures Handbook*[21] recommends reporting PSAE if present in significant amounts, even if not predominant, and SA if it is present in significant amounts and is the predominant organism in culture, particularly if gram-positive cocci in clusters are seen in a Gram-stained smear. Musgrove and colleagues[22] reported how a simple change in culture reporting verbiage for patients with suspected respiratory tract infections influenced empiric antimicrobial therapy. Before their intervention, cultures with no dominant organism and no *P aeruginosa* or SA were reported as "commensal respiratory flora." After the intervention, these cultures were reported as "commensal respiratory flora: No S aureus/MRSA or P aeruginosa." This minor but valuable modification in verbiage resulted in deescalation and discontinuation of unnecessary broad-spectrum antibiotics. Therefore, protocols should include methods to rapidly recognize SA/PSAE from media used for respiratory cultures, preferably including the use of selective and differential agars to enhance early detection, similar to the approach commonly used for respiratory specimens from patients with cystic fibrosis.[23–25]

Once presumptive colonies are recognized, the most rapid and reliable identification is achieved using MALDI-TOF MS, but identification by any method ultimately depends on the recognition of an SA or PSAE colony on an agar plate; when specimens are heavily mixed or colony phenotypes are atypical, sensitivity and time to identification can suffer. NAAT methods can mitigate these obstacles, offering the most sensitive and specific detection of SA, PSAE, and other lower respiratory tract (LRT) pathogens, either individually or as a part of a panel of organisms. Recently, NAAT panels tailored for the rapid detection of LRT pathogens have been designed to provide semiquantitative polymerase chain reaction (PCR) results reflecting the relative organism prevalence within LRT specimens. This information is a crucial component in distinguishing among true pathogens, such as SA and PSAE that are relevant in any quantity, from those organisms whose role in LRT disease may vary from oropharyngeal contaminant to opportunistic pathogen, depending on the quantity detected.[26–29]

CATHETER-ASSOCIATED URINARY TRACT INFECTIONS

Management of CAUTIs has not changed in the last decade from a perspective of technology in the CML. The primary support a CML can offer to the IPP in managing CAUTIs is in providing efficient and accurate mechanisms to help prevent unnecessary culture of specimens from patients with asymptomatic bacteriuria. Close collaboration is needed between the CML and the IPP and hematology laboratory to develop a reflexive ordering system designed to allow culture only after certain urinalysis thresholds are met, such as thresholds for quantitative urine white blood cell count greater than 10 cells/μL and/or abnormal levels of leukocyte esterase or nitrite. The effectiveness of this strategy alone is controversial in reducing CAUTI rates and it should be paired with an IPP-driven strategy to limit the collection of urine in patients with indwelling catheters for the purpose of performing urinalysis and/or culture only if clinically indicated (eg, if the patient has symptoms of urinary tract infection).[30–35] Furthermore, the CML should work closely with IPP and other appropriate providers to develop clinically relevant organism-reporting algorithms for urine cultures, designed to prevent the over-reporting of urogenital commensal organisms, thereby resulting in a more accurate assessment of true CAUTI rates.

CLOSTRIDIOIDES DIFFICILE INFECTION

The role of the CML in supporting IPP reduction of CDI revolves around not only the accurate and rapid detection of C difficile toxin and toxigenic organisms but, most importantly, differentiating between the significance of the detection of either. The detection of toxigenic C difficile in the CML is a process that has evolved drastically in the past 10 years. Early in the 2010s it was common practice in most CMLs to use antigen tests for the detection of C difficile toxin as the primary methodology for the detection of CDI. Although specificity of the antigen test was generally reliable, its sensitivity in the detection of CDI has always been poor,[36] reflected by the practice of requiring as many as 3 serial negative antigen tests in order to rule out CDI. The development of PCR assays targeting the toxin gene locus improved the sensitivity for CDI detection, but at the cost of decreased clinical specificity, because it quickly became apparent that many mildly and asymptomatic patients carried detectable amounts of toxigenic C difficile nucleic acid in their stool.[37] Institutions that switched from toxin antigen to toxin gene PCR saw their rates increase by ~50% to 200%,[38–40] warranting reexamination of testing strategies and algorithms to appropriately manage apparent drastic increases in rates of CDI. Ultimately, this resulted in the development of new testing algorithms using toxin/glutamate dehydrogenase (GDH) combination antigen tests, followed by a toxin gene PCR confirmatory test if toxin/GDH antigen test results were discrepant. Alternatively, and more commonly used in Europe, an algorithm with PCR used first followed by a toxin antigen test (if PCR is positive) has helped discriminate between patients with indisputable CDI (PCR+tox+) and those whose diagnosis between C difficile carriage and true CDI requires clinical judgment (PCR+tox−).[41] IPP teams must also work closely with CMLs to develop stewardship criteria regarding appropriate test criteria to help enforce IDSA guidelines that advise limiting CDI testing to only those patients who have had 3 or more unexplained and new-onset unformed stools within a 24-hour period. These guidelines are particularly important if an NAAT-only testing option is used.

MULTIDRUG-RESISTANT ORGANISMS AND PATHOGEN SCREENING

The CDC has identified the control and management of multidrug-resistant organisms (MDROs) as a strongly recommended priority for health care institutions and their IPPs. The MDRO category contains a variety of organisms, including MRSA, VRE, ESBL, carbapenemase-producing carbapenem-resistant Enterobacteriaceae (CP-CRE), carbapenemase-producing *Acinetobacter* and *Pseudomonas* (CP-CRO), as well as multidrug resistant (MDR) and extensively drug-resistant *Acinetobacter* and *Pseudomonas* strains. The role of the CML is to provide rapid and accurate detection of these organisms via a combination of molecular identification platforms and broad antimicrobial susceptibility testing with drug panels developed in cooperation with the institutional IPP and antimicrobial stewardship committee (ASC). Detection of many of these MDROs within hours of specimen submission has been facilitated by the development of multiplex PCR panels that include targets specific for both the organism and resistance genes of importance, such as *mec*A (MRSA), *van*A/B (VRE), *ctx*M (ESBL) and KPC, NDM, VIM, IMP, and OXA (CP-CRE and CP-CRO). Although the detection and control of these MDROs is essential from clinical specimens in patients with acute disease, many IPPs also see value in the potential of active surveillance of at-risk patient populations for the MDROs mentioned earlier[42–48] and other high-risk organisms such as *Candida auris*,[49] *C difficile*,[50] *Klebsiella pneumoniae*,[51] and, most notably as of late, severe acute respiratory syndrome coronavirus-2 (SARS-CoV-2).[52] Specifically, the ability to rapidly screen for SA and MRSA in high-risk preoperative groups has contributed greatly to the IPPs mission to reduce SSIs.[53,54] Direct IPP management of SSIs typically does not involve the CML and is primarily related to the development of IPP policies directed toward the prevention of SSIs during the procedure. However, the CML can take on an integral role in infection prevention by implementing preprocedural patient screening tests to detect high-risk pathogens, including MDROs, to ultimately assist in targeted prophylactic therapy and risk management strategies. Because the available molecular assays are not sufficient to cover all possible mechanisms or specimen sources of infection caused by these suspect pathogens, traditional methods of culture and susceptibility testing must be maintained, and protocols continually developed to improve their time to detection. Improvements in rapid detection of MDROs directly from culture include the development of MALDI-TOF MS technology to categorized MRSA or KPC-type strains at the time of organism identification, chromogenic culture media for the rapid detection of a wide variety of MDROs, or the use of inexpensive antigen tests to rapidly screen gram-negative organisms from culture for the presence of carbapenemase proteins.[55–59]

ANTIMICROBIAL SUSCEPTIBILITY TESTING

Antimicrobial susceptibility testing (AST) has long proved to be the most stubborn bottleneck in the race to placing patients on the most effective therapy, because phenotypic detection of true minimum inhibitory concentration (MIC) levels of antimicrobial resistance is difficult to expedite on a large scale. A notable exception has used automated microscopic measurement of the effect of select antimicrobials on nanocolony development of individual organisms from blood cultures; however, even this revolutionary technology has only reduced the time of reporting AST results from 18 to 24 hours to 7 hours for a limited set of organism and antibiotic combinations.[60–62] Performance of AST on isolates directly from blood culture using traditional disc diffusion methods can provide an accurate and more rapid AST result compared with conventional methods; however, the utility of this information in the context of antimicrobial stewardship is limited because it does not provide an MIC value and is only successful with monomicrobic cultures.[63] With almost all CMLs still beholden to AST instrumentation that requires 12 to 24 hours of growth to establish an accurate MIC value, efforts to improve time to AST result are best focused on maximizing laboratory efficiencies.[64] With appropriately trained CML staff on all shifts (and, equally important, clinical and IPP staff available and trained to respond to relevant AST released at any time during the day), the time from availability of organism identification and full susceptibility report that can be acted on clinically can be reduced significantly.

INFECTION PREVENTION IN MYCOBACTERIOLOGY, MYCOLOGY, AND VIROLOGY

The role of the CML in enabling effective infection control practices by the IPP extends beyond the realm of traditional bacteriology in those facilities that maintain in-house testing for mycobacteria, fungi, and viruses. The rapid and accurate detection of *Mycobacterium tuberculosis* (MTB) is a critical support role for the CML, enabling rapid implementation of IPP-directed isolation precautions and contact tracing for any potential health care–related exposures. Acid-fast bacilli (AFB) staining typically serves as the first line of defense in the CML for the detection of MTB and other *Mycobacterium* species, with current recommendations advising serial analysis of 3 sputum smears to rule out disease in suspect cases.[65] The technical expertise required in a CML to safely handle, perform, and interpret these smears makes it common for turnaround times of this first-line test to be monitored and maintained at less than 24 hours as a standard laboratory quality control indicator. CML facilities that do not have the capacity to perform AFB staining or culture processing typically use their state health department laboratory or commercial reference laboratory for this testing. Although molecular probes have long been used to identify MTB and other mycobacteria from culture isolates, NAAT techniques for the direct detection of MTB in respiratory specimens have emerged as a faster, more sensitive option than traditional smear,[66,67] and are already routinely used to confirm MTB from AFB smear–positive specimens.[68] MALDI-TOF MS technology has also recently been developed for use with identification of both rapid-growing and slow-growing mycobacteria, including MTB.[69–72]

Management of health care–associated (HCA) fungal infections in the CML ranges from the importance of rapidly detecting candidemia to assisting in the detection and deciphering of hospital outbreaks caused by airborne molds, primarily *Aspergillus* spp but also including *Zygomycetes* spp, *Fusarium* spp, and *Scedosporium* spp. Rapid detection of candidemia in the CML has been made possible by the use of selective and differential chromogenic agars,[73] inclusion of *Candida* species targets on multiplex PCR panels,[74] and direct detection of *Candida* in blood without the need for culture (which is only suitable for patients at the highest risk of developing candidemia).[75] Identification of other HCA fungal infections is routinely accomplished by traditional microscopic identification of unique morphologic structures of culture-grown isolates. This identification requires not only a high level of technical expertise but also time and multiple types of culture media to enhance formation of diagnostic structures. The application and adaptation of MALDI-TOF technologies has significantly improved the ability of the CML to accurately identify filamentous fungi and is particularly accurate in differentiating among *Aspergillus* spp.[76]

Detection of HCA viral infections, primarily in the respiratory tract, is another area of the CML that has undergone significant changes in the last decade. In the early 2010s, respiratory viral culture was still being performed by some CMLs, although the typical time to result (even the 1–2 days required for more rapid shell culture methodologies) limited its utility from a clinical and IPP management perspective. In many CMLs, viral culture was eventually phased out and replaced by rapid antigen detection methodologies, which then were subsequently replaced by significantly more sensitive and specific PCR assays. The most relevant HCA respiratory viral infections are those caused by influenza A and B; respiratory syncytial virus (RSV); and less frequently adenovirus, parainfluenza, and human metapneumovirus. Rapid and accurate screening for these pathogens in symptomatic patients is an essential part of IPP management, with implementation of appropriate precautions indicated by the virus detected and the risk level of the patient. At our institution, droplet precautions are required for all patients with infections caused by adenovirus, human metapneumovirus, influenza A virus, influenza B virus, and RSV. Furthermore, droplet precautions are also required for select groups of other high-risk patients that are positive for coronavirus (229e, OC43, HKU1, NL63), rhinovirus-enterovirus, and parainfluenza virus. The emergence of novel respiratory viruses causing the swine flu pandemic of 2009 and the COVID-19 pandemic in 2020 highlights the diagnostic challenges CMLs face in urgently developing new, rapid, and accurate diagnostic assays. Such assays are critical not only for diagnosis of acute disease but also to enable the implementation of special pathogen and airborne precautions required for patient management. The broad range of viruses, with overlapping clinical presentations and requiring unique contact precautions, necessitates the use of a multiplexed respiratory virus PCR panel in the CML to support IPP practices in most, if not all, acute care hospitals.

OUTBREAK INVESTIGATION

Aside from the CML's role in providing the IPP with the most accurate and efficient pathogen identification to help control HAIs, the CML also contributes to the further investigation and identification of outbreaks and epidemiologic tracking of infections within its institution. Tools available to accomplish these tasks include restriction fragment length polymorphism analysis,[77,78] pulsed field gel electrophoresis,[79,80] repetitive element sequence-based PCR,[81,82] and infrared spectroscopy technology.[83,84] The difficulty in implementing these tools in a CML is the requirement for specialized training that may not be widely available, and the resource intensiveness of these methods compared with methods commonly used in CMLs. Furthermore, because the volume of testing is low and results are not reimbursable, implementing these tools may not be a cost-effective use of hospital laboratory resources. As a result, these methodologies are frequently only available from public health or reference laboratories and may not provide results in a time frame that can affect efficient outbreak management. Cost sharing between the CML and the IPP of the resources required to implement these epidemiologic technologies in the CML offers an ideal solution to acquire the ability to perform detailed and timely epidemiologic studies, relevant to acute patient management.

Whether detection of an MDRO by molecular methods within hours of specimen collection or identification by traditional AST methods days after culture positivity, the final piece of the puzzle is that it is essential that the CML cooperates with the IPP and ASC to develop reliable and automated reporting and notification mechanisms. These mechanisms should be designed to not only notify clinicians in direct care of the patient but also be sent to (1) the infectious diseases pharmacist, with the expertise to assess and modify therapy as appropriate, and (2) to the infection preventionist, who can initiate any contact precaution or reporting protocols that have been established by the IPP. Numerous studies have shown that simply relying on updating the CML capabilities through incorporation of novel technologies alone is not enough to result in improved patient care.[85–88] Significant attention by the CML, in collaboration with the IPP and ASC, must be paid to the development of interpretative guidelines and clinician education whenever improving the quality and speed to a result.[89] In the end, only by continual attention to strengthening the collaboration and relationship between the IPP and the CML, in all facets of infection control and prevention, is the ultimate goal of the best in patient care realized in a health care system.

DISCLOSURE

The authors have nothing to disclose.

REFERENCES

1. Diekema DJ, Saubolle MA. Clinical microbiology and infection prevention. J Clin Microbiol 2011;49(9 Suppl):S57–60.
2. Garcia E, Kundu I, Kelly M, et al. The American Society for clinical pathology's 2018 vacancy survey of medical laboratories in the United States. Am J Clin Pathol 2019;152(2):155–68.
3. Patel TS, Kaakeh R, Nagel JL, et al. Cost analysis of implementing matrix-assisted laser desorption ionization-time of flight mass spectrometry plus real-time antimicrobial stewardship intervention for bloodstream infections. J Clin Microbiol 2017;55(1):60–7.
4. Patel R. MALDI-TOF MS for the diagnosis of infectious diseases. Clin Chem 2015; 61(1):100–11.
5. Dingle TC, Butler-Wu SM. Maldi-tof mass spectrometry for microorganism identification. Clin Lab Med 2013;33(3):589–609.
6. Clark AE, Kaleta EJ, Arora A, et al. Matrix-assisted laser desorption ionization–time of flight mass spectrometry: a fundamental shift in the routine practice of clinical microbiology. Clin Microbiol Rev 2013;26(3):547–603.
7. Huang HS, Tsai CL, Chang J, et al. Multiplex PCR system for the rapid diagnosis of respiratory virus infection: systematic review and meta-analysis. Clin Microbiol Infect 2018;24(10):1055–63.
8. Ramanan P, Bryson AL, Binnicker MJ, et al. Syndromic panel-based testing in clinical microbiology. Clin Microbiol Rev 2018;31(1). e00024-17.
9. Caliendo AM. Multiplex PCR and emerging technologies for the detection of respiratory pathogens. Clin Infect Dis 2011;52 Suppl 4(Suppl 4):S326–30.
10. Duncan R, Kourout M, Grigorenko E, et al. Advances in multiplex nucleic acid diagnostics for blood-borne pathogens: promises and pitfalls. Expert Rev Mol Diagn 2016;16(1):83–95.
11. Thomson RB Jr, McElvania E. Total laboratory automation: what is gained, what is lost, and who can afford it? Clin Lab Med 2019;39(3):371–89.
12. Bailey AL, Ledeboer N, Burnham CD. Clinical microbiology is growing up: the total laboratory automation revolution. Clin Chem 2019;65(5):634–43.
13. Bourbeau PP, Ledeboer NA. Automation in clinical microbiology. J Clin Microbiol 2013;51(6):1658–65.

14. Dauwalder O, Landrieve L, Laurent F, et al. Does bacteriology laboratory automation reduce time to results and increase quality management? Clin Microbiol Infect 2016;22(3):236–43.

15. Novak SM, Marlowe EM. Automation in the clinical microbiology laboratory. Clin Lab Med 2013;33(3):567–88.

16. Gonzalez MD, Chao T, Pettengill MA. Modern blood culture: management decisions and method options. Clin Lab Med 2020;40(4):379–92.

17. Kirn TJ, Weinstein MP. Update on blood cultures: how to obtain, process, report, and interpret. Clin Microbiol Infect 2013;19(6):513–20.

18. Garcia RA, Spitzer ED, Beaudry J, et al. Multidisciplinary team review of best practices for collection and handling of blood cultures to determine effective interventions for increasing the yield of true-positive bacteremias, reducing contamination, and eliminating false-positive central line-associated bloodstream infections. Am J Infect Control 2015;43(11):1222–37.

19. Magill SS, O'Leary E, Janelle SJ, et al. Changes in prevalence of health care-associated infections in U.S. hospitals. N Engl J Med 2018;379(18):1732–44.

20. Metlay JP, Waterer GW, Long AC, et al. Diagnosis and treatment of adults with community-acquired pneumonia. An official clinical practice guideline of the American Thoracic Society and Infectious Diseases Society of America. Am J Respir Crit Care Med 2019;200(7):e45–67.

21. Leber AL. Clinical microbiology procedures handbook. 4th edition. Washington, DC: ASM Press; 2016.

22. Musgrove MA, Kenney RM, Kendall RE, et al. Microbiology comment nudge improves pneumonia prescribing. Open Forum Infect Dis 2018;5(7):ofy162.

23. Sharp SE, Searcy C. Comparison of mannitol salt agar and blood agar plates for identification and susceptibility testing of Staphylococcus aureus in specimens from cystic fibrosis patients. J Clin Microbiol 2006;44(12):4545–6.

24. Flayhart D, Lema C, Borek A, et al. Comparison of the BBL CHROMagar Staph aureus agar medium to conventional media for detection of Staphylococcus aureus in respiratory samples. J Clin Microbiol 2004;42(8):3566–9.

25. Dahal M, Schwan WR. Management of methicillin-resistant Staphylococcus aureus mediated ventilator-associated pneumonia. Curr Trends Microbiol 2018; 12:95–107.

26. Cercenado E, Marín M, Burillo A, et al. Rapid detection of Staphylococcus aureus in lower respiratory tract secretions from patients with suspected ventilator-associated pneumonia: evaluation of the Cepheid Xpert MRSA/SA SSTI assay. J Clin Microbiol 2012;50(12):4095–7.

27. Buchan BW, Windham S, Balada-Llasat J-M, et al. Practical comparison of the BioFire FilmArray pneumonia panel to routine diagnostic methods and potential impact on antimicrobial stewardship in adult hospitalized patients with lower respiratory tract infections. J Clin Microbiol 2020;58(7):e00135–220.

28. Smith MN, Erdman MJ, Ferreira JA, et al. Clinical utility of methicillin-resistant Staphylococcus aureus nasal polymerase chain reaction assay in critically ill patients with nosocomial pneumonia. J Crit Care 2017;38:168–71.

29. Leone M, Malavieille F, Papazian L, et al. Routine use of Staphylococcus aureus rapid diagnostic test in patients with suspected ventilator-associated pneumonia. Crit Care 2013;17(4):R170.

30. Trautner BW. Management of catheter-associated urinary tract infection. Curr Opin Infect Dis 2010;23(1):76–82.

31. Chenoweth CE, Gould CV, Saint S. Diagnosis, management, and prevention of catheter-associated urinary tract infections. Infect Dis Clin North Am 2014; 28(1):105–19.

32. Sampathkumar P. Reducing catheter-associated urinary tract infections in the ICU. Curr Opin Crit Care 2017;23(5):372–7.

33. Lynch CS, Appleby-Sigler A, Bork JT, et al. Effect of urine reflex culturing on rates of cultures and infections in acute and long-term care. Antimicrob Resist Infect Control 2020;9(1):96.

34. Drekonja DM, Grigoryan L, Lichtenberger P, et al. Teamwork and safety climate affect antimicrobial stewardship for asymptomatic bacteriuria. Infect Control Hosp Epidemiol 2019;40(9):963–7.

35. Watson KJ, Trautner B, Russo H, et al. Using clinical decision support to improve urine culture diagnostic stewardship, antimicrobial stewardship, and financial cost: a multicenter experience. Infect Control Hosp Epidemiol 2020;41(5): 564–70.

36. Tenover FC, Baron EJ, Peterson LR, et al. Laboratory diagnosis of Clostridium difficile infection can molecular amplification methods move us out of uncertainty? J Mol Diagn 2011;13(6):573–82.

37. Bagdasarian N, Rao K, Malani PN. Diagnosis and treatment of Clostridium difficile in adults: a systematic review. JAMA 2015;313(4):398–408.

38. Moehring RW, Lofgren ET, Anderson DJ. Impact of change to molecular testing for Clostridium difficile infection on healthcare facility-associated incidence rates. Infect Control Hosp Epidemiol 2013;34(10):1055–61.

39. Murad YM, Perez J, Nokhbeh R, et al. Impact of polymerase chain reaction testing on Clostridium difficile infection rates in an acute health care facility. Am J Infect Control 2015;43(4):383–6.

40. Akbari M, Vodonos A, Silva G, et al. The impact of PCR on Clostridium difficile detection and clinical outcomes. J Med Microbiol 2015;64(9):1082–6.

41. Wilcox MH. Overcoming barriers to effective recognition and diagnosis of Clostridium difficile infection. Clin Microbiol Infect 2012;18(Suppl 6):13–20.

42. Carr AL, Daley MJ, Givens Merkel K, et al. Clinical utility of methicillin-resistant Staphylococcus aureus nasal screening for antimicrobial stewardship: a review of current literature. Pharmacotherapy 2018;38(12):1216–28.

43. Parente DM, Cunha CB, Mylonakis E, et al. The clinical utility of methicillin-resistant Staphylococcus aureus (MRSA) nasal screening to rule out MRSA pneumonia: a diagnostic meta-analysis with antimicrobial stewardship implications. Clin Infect Dis 2018;67(1):1–7.

44. MacDougall C, Johnstone J, Prematunge C, et al. Economic evaluation of vancomycin-resistant enterococci (VRE) control practices: a systematic review. J Hosp Infect 2020;105(1):53–63.

45. Zahar JR, Blot S, Nordmann P, et al. Screening for intestinal carriage of extended-spectrum beta-lactamase-producing enterobacteriaceae in critically ill patients: expected benefits and evidence-based controversies. Clin Infect Dis 2019; 68(12):2125–30.

46. Vink J, Edgeworth J, Bailey SL. Acquisition of MDR-GNB in hospital settings: a systematic review and meta-analysis focusing on ESBL-E. J Hosp Infect 2020; 106(3):419–28.

47. Saliba R, Aho-Glélé LS, Karam-Sarkis D, et al. Evaluation of polymerase chain reaction assays for direct screening of carbapenemase-producing Enterobacteriaceae from rectal swabs: a diagnostic meta-analysis. J Hosp Infect 2020; 104(3):381–9.

48. Richter SS, Marchaim D. Screening for carbapenem-resistant enterobacteriaceae: who, when, and how? Virulence 2017;8(4):417–26.
49. Tsay S, Kallen A, Jackson BR, et al. Approach to the investigation and management of patients with candida auris, an emerging multidrug-resistant yeast. Clin Infect Dis 2018;66(2):306–11.
50. Linsenmeyer K, O'Brien W, Brecher SM, et al. Clostridium difficile screening for colonization during an outbreak setting. Clin Infect Dis 2018;67(12):1912–4.
51. Collingwood A, Blostein F, Seekatz AM, et al. Epidemiological and microbiome associations between klebsiella pneumoniae and vancomycin-resistant enterococcus colonization in intensive care unit patients. Open Forum Infect Dis 2020;7(1):ofaa012.
52. Aslam A, Singh J, Robilotti E, et al. SARS CoV-2 surveillance and exposure in the perioperative setting with universal testing and personal protective equipment (PPE) policies. Clin Infect Dis 2020. [Epub ahead of print].
53. Humphreys H, Becker K, Dohmen PM, et al. Staphylococcus aureus and surgical site infections: benefits of screening and decolonization before surgery. J Hosp Infect 2016;94(3):295–304.
54. Ling ML, Apisarnthanarak A, Abbas A, et al. APSIC guidelines for the prevention of surgical site infections. Antimicrob Resist Infect Control 2019;8(1):174.
55. Sogawa K, Watanabe M, Ishige T, et al. Rapid discrimination between methicillin-sensitive and methicillin-resistant staphylococcus aureus using MALDI-TOF mass spectrometry. Biocontrol Sci 2017;22(3):163–9.
56. Hu Y, Huang Y, Lizou Y, et al. Evaluation of Staphylococcus aureus subtyping module for methicillin-resistant staphylococcus aureus detection based on matrix-assisted laser desorption ionization time-of-flight mass spectrometry. Front Microbiol 2019;10:2504.
57. Cordovana M, Pranada AB, Ambretti S, et al. MALDI-TOF bacterial subtyping to detect antibiotic resistance. Clin Mass Spectrom 2019;14:3–8.
58. Perry JD. A decade of development of chromogenic culture media for clinical microbiology in an era of molecular diagnostics. Clin Microbiol Rev 2017;30(2):449–79.
59. Tamma PD, Simner PJ. Phenotypic detection of carbapenemase-producing organisms from clinical isolates. J Clin Microbiol 2018;56(11). e01140-18.
60. Charnot-Katsikas A, Tesic V, Love N, et al. Use of the accelerate pheno system for identification and antimicrobial susceptibility testing of pathogens in positive blood cultures and impact on time to results and workflow. J Clin Microbiol 2018;56(1). e01166-17.
61. Humphries R, Di Martino T. Effective implementation of the Accelerate Pheno™ system for positive blood cultures. J Antimicrob Chemother 2019;74(Suppl 1):i40–3.
62. Pantel A, Monier J, Lavigne J-P. Performance of the Accelerate Pheno™ system for identification and antimicrobial susceptibility testing of a panel of multidrug-resistant Gram-negative bacilli directly from positive blood cultures. J Antimicrob Chemother 2018;73(6):1546–52.
63. Chandrasekaran S, Abbott A, Campeau S, et al. Direct-from-blood-culture disk diffusion to determine antimicrobial susceptibility of gram-negative bacteria: preliminary report from the clinical and laboratory standards institute methods development and standardization working group. J Clin Microbiol 2018;56(3). e01678-01617.
64. Idelevich EA, Becker K. How to accelerate antimicrobial susceptibility testing. Clin Microbiol Infect 2019;25(11):1347–55.

65. Caulfield AJ, Wengenack NL. Diagnosis of active tuberculosis disease: From microscopy to molecular techniques. J Clin Tuberc Other Mycobact Dis 2016;4: 33–43.

66. Luetkemeyer AF, Firnhaber C, Kendall MA, et al. Evaluation of Xpert MTB/RIF versus AFB Smear and culture to identify pulmonary tuberculosis in patients with suspected tuberculosis from low and higher prevalence settings. Clin Infect Dis 2016;62(9):1081–8.

67. Chaisson LH, Duong D, Cattamanchi A, et al. Association of rapid molecular testing with duration of respiratory isolation for patients with possible tuberculosis in a US hospital. JAMA Intern Med 2018;178(10):1380–8.

68. Tukvadze N, Kempker RR, Kalandadze I, et al. Use of a molecular diagnostic test in AFB smear positive tuberculosis suspects greatly reduces time to detection of multidrug resistant tuberculosis. PLoS One 2012;7(2):e31563.

69. Alcaide F, Amlerová J, Bou G, et al. How to: identify non-tuberculous Mycobacterium species using MALDI-TOF mass spectrometry. Clin Microbiol Infect 2018;24(6):599–603.

70. Buchan BW, Riebe KM, Timke M, et al. Comparison of MALDI-TOF MS with HPLC and nucleic acid sequencing for the identification of mycobacterium species in cultures using solid medium and broth. Am J Clin Pathol 2014;141(1):25–34.

71. Rodriguez-Temporal D, Rodríguez-Sánchez B, Alcaide F. Evaluation of MALDI biotyper interpretation criteria for accurate identification of nontuberculous mycobacteria. J Clin Microbiol 2020;58(10):e01103–20.

72. Gonzalo X, Broda A, Drobniewski F, et al. Performance of lipid fingerprint-based MALDI-ToF for the diagnosis of mycobacterial infections. Clinical microbiology and infection : the official publication of the European Society of Clinical Microbiology and Infectious Diseases 2021;27(6). 912 e911–912 e915.

73. Ghelardi E, Pichierri G, Castagna B, et al. Efficacy of chromogenic candida agar for isolation and presumptive identification of pathogenic yeast species. Clin Microbiol Infect 2008;14(2):141–7.

74. Simor AE, Porter V, Mubareka S, et al. Rapid identification of Candida species from positive blood cultures by use of the FilmArray blood culture identification panel. J Clin Microbiol 2018;56(12). e01387-01318.

75. Clancy CJ, Nguyen MH. Diagnosing invasive candidiasis. J Clin Microbiol 2018; 56(5):e01909–17.

76. Patel R. A moldy application of MALDI: MALDI-ToF mass spectrometry for fungal identification. J Fungi (Basel) 2019;5(1):4.

77. Wichelhaus TA, Hunfeld K-P, Böddinghaus B, et al. Rapid molecular typing of methicillin-resistant staphylococcus aureus by PCR-RFLP. Infect Control Hosp Epidemiol 2001;22(5):294–8.

78. O'Halloran F, Lynch M, Cryan B, et al. Application of restriction fragment length polymorphism analysis of VP7-encoding genes: fine comparison of irish and global rotavirus isolates. J Clin Microbiol 2002;40(2):524–31.

79. Jenney A, Liolios L, Spelman D, et al. Use of pulsed-field gel electrophoresis in infection control issues concerning Burkholderia cepacia. Infect Control Hosp Epidemiol 2003;24(8):624–6.

80. Neoh H-m, Tan X-E, Sapri HF, et al. Pulsed-field gel electrophoresis (PFGE): a review of the "gold standard" for bacteria typing and current alternatives. Infect Genet Evol 2019;74:103935.

81. Tenover FC, Gay EA, Frye S, et al. Comparison of typing results obtained for methicillin-resistant Staphylococcus aureus isolates with the

DiversiLab system and pulsed-field gel electrophoresis. J Clin Microbiol 2009; 47(8):2452–7.

82. Healy M, Reece K, Walton D, et al. Use of the DiversiLab system for species and strain differentiation of Fusarium species isolates. J Clin Microbiol 2005;43(10):5278–80.

83. Martak D, Valot B, Sauget M, et al. Fourier-transform infrared spectroscopy can quickly type gram-negative bacilli responsible for hospital outbreaks. Front Microbiol 2019;10:1440.

84. Rakovitsky N, Frenk S, Kon H, et al. Fourier transform infrared spectroscopy is a new option for outbreak investigation: a retrospective analysis of an extended-spectrum-beta-lactamase-producing Klebsiella pneumoniae outbreak in a neonatal intensive care unit. J Clin Microbiol 2020;58(5):e00098–120.

85. Morency-Potvin P, Schwartz DN, Weinstein RA. Antimicrobial stewardship: how the microbiology laboratory can right the ship. Clin Microbiol Rev 2017;30(1): 381–407.

86. Das S, Shibib DR, Vernon MO. The new frontier of diagnostics: molecular assays and their role in infection prevention and control. Am J Infect Control 2017;45(2): 158–69.

87. Diekema DJ. Rising stakes for health care-associated infection prevention: implications for the clinical microbiology laboratory. J Clin Microbiol 2017;55(4): 996–1001.

88. Sullivan KV. Advances in diagnostic testing that impact infection prevention and antimicrobial stewardship programs. Curr Infect Dis Rep 2019;21(6):20.

89. Manning ML, Septimus EJ, Ashley ESD, et al. Antimicrobial stewardship and infection prevention—leveraging the synergy: a position paper update. Am J Infect Control 2018;46(4):364–8.

Updates on Infection Control in Alternative Health Care Settings

Lisa Sturm, MPH, CIC, FAPIC[a], Michelle Flood, RN, MSN, CIC, FAPIC[b],
Ana Montoya, MD, MPH, CMD[c], Lona Mody, MD, MSc[c,d],
Marco Cassone, MD, PhD[e,*]

KEYWORDS

- Long-term care • Nursing homes • Infection prevention
- Multidrug-resistant organisms • Antibiotic stewardship • Disinfection • Ambulatory
- Outpatient settings

KEY POINTS

- Ongoing changes in care delivery include more time spent in NHs and outpatient settings, where delivery of specialized care and attention to quality of life are increasing rapidly.
- This changing care landscape entails new challenges in infection prevention and control for NH residents, whose number surpasses that of hospital patients in many developed countries including the US.
- The number of NH residents acquiring infection during stay remains stubbornly high, in part due to residents' characteristics, in part due to challenges inherent of this setting such suboptimal staffing, frequent leadership changes and paucity of resources.
- As infection prevention programs become a key common feature in NH practice, and interventional studies are performed, effective measures to curb infections are starting to be established.
- Keystone infection control practice include, but are not limited to, improved use of protective equipment/hand hygiene, infection surveillance, antimicrobial stewardship, worker education and feedback.

[a] Sr. Director-Infection Prevention, Quality, Clinical & Network Services, Ascension, 4600 Edmundson Road, St. Louis, MO 63134, USA; [b] Ascension St John Hospital Detroit, 19251 Mack Avenue Suite 190, Grosse Pointe Woods, MI 48236, USA; [c] East Ann Arbor Geriatrics Center, 4260 Plymouth Road, Room B1337, Ann Arbor, MI 48109, USA; [d] University of Michigan Geriatrics, 300 North Ingalls Street, Room 914, Ann Arbor, MI 48109-2007, USA; [e] Department of Internal Medicine, Michigan Medicine BSRB Building, Room 3023. 109 Zina Pitcher place, Ann Arbor, MI 48109, USA
* Corresponding author. 3023 BSRB, 109 Zina Pitcher Place, Ann Arbor, MI 48109.
E-mail address: mcas@med.umich.edu

Infect Dis Clin N Am 35 (2021) 803–825
https://doi.org/10.1016/j.idc.2021.04.013
0891-5520/21/© 2021 Elsevier Inc. All rights reserved.

id.theclinics.com

BACKGROUND

Delivery of health care in the United States is undergoing profound logistic changes, with a progressive shift of the burden of care from acute care facilities to rehabilitation units, nursing homes (NHs), assisted living facilities, home, and outpatient settings. A drive to contain the cost of health care, coupled with increasing attention to the patients' quality of life, has led to a decreased number of hospitalizations and shorter inpatient stays along with increased outpatient and home care services' use as well as NH stays for older adults.[1–3] This article focuses on infection control issues in NHs and outpatient settings.

INFECTION PREVENTION PROGRAMS IN NURSING HOMES

In the United States, NHs host more than 1.7 million residents, which is more than the total number of beds occupied in all acute care hospitals and centers. Up to 15% of nursing home residents may acquire an infection while staying in these facilities (1.8–13.5 infections per 1000 patient-care days). A mix of patient vulnerability and a high number of daily interaction opportunities with health care workers (HCWs), other patients, and visitors accounts for a high likelihood of epidemics, as exemplified by the numerous deadly outbreaks in NHs during the currently ongoing coronavirus disease 2019 (COVID-19) pandemic.[4] Infections are among the top 5 causes of death in NHs[5] and rank even higher among preventable causes. It is no surprise then that NH residents are more likely to be prescribed antimicrobial therapy than any other drug class, even though they are responsible for more than one-fifth of all adverse drug reactions.[6,7] Every year there are more than 2 million discharges from NHs, including planned and unplanned transfers to hospitals, and these numbers will likely grow.[2] Most discharged patients are likely to use several different health care settings in the near future, including NHs. This frequent movement of patients across various health care facilities is a major driver of transmission of pathogens in NHs.

A steady aspect of the NH role during the recent and ongoing US health care system changes is the dual importance of NHs as keystone institutions delivering health care to people who are unable to manage independently in the community in 2 different circumstances: for chronic care management, and for short-term rehabilitative services following an acute care hospital stay. Because hospitalized patients are being discharged sooner than in previous years, NHs face an influx of increasingly complex patients from acute care settings, and infection prevention protocols become critical to prevent pathogen transmission. Previously a grossly underinvestigated field, infection prevention in NHs has been the subject of intense research more recently, leading to a much better understanding of the many challenges specific to this setting and the development of efficacious interventions. Because of the structural peculiarities of NHs, the changing dynamics and characteristics of their resident population, and the continually evolving epidemiology of pathogens and their antimicrobial susceptibility profiles, infection prevention strategies in NHs have to be more individualized than in hospital settings, and residents' social well-being remains paramount.

Implementing an infection prevention program in NHs involves additional challenges because of the unique characteristics of this setting. First, securing the needed human and capital investment can be difficult, as is finding personnel with adequate experience. Second, it is well known that NH residents are especially susceptible to infection, because of the presence of comorbidities, greater severity of illness, functional and cognitive impairment, incontinence, and short-term and long-term indwelling device use such as urinary catheters and feeding tubes. These factors also make the diagnostic process more challenging, especially when cognitive deficit is present or when fever response is atypical. Third, NH residents may be persistently colonized by antimicrobial-resistant organisms (MDROs), such as methicillin-resistant *Staphylococcus aureus* (MRSA, which in the United States accounts for more than half of all *S aureus* isolates) and vancomycin-resistant enterococci (VRE). These MDROs present an infection risk to residents who are colonized with them but also present risk to the general NH population because they can be transmitted to other residents. A previous stay in an NH is now considered to be a risk factor for MDRO colonization. Because inpatient hospital stays before transfer to a nursing home tend to be shorter than in previous years, patients sometimes present to the short-term care nursing unit with a higher degree of acuity, leading in turn to more frequent transfers back to acute care. This vicious transfer cycle, coupled with increased use of ambulatory and other specialty services, leads over time to a network of pathogen transmission between different types of health care environments. Fourth, the diagnostic work-up in NH residents may be challenging, with difficult to obtain and/or low-quality specimens caused by patient compliance and functional challenges (for example, obtaining a sputum sample or clean-catch urine sample). Although available, staple diagnostic aids such as ultrasonography and radiographs, as well as laboratory analyses, may have a longer turnaround time, ultimately delaying management decisions. In addition, uncertainty and lack of information on recent work-ups performed by providers in other facilities (such as the hospital) is a further challenge, leading to risk-aversion practices such as unnecessary and/or prolonged empiric antibiotic therapy. Over time, these practices lead to increased prevalence of MDROs, and consequently to further overuse of broad-spectrum antibiotics.

New, specific challenges are always around the corner: for example, high staff turnover and the prevalence of multiple-occupancy rooms have greatly complicated efforts to contain COVID-19 outbreaks. In turn, the countermeasures adopted to prevent or contain outbreaks have posed an enormous strain on NH patients' quality of life, such as restrictions to using common areas and receiving visits from family members.

To help navigate through those challenges, criteria for the diagnosis of infection in the NH were developed and updated according to the increasing body of evidence and improvements in diagnostic tools available.[8] Loeb and colleagues'[9] minimum criteria should be used to help determine when it is appropriate to initiate antimicrobial therapy. However, adherence to these criteria still seems to be suboptimal,[10,11] increasing the risk for MDRO spread and making infection prevention programs even more crucial.

INFECTION PREVENTION PROGRAMS IN NURSING HOMES: FUNCTIONS, COMPONENTS AND OVERSIGHT

Infection prevention programs in NHs are formally similar to those in hospitals (discussed in article: "Infection Control in Hospitals," in this issue), but present unique practical challenges. For example, many NH residents are often transported to therapy sessions and specialists' visits at other locations, raising the challenge of effective coordination with other health care facilities, public health officials, and peers in the area. Effective communication is critical so that NHs are not operating in silos, with the risk of missing critical information and of performing redundant procedures. In addition, because most NHs host a limited number of patients (generally between 50 and 200) and many key personnel are required to have multiple roles, infection preventionists (IP)can rarely devote their full attention to infection prevention.

Interventions using novel and proven infection prevention measures are a key tool to decrease the burden of infections, and the IP is a key coordinating figure. The last decade has witnessed the emergence of complex interventions in NHs using multiple proven strategies in order to improve the chances and degree of success, while optimizing the effort and time required. These multicomponent interventions, or bundles of interventions, enable better engagement of the entire facility's personnel; creation of a culture of safety, quality, and accountability (with lasting benefits); and also an effective use of monetary and human resources, a critical advantage in settings where knowledge and needs are continuously evolving in the face of limited resources. Disadvantages of bundles are mostly limited to the research realm, including difficulty in establishing which (if any) of the several components is most effective. A potential disadvantage that may challenge the development of a multicomponent intervention is that, in certain unique health care settings and patient populations, no single intervention may have been proved to be effective already, before being included as part of a bundle.

Recent examples of successful protocols using bundles in NHs include:

- A multimodal intervention including preemptive barrier precautions, active surveillance for MDROs and infections, and NH staff education, leading to a decrease in overall MDRO prevalence density and catheter-associated urinary tract infection.[12]
- A nationwide initiative in 133 VA NHs, consisting of universal nasal surveillance for MRSA, contact precautions for patients colonized or infected with MRSA, hand hygiene (HH), and direct accountability for everyone who had contact with patients, leading to a 36% decrease in MRSA health care–associated infections.[13]
- An active protocol of decolonization with nasal mupirocin and chlorhexidine bathing, coupled with enhanced environmental cleaning, which reduced MRSA colonization from 16% to 10% in a high-risk population.[14]
- A comprehensive protocol based on the World Health Organization (WHO) multimodal HH improvement strategy, which includes use of alcohol-based hand rub placed at point of care on dedicated racks, pull reels, HH posters and reminders, educational programs, and performance feedback, which resulted in both compliance improvement and reduction in respiratory outbreaks and MRSA infections requiring hospital admission.[15]
- A multimodal protocol targeted at HCWs, which reduced hand colonization and resolved long-standing issues of enteral feed contamination.[16]
- A multicomponent cluster randomized trial of 26 NHs focused on HH interventions, including increased availability of alcohol-based hand rub, HH promotion, staff education, and local work groups, resulting in lower antibiotic prescription rates and also in lower mortality.[17]

Information Transfer During Care Transitions

Transitional care is defined as "a set of actions designed to ensure the coordination and continuity of health care as patients transfer between different locations or different levels of care in the same location."[18] Older adults typically use several services within primary care locations, hospitals, NHs (including skilled nursing facilities), rehabilitation facilities within short-term or long-term care environments, assisted living, inpatient hospices, outpatient specialty clinics, and also home care. Transitions between these environments place patients at risk of care fragmentation, potentially leading to omissions and errors, and also represent a key pathway for pathogen spread between different settings, especially when chronic wounds and invasive devices are present.[19] To prevent this risk, it is necessary that admitting facilities contact the transferring entity to obtain records of microbiological cultures and their findings, in particular if they uncovered the presence of MDROs. This action is easier to perform when the discharging and admitting facilities belong to the same ownership or management, a recently increasing trend. In this scenario, facilities may share compatible electronic health record systems and, in some cases, also caregiver personnel, especially physicians. Availability of previous records enables physician providers and HCWs to determine the nursing care interventions necessary to meet the resident's needs and to prevent the spread of pathogens in the facility. The optimal solution to the challenges of care transitions, from the infection prevention point of view, is still to perform screening cultures for MDROs before a patient is transferred to a new facility, accounting for turnaround time, so that the results can be included in the discharge packet. Timing is of the essence because many decisions, such as isolating the patient, are much more effective if they are implemented at the time of admission rather than days later. In addition to records of current patient colonization status, it is very useful to include in every patient's discharge information a list of that patient's risk factors for infections, recent antibiotic regimens, and known history of MDRO colonization or infection. The use of standardized reporting methods makes these important data easy to retrieve and consult. The advantages of such practices go beyond a decrease in colonization and subsequent infections in adopting facilities, because it enables the building of knowledge and awareness about the epidemiology of MDRO transmission between different care settings. A slow but progressive movement toward compatibility and communication in electronic records should greatly facilitate care transitions and reduce associated patient risks.

Hand Hygiene

Despite their effectiveness,[20,21] adoption of proper HH practices among HCWs is still grossly insufficient, generally ranging from 30% to 50%.[8,22–25]

In NHs specifically, HH has a major role in infection prevention,[26,27] leading to up to 80% decrease of respiratory infections and influenza (80%), 76% for infections caused by gram-positive bacteria, and 44% for infections caused by gram-negative bacteria.[29,28] Formal policies for monitoring staff compliance are often lacking. Alcohol-based hand rubs are a cost-effective way to improve HH compliance in NHs,[30] where their use is intended as a complement to staff education,[23] although they are not a substitute for handwashing when hands are visibly soiled. A study reported that the cost of purchasing and promoting hand rub was 100 times lower than the expected cost of the infections prevented.[24] For more information on HH, see the John M. Boyce's article, "Hand Hygiene, An Update," in this issue.

Gowns and gloves are another staple in infection prevention, and consistent use must be promoted in the face of suboptimal levels of compliance. Also, staff must be knowledgeable of all cases where glove and gown changes are required, otherwise unacceptable rates of contamination will result. Research in this field has now led to a good understanding of which situations require immediate equipment change to avoid contamination, to the point of calculating contamination rates for each activity.[31] This knowledge must supersede norms based on habit or personal judgment. Along with activities that are obvious candidates for equipment change (diapering, linen change), there are others with similar risk, such as dressing, and even transferring the resident.[31]

Multidrug-Resistant Organisms

A critical challenge NHs face is the high burden of colonization with pathogens often resistant to multiple antibiotics, leading to infections that are difficult to treat. This challenge results from a combination of patient-level factors (frailty, functional impairment, predisposing comorbidities such as diabetes, use of indwelling devices) and health care–related factors (widespread use of empiric antibiotics, limited adherence to HH programs among HCWs, cross-transmission during group activities and/or therapeutic sessions). These factors are not specific to the NH setting, but it is this setting where they may pose the most difficult challenges; for example, because of limited resources. NHs frequently find themselves at the tail end of a complex health care process where the patient undergoes a series of care transitions, and this may lead to a confluence of risk factors coming to a head of increased MDRO risk. Note that, for some MDROs, and especially in the case of MRSA, the overall burden is currently undergoing a gradual reduction in hospitals, thanks to the implementation of ambitious prevention programs. However, the burden related to MDROs has not notably changed in NHs. In 2019, the US Centers for Disease Control and prevention (CDC) updated its list of the antimicrobial-resistant organisms of highest clinical concern.[32–34] More than half of the pathogens included (11 out of 18) often affect NH residents.

In the NH setting, key risk factors for infections with MDROs are functional disability, presence of wounds[35] or indwelling devices, recent hospitalization (especially in the prior 30 days), and previous antimicrobial use.[36] There is heightened interest in devising methods to estimate the likelihood of infection of newly admitted patients, and it is no surprise that, in the interconnected world of clinical care, some methods developed for other primary purposes may also prove useful toward this specific aim. There are familiar prognostic algorithms intended to establish comorbidity and disability levels in patients and that have been found to also provide useful information to estimate risk of infection[37] (for example, the Charlson's Comorbidity index and the Physical Self Maintenance Score). Among strategies to abate MDRO infection rates by focusing on the patient's colonization burden, key roles belong to the establishment of antimicrobial stewardship programs, HH promotion, developing an infection prevention program tailored to the facility's specific challenges, and reinforcing evidence-based approaches for diagnosis and treatment of residents with a suspected infection. Guidelines and expert reviews to control MRSA and VRE are a source of solid and reliable tools for implementing facility-specific policies.[1,38–40]

Active surveillance cultures are a powerful tool in infection prevention; however, there is not a full agreement yet on when they should be performed. Although the Society for Healthcare Epidemiology of America (SHEA) advocates their use to prevent nosocomial transmission of MDROs,[41] the CDC's Healthcare Infection Control and Prevention Advisory Committee (HICPAC) suggests that the choice of performing surveillance cultures should depend on a facility's assessment of its own needs.[42] It is important to point out that these guidelines are intended for hospitals, where patients generally present requiring a higher acuity of care than in NHs.

In a study conducted within a relatively isolated health care network consisting of a hospital, its 5 affiliated NHs, and an outpatient facility, active surveillance cultures were very effective, leading to a large decrease of both MRSA colonization burden (in NHs) and infection rates (in hospital patients).[43] In high-density urban areas hosting multiple interconnected health care networks, it may be more challenging to obtain statistical proof of the efficacy of active surveillance on clinically measurable outcomes, unless most of the facilities adopt a coordinated effort.

Isolation Precautions

HICPAC suggests the adoption of 1 or both of 2 separate isolation precautions tiers, depending on the NH patient status. The first tier consists of standard precautions, which apply to all patients, including those who do not have a diagnosis of infection or known colonization status, and is the main strategy to prevent pathogen transmission between patients and HCWs. The second tier consists of transmission-based precautions, to be adopted when caring for patients suspected or known to be infected with pathogens of epidemiologic importance (including MDROs) that have been acquired, and may be transmitted, through physical contact, airborne transmission, or droplet transmission.[44]

Standard precautions apply to acute care settings but also to NHs, and are intended to prevent pathogen transmission from potential sources of infection. These precautions include use of gloves and HH, and wearing a gown, a mask, and eye protection or face shield any time there is a possibility of coming in contact with nonintact skin, blood and body fluids, mucous membrane material, or secretions and excretions regardless of whether they contain visible blood. Also, they include safe injection practices and practices to prevent sharps injuries, as well as respiratory hygiene/cough etiquette. Specifically, education in respiratory hygiene/cough etiquette must not be limited to HCWs, but must be extended to all staff, patients, and visitors and includes use of posters and signs. The measures to be promoted include sneezing with a tissue to be then disposed of immediately, and sneezing into the elbow area rather than the hand if tissues are not available; practicing HH after contact with respiratory secretions; and keeping a distance of more than 1 m (3 feet) from others when in common areas, unless closer distance is necessary. Safe injection practices are based on using sterile disposable needle and syringes, as well as practices ensuring that no contamination of medications or injection equipment is possible.[44] Needle and sharps injuries are a proven cause of hepatitis B and C virus and human immunodeficiency virus (HIV) transmission.

Transmission-based precautions are mandatory when caring for residents who are carriers or who have a known or potential infection with any highly transmissible or epidemiologically significant microorganism but also for all residents who need daily care assistance or who have difficult-to-control drainage or secretions. Transmission precautions may have 1 or more of the following 3 main focuses, depending on the transmission route of the pathogen of concern: (1) airborne (mandated for tuberculosis and COVID-19, as an example); (2) droplet (eg, influenza, COVID-19), and (3) contact (eg, MRSA, *Clostridium difficile*). Coughing patients, those known to be colonized with highly transmissible pathogens, and patients with compromised skin integrity should be in single occupancy rooms, or, if this is not possible, should have 1 m of space between beds or more. The current strategy regarding the choice of roommate for such patients is to have roommates with the lowest possible risk of acquiring the pathogens of concern. In general, these types of roommates are immunocompetent and independent patients with no wounds or indwelling devices.[44] When airborne transmission is not a concern, reasonable arrangements may be made to allow the use of common dining spaces and taking part in activities as much as possible, as long as HH is performed consistently and especially before leaving the room, and any wounds or device insertion sites are covered and clean. Note that these are general guidelines intended for all health care settings, and that each facility needs to adjust them according to its particular situation.

Surveillance for Infections and Antimicrobial Usage

Excessive use of antibiotics and inappropriate prescription of wide-spectrum antibiotics are common and important issues in NHs, because of their potential to increase rates of MDRO infections. Because of the high prevalence of MDROs in NHs, this risk is also shared by residents who are not treated with antibiotics, because of person-to-person transmission.[36,45–48] In Europe, as an example, 80% of all antimicrobial regimens administered to NH residents are not prescribed to cure a diagnosed infection, but consist of empiric and prophylactic antibiotics. Among the different regulatory and epidemiologic scenarios found in different areas of the world, a few common issues can be identified, including unnecessary treatment of bacteriuria as the most widely diffused concern, calling for structured and sustained surveillance practices.[49,50]

Infection surveillance in NHs involves collection of data on facility-acquired infections. Surveillance can be limited based on a particular objective, a particular ward, or an unusual organism, or may be facility-wide. For surveillance to be conducted correctly, use of standardized NH-appropriate definitions of infections is crucial.[51,52] Besides using valid surveillance definitions, a facility must have clear goals and aims for setting up a surveillance program. These goals, as with other elements of an infection control program, have to be reviewed periodically to reflect changes in the facility's population, pathogens of interest, and changing antimicrobial resistance patterns. Plans to analyze the data and use of these data to design and implement proven preventive measures must also be clearly delineated in advance. The analysis and reporting of infection rates in NHs are typically conducted monthly, quarterly, and annually to detect trends. Infection rates (preferably reported as infections per 1000 resident-days) can be calculated by using as the denominator resident-days or average resident census for the surveillance period.

These data can then be used to establish endemic baseline infection rates, and to recognize variations from the baseline that could represent an outbreak. This information should eventually lead to specific, targeted infection control initiatives and to evaluation of the success of the changes. In addition, a facility's surveillance system should include monitoring for appropriate antibiotic use. For example, a positive culture in a person without clinical symptoms rarely requires treatment with antibiotics. Surveillance strategies may alternatively focus the effort on screening for MDROs in high-risk patients, such as those with indwelling devices or functional disability.[53,54] Evidence on the optimal strategy to screen for MDROs in NHs is not yet clear. Screening in research studies has included screening of multiple anatomic sites, which greatly improves not just sensitivity but also the quality of screening data and allows the uncovering of important strain-specific epidemiology.[55,56] In addition, a focus on repeating active surveillance cultures over time may allow the defining of colonization as transient versus persistent (2 or more positive cultures separated by fewer than 2 negative cultures),[57] the latter of which could play a more important role in transmission of organisms.

For high-risk groups, surveillance could be conducted using the PRECEDE [Predisposing, Reinforcing, and Enabling Constructs in Educational Diagnosis and Evaluation] model, which follows 4 stages. The starting stage is defining predisposing factors, by assessing the local, current epidemiology of infection and colonization with MDROs, and the relevant attitude, practices, and knowledge of HCWs. The second stage focuses on enabling HCWs using education, involvement in leadership and promotion of prevention practices, HH campaigns, and by making related products and infrastructure available. Reinforcement is then provided to NH staff using simple, regular feedback on infection and colonization rates. The fourth stage, which is intended to feed back into the first, consists of outcome evaluation by knowledge and adherence assessment and by determining how rates of infection and colonization have been affected.[53]

Outbreak Management

It is vital that the NH IP, in conjunction with physician support, has the skills to recognize an outbreak; conduct appropriate data collection methods; analyze and interpret data using simple epidemiologic measures; conduct an initial outbreak investigation efficiently; and institute emergent, effective, and appropriate outbreak control measures. Although local health departments are available for counseling, it may also be beneficial for the IP to have access to a hospital epidemiologist for consultation. For more information about outbreak investigations, see the Geeta Sood and Trish M. Perl's article, "Outbreaks in Healthcare Settings," in this issue.

Rehabilitation Services

NHs also provide post–acute care rehabilitation, including physical therapy (PT), occupational therapy (OT), and wound care with or without hydrotherapy. Therapists in these settings, like other clinical staff such as nurses and nurses' aides, frequently come into contact with residents and thus have many opportunities to transmit pathogens. In an NH, PT and OT services can be provided either at the bedside or in a central therapy unit. For bedside therapy, therapists may move between rooms and units and do not routinely wear gloves and gowns but always must practice appropriate HH. For care in a central therapy unit, residents are transported to an open unit, where handwashing sinks may not be readily available. Although therapists are seldom directly linked to hospital outbreaks,[58] it is important to be aware that some specific procedures (for example, hydrotherapy for wounds) have been shown to facilitate outbreaks with resistant pathogens.[59]

A detailed infection control program for rehabilitation services should be prepared and focus on facility design to promote HH compliance, including convenient and easy access to sinks and the use of alcohol-based hand rub. Patients who have the potential to transmit pathogens to others (for example, patients infected with respiratory viruses) should not be treated at the central facility. Patients infected or colonized with contact-transmissible pathogens, such as MRSA, should not share equipment and should only be provided with one-on-one care. Facilities providing hydrotherapy should consider providing the service in a dedicated room with a separate resident entrance.

Environmental Hygiene

Cleaning and disinfection of frequently touched surfaces reduces the risk of transmission of MDROs and C difficile. NH residents share common areas such as rehabilitation rooms, dining areas, common halls, and activity rooms, offering opportunities for pathogen exchange.[60] Staff should be educated on the use of approved disinfectants, and annual competencies are recommended to be required for specific disinfection procedures in compliance with CDC guidelines.[61]

Resident and Employee Health Program

The resident health program should focus on immunizations, tuberculin testing, and infection control policies to prevent specific infections. The program should include areas such as skin care, oral hygiene, prevention of aspiration, and catheter care to prevent urinary tract infections. Adults more than 65 years of age should receive pneumococcal vaccination at least once and influenza vaccination every year. New pneumococcal vaccinations covering additional serotypes should be also considered in residents who received previous formulations. Standing orders for pneumococcal vaccination have improved vaccination rates in NHs.[62] Tdap vaccination is also recommended among older adults in NHs.

The employee health program mainly concerns employees with potentially communicable diseases, policies for sick leave, immunizations, and Occupational Safety and Health Administration (OSHA) regulations to protect them from blood-borne pathogens. It is a requirement that NHs bar employees with known communicable diseases or infected skin lesions from providing direct contact with the residents, and that employees with infected skin lesions or infectious diarrhea be prevented from having direct contact with residents' food. Moreover, when hiring new employees, an initial medical history must be obtained along with a physical examination and screening for tuberculosis. Also, immunization status should be assessed.

Infection control policies and measures in NHs must be in place to address postexposure prophylaxis for infections such as HIV and hepatitis B. Varicella vaccine should be given to employees not immune to the virus. Employees are expected to be up to date with their tetanus boosters and to receive influenza vaccinations every year. Influenza vaccination of HCWs has been associated not only with decreased influenza mortality in NH residents but also with decreased absenteeism among HCWs.[63,64] Annual influenza vaccination campaigns play a central role in deterring and preventing nosocomial transmission of the influenza virus and should be promoted by the IP and

---

Box 1
Resources for infection preventionists

1. SHEA and the Association for Professionals in Infection Control (APIC) both have long-term care committees that publish and approve NH infection guidelines and publish periodic position papers related to pertinent infection control issues. Their Web sites have several educational resources for staff education and in-services. In addition, APIC also publishes a quarterly long-term care newsletter.

2. Local APIC chapters provide a network for infection control practitioners to socialize, discuss infection control challenges and practical solutions to overcome them, and provide access to educational resources and services. Infection control practitioners should become members of APIC at both the local and national level to remain up to date with practice guidelines, position statements, information technology resources, and changes in policies and regulations.

3. Hospital Epidemiology and Infection Control, 5th Edition; C. Glen Mayhall, editor: Lippincott Williams & Wilkins: Philadelphia, PA.

4. Selected On Line Resources and Web sites:
   a. CDC: http://www.cdc.gov
   b. SHEA: http://www.shea-online.org/
   c. APIC: http://www.apic.org
   d. OSHA: http://www.osha.gov
   e. Joint Commission on Accreditation of Healthcare Organizations–Infection Control Initiatives: https://www.jointcommission.org/resources/patient-safety-topics/infection-prevention-and-control/
   f. Association for the Advancement in Medical Instrumentation (AAMI) Standards and Recommended Practices Sterilization in Health Care Facilities, 2017 Edition: www.aami.org and https://webstore.ansi.org/Standards/AAMI/ANSIAAMIST792017?source=blog&_ga=2.90169363.98205541.1611667716-2120631435.1611667716
   g. Guidelines for Perioperative Practice, 2015 Edition: www.aorn.org
   h. CDC Guide to Infection Prevention for Outpatient Settings: Minimum Expectations for Safe Care Web site: https://www.cdc.gov/HAI/settings/outpatient/outpatient-care-guidelines.html

NH leadership. Employee immunization records should reflect immunity status for indicated vaccinations and those administered during employment, and should be easily accessible in the event of an outbreak situation.[65]

Role of the Infection Preventionist

An IP, usually a staff nurse, is assigned the responsibility of directing infection control activities in an NH. The IP is responsible for implementing, monitoring, and evaluating the infection control program. To maintain compliance with regulations, NHs are increasing the rate of NH IP employment, which went up from 8.1% in 2003 to 44% in 2008,[66] and is expected to increase further as new mandates regarding the presence of an infection control and surveillance program are adopted.[67] However, IPs often share other responsibilities, such as employee health or staff education.[68] For an infection control program to succeed, the IP should be empowered with sufficient time and resources to perform infection control activities. The IP should also be familiar with the federal, state, and local regulations regarding infection control. Collaborating with an infectious diseases epidemiologist and/or physician should be encouraged. Such collaborations could also provide assistance with outbreak investigations, emergency preparedness in the event of bioterrorism and vaccine shortages, and the use of microbiologic and molecular methods for infection prevention. Examples of authoritative resources available to IPs are listed in **Box 1**.

Environmental rounds

IPs should conduct walk-rounds on a regular basis to make observations regarding equipment decontamination and cleaning procedures in bathroom/tub areas, and adherence to infection control guidelines by PTs in medication/treatment rooms, and in kitchen and laundry areas. Observations should be made regarding availability of soap and paper towels; handling of sharps and infectious waste; and storage of health care supplies, medications, and food.

Staff education

IPs play a vital role in educating NH personnel on various infection control measures, as the persons responsible for implementing infection prevention education programs and as the reference point for all personnel in case of any infection control issues. This effort is always ongoing as evidence-based updates are introduced, and also in view of rapid staff turnover in many NHs. A lack of understanding of key infection prevention concepts among NH staff has been reported.[69] A recent study on nursing assistants reported language barrier, lack of knowledge, part-time status, workload demands, and accountability as barriers to appropriately using infection prevention and control (IPC) practices, and proposed translating in-services, hands-on training, on-the-spot training for part-time staff, increased staffing ratios, and inclusion and empowerment as strategies to overcome these barriers.[70] Informal education during infection control and quality improvement meetings as well as during infection control walk-rounds should be complemented with in-service education on HH, appropriate and early diagnosis of infections, indications for appropriate antibiotic usage, antimicrobial resistance, and isolation precautions and policies. Several technological supports are available for conducting both formal and informal educational activities, and new ones are continuously developed and need not be limited strictly to classroom or meeting room settings. Instead, a portion of this knowledge may be delivered as online packages in a manner that fits well with flexible and varying schedules. Personnel are generally receptive to, and often favor, new approaches, especially interactive approaches that keep them focused and engaged at the same time.

Ongoing staff education is important because of the new research and guidelines published every year, advancements in technology, and regulatory demands. The Joint Commission on Accreditation of Healthcare Organizations (JCAHO) expects new employee orientation to include education about the facility's infection prevention program; and the employee's individual responsibility to prevent infections. In addition, the OSHA requires training for blood-borne pathogens and tuberculosis for any employee expected to potentially come into contact with infectious agents.

The Infection Control Committee at Nursing Homes

The Federal Nursing Home Reform Act from the Omnibus Budget Reconciliation Act of 1987 mandated the formation of a formal infection control committee to evaluate infection rates, implement infection control programs, and review policies and procedures. This mandate has been dropped by Omnibus Budget Reconciliation Act at the federal level. However, some states may still require it. A small subcommittee or a working group composed of the medical director, administrator or nursing supervisor, and IP should evaluate NH infection rates on a regular basis and present the data at quality control meetings, review policies and any relevant research, and make decisions regarding infection control changes. This subcommittee can review and analyze the surveillance data, ensure that these data are presented to the nursing and physician staff, and approve targeted recommendations to reduce the incidence of infections. Records pertaining to these activities and infection data should be kept for future reference. Given that infection control involves multiple disciplines, the participation of representatives from food services, maintenance, housekeeping, laundry services, clinical services, resident activities, and employee health should be considered. It is recommended that the infection control committee meet at least quarterly throughout the year and on an emergent basis as needed.

AMBULATORY CARE CENTERS

Ambulatory care settings have many of the same infection prevention and control requirements as inpatient hospital settings. However, the method of application to comply with the standards vary depending on the type of care provided by the clinic. These settings can range from primary to specialized care, to clinics where hemodialysis or invasive procedures such as endoscopy or surgery are performed. There are many challenges in ambulatory care to reduce infection risk and improve patient safety. Infection prevention oversight and accountability are often lacking, especially if the clinics are not part of a hospital or system. The CDC provides a comprehensive resource outlining the minimum expectations of care, as well as a checklist appropriate for the outpatient setting.[71]

Communicable Disease and Isolation Management

Patients and staff may unknowingly be exposed to infectious diseases in the ambulatory care setting. HCWs need to follow standard precautions in the care of all patients, but patients showing communicable disease symptoms should be managed using the CDC transmission-based precautions.[42] Because transmission of communicable disease can occur in waiting rooms and other shared spaces, a triage policy should be followed. The goal is to promptly identify and process patients with symptoms compatible with communicable disease in order to protect other patients and ambulatory care staff from exposure or infection. Tuberculosis is one example of an airborne disease whose symptoms can include cough, bloody sputum production, night sweats, weight loss, anorexia, and fever. Symptoms of other communicable diseases might include rashes or persistent cough. Patients with respiratory symptoms should be given a mask to wear and be promptly processed to a separate waiting area or examination room away from other patients.

During the COVID-19 pandemic, telehealth and telemedicine saw an increase in use as a way to assess patients and give guidance while preventing unnecessary exposure to patients or staff. Telehealth can have multiple benefits by expanding access to care, reducing disease exposure for staff and patients, preserving scarce supplies of personal protective equipment, and reducing patient demand on facilities.[72] Telehealth or virtual visits are especially critical for those ambulatory sites that are without access to or means to provide airborne precautions.

Patients with suspected tuberculosis or other communicable diseases transmitted by the airborne route should be masked immediately and triaged to a negative pressure room, also known as an airborne infection isolation room, if available.[73] When entering the room of a patient with suspected or confirmed tuberculosis or other airborne disease, all ambulatory staff should wear a fit-tested particulate respirator. Cough-inducing procedures such as aerosol administration of medication, bronchoscopy, and sputum inductions on patients with a respiratory illness pose a high risk of aerosolization of organisms and infection of staff and other patients. Rooms where these aerosol-producing procedures are performed must be modified to meet airborne isolation standards to protect ambulatory care staff and other patients. Ambulatory surgery centers (ASCs) must provide respirators to staff caring for patients who require airborne precautions. Dental clinics should defer treatment on a patient with known or suspected active *Mycobacterium tuberculosis*, COVID-19, or other potentially communicable airborne disease unless it is determined that the procedure is an emergency.

Respiratory hygiene/cough etiquette is an infection control component of the CDC standard precautions in the care of patients. The protocol is optimized by giving patients tissues and instructions to cover the mouth and nose when coughing or sneezing and disposing of tissues in the trash. Handwashing must be reinforced with accessible handwashing facilities or waterless HH agents. Patients with a cough are to be given a medical face mask while in a waiting room or other common areas and instructed to ask for a new mask if the old mask becomes soiled or moistened. Respiratory etiquette signage is a Joint Commission requirement for ambulatory centers within hospital institutions but is encouraged to be used in all ambulatory centers, especially during flu season.

Beyond routine respiratory hygiene and cough etiquette measures, more advanced respiratory prevention plans should be considered as well. The COVID-19 pandemic has underscored the importance of all settings of health care having a robust respiratory viral pathogen (RVP) preparedness plan. This plan should, at a minimum, include the following 5 basic elements, and may be a part of the facility's bioterrorism/disaster plan:

- Identify: measures are in place to quickly and accurately identify patients that potentially have the infection. It is recommended that a screening tool be put into place.
- Isolate: there is a process in place to ensure that the patient is masked and room accommodations are available to isolate the patient away from other patients or unprotected staff members.
- Act: there is a process in place to communicate to the clinicians providing care to the patient the need for isolation and that proper personal protective equipment must be donned before entering the room.

- Notify: if the patient meets criteria, call the public health department for reporting purposes or to request laboratory confirmation testing. Notify the local infection prevention department per policy.
- Resolve: consider testing for other respiratory diseases; consider home isolation if appropriate; admit if clinical symptoms support the need for hospitalization. Ensure communication to receiving facility.

The RVP preparedness plan needs to take into consideration the following components to support the elements of control and prevention:

- A written plan minimally outlining the 5 elements listed earlier.
- Adequate personal protective equipment (eg, gowns, gloves, masks, face shields/goggles) and disinfecting solution/wipes availability.
- Signage for entrances, waiting rooms, and areas where patients will be isolated.
- A communication plan, both internally for employees and externally for patients and the public, if necessary.
- A contact list of important phone numbers, including administration, medical director, office manager, local and state public health department phone numbers, local IPs.
- Contingency staffing plans, taking into account that employees may become ill as well.

Environmental Hygiene: Cleaning, Disinfection, and Sterilization

Cleaning and disinfection of frequently touched surfaces reduces the risk of healthcare associated infection (HAI) transmission, including those caused by MDROs and *C difficile*. Ambulatory settings need to standardize cleaning procedures and the types of chemicals used, and to establish a monitoring system to ensure that the patient-care equipment and environment is cleaned, disinfected, and stored appropriately so that patient safety is optimized.[74] Staff should be educated on the use of the chemicals and contact time, and annual competencies are recommended to be required for specific disinfection and sterilization procedures. All cleaning, disinfection, and sterilization processes should comply with the CDC guidelines and the disinfectant and equipment manufacturers' instructions for use (IFU).[75] New technologies in disinfection include area decontamination/disinfection systems, antimicrobial surfaces, ultraviolet light, no-touch spray products, and others that are intended to reduce surface contamination and prevent HAIs. It is important not only to review the manufacturer's technical data but also to inquire whether there are any third-party clinical outcomes data when investigating purchasing these types of supplemental products.

High-level disinfection and sterilization of patient-care equipment is an important area of infection control in many ambulatory settings and is discussed later and also in the William A. Rutala and David J. Weber's article, "Disinfection and Sterilization in Health-Care Facilities: An Overview and Current Issues," in this issue.

All IFUs should be reviewed before purchasing a new piece of equipment or whenever changing hospital disinfectant products, to ensure consistency in practice with manufacturer recommendations. Failing to follow those recommendations may result in a range of undesired outcomes, including insufficient disinfection and patient harm, as well as causing damage to the equipment.

Ambulatory Surgical Centers

The same aseptic technique and environmental standards apply to all surgical settings. In 2017, there were more than 5600 Medicare-certified ASCs, which represents nearly 17,000 operating rooms (ORs).[76] The National Patient Safety Goals (NPSGs) for ambulatory and office-based surgery provide the elements of performance to achieve safe patient care.[77] One of the NPSG elements is to set goals for improving HH and using the goals to improve compliance. ASCs also must abide by local and state licensing rules. These rules can include requiring infection prevention and control performance improvement activities that are continuous and ongoing based on surveillance data results. Monitoring in the ambulatory setting can pose a challenge and may include follow-up with patients after discharge to gather evidence regarding whether the patient has developed an infection associated with the surgery.

The IP can provide guidance to improve surgical outcomes. In 2017, the CDC published guidelines for the prevention of surgical site infection (SSI). This guideline provides new and updated evidence-based recommendations for the prevention of SSI. Major components include glycemic control, normothermia, prophylactic antimicrobials, alcohol-based skin antiseptic agents, and supplemental oxygen.[78] Process and outcome measures need to be documented and reviewed as determined by the ambulatory site's risk assessment. These measures might include incidence of SSI, compliance with antibiotic prophylaxis, time-out practices by the OR team, preoperative chlorhexidine bathing, surgical skin prep compliance, use of wound protectors, use of supplemental oxygen, or compliance with hair removal methods. The IP can collaborate with the surgery team in identifying the high-risk or most frequent surgical procedures performed, so that the surveillance program can be targeted to address key components of operative care.

ASCs now have the option of using the Outpatient Procedure Component (OPC) for surveillance of SSI events through the National Healthcare Safety Network (NHSN). The OPC includes 2 modules that focus on adverse events associated with surgical procedures performed in . The 2 modules include Same Day Outcome Measures and SSIs. Like the SSI module in the Patient Safety Component, once the denominator and event data are entered in to the NHSN OPC module, analysis reports for both denominator and numerator data and the Standardized Infection Ratio reports can be generated. The OPC manual also contains a toolkit for postdischarge surveillance that can assist IPs in developing individualized surgeon letters, worksheets, and procedure line lists. Any ASC as defined in the Code of Federal Regulations 42 CFR § 416.2 is eligible to join NHSN and use this protocol for surveillance of surgical patients receiving an eligible NHSN outpatient procedure.[79]

IPs and other HCWs who clean and process patient-care equipment should be familiar with the basic principles for sterilization and disinfection outlined by Spaulding,[80] which classify patient-care items and equipment into 3 categories based on the degree of risk of infection involved in the use of the items: critical, semicritical, and noncritical. This classification provides guidance for determining the level of disinfection required and items requiring sterilization. According to the Association for the Advancement in Medical Instrumentation (AAMI) guidelines, immediate-use steam sterilization (IUSS) must be kept to a minimum, and avoiding equipment shortages and back-to-back procedures helps to minimize IUSS.[74] After IUSS, biological monitoring is required before use. The Joint Commission Infection Control Standards have now placed a focus on IUSS procedures in the OR to ensure optimal procedural compliance.[74]

A major challenge to ambulatory surgical centers and IPs is to remain current with changes in sterilization technology and disinfectant products. New surgical equipment is frequently becoming available and manufacturer processing guidelines need to be followed to prevent damage to the instruments as well as adequate disinfection or sterilization. The Joint Commission and Centers for Medicare, Medicaid services

(CMS) require documentation of staff competencies and knowledge of the manufacturer guidelines for management of surgical equipment in their surveys. Endoscopy centers must comply with Society of Gastroenterology Nurses and Associates (SGNA) and or AAMI standards for flexible and semirigid endoscope cleaning and disinfection processing to prevent cross contamination between patients.[75]

Safe Injection Practices

The CDC has implemented recommendations relating to safe injection practices as part of their standard precautions to provide safety to both HCWs and patients. Injuries caused by needles and other sharps have been associated with the transmission of hepatitis B virus, hepatitis C virus, and HIV. The federal Needlestick Safety and Prevention Act signed into law in November 2000 authorized OSHA's revision of its Bloodborne Pathogens Standard to require the use of safety-engineered sharp devices.[81] Ambulatory care centers need to educate and monitor staff on safe injection practices and the correct management of sharps and medication vials in patient-care areas. Additional risks related to potential transmission of blood-borne pathogens can be present because of drug diversion. Drug diversion is the practice of HCWs stealing narcotics for their personal use from the patient supply. Securing and close monitoring of narcotics, as well as wasting practices, are important strategies to mitigate this risk.

Syringes and needles are single-use devices; changing a needle or cannula and using the same syringe can lead to transmission of pathogens or viruses. Fluid infusion and administration sets should be single use.[82] Single-dose vials should be used whenever possible and clearly dedicated to a single patient. If multiple-dose vials are used, they should be dedicated to a single patient whenever possible. If a multidose vial must be used for more than 1 patient, it should only be accessed in a clean medication preparation area and not entered or stored in an immediate patient treatment space. Bags or bottles of intravenous solution used for multiple patients is an unsafe practice and has been associated with outbreaks.[83]

Large outbreaks have occurred in ambulatory care facilities across the United States associated with the reuse of needles/syringes and the contamination of medications administered to multiple patients. Examples include a hepatitis B outbreak in New York City associated with the contamination of multiple-dose vials used for injections on multiple patients. Contaminated syringes had also been found left on a table where medications were prepared, possibly also contributing to the outbreak.[84] Another outbreak occurred in a Nevada Endoscopy clinic in 2007 with hepatitis C caused by reuse of the same syringe for propofol administration.[85] The CDC's One and Only Campaign emphasizes the importance of "1 needle, 1 syringe, only 1 time."[86] Other outbreaks have occurred related to the reuse of glucometers and insulin pens on multiple patients resulting in hepatitis B and C transmission.[87]

Bioterrorism and Disaster Planning

A risk assessment of the clinic location and the community it services provides guidance for emergency preparedness emergency plans. Factors to consider in planning are the socioeconomic level and vaccine status of the population, natural disasters the area may be prone to, and access routes to the clinic. Clinics associated with health systems should be included in the emergency plans of the health system. Independent clinics need to collaborate with a local hospital, public health department, and government agencies and have a generic screening form for infectious disease disasters. The plans should provide a process by which the facility can use mitigation strategies to become prepared to respond to and recover from all types of disasters. IPs should actively participate in the planning process.[88]

SUMMARY

Outpatient services are continually increasing and changing with expansion of new technologies, and, in the past year, the emergence of a novel virus changed the way services were delivered to patients. Some of these changes, such as the increase in use of telemedicine, will likely be permanent. Increased use of invasive devices and procedures provides new and challenging risks for infection. Risks associated with contaminated equipment can be decreased by HCW knowledge and maintenance of aseptic technique and disinfection practices. The challenge to infection control and ambulatory staff is to remain updated and familiar with emerging technologies to increase the likelihood of preventing health care–associated infection and providing safe patient care. More patients with a high acuity of illness are now being seen in ambulatory instead of inpatient settings, and these patients often spend prolonged periods in waiting rooms, in close proximity to others. The risk of communicable disease transmission and the high prevalence of some MDROs in health care and community settings necessitates standard and transmission-based precautions for all patient-care settings, including ambulatory settings. HCWs, patients, and family members of patients need to be provided education to support patient safety and minimize infection risk. IPs have unique challenges in providing ambulatory clinics with both infection prevention and regulatory strategies.

CLINICS CARE POINTS

- NHs must establish and coordinate consistent practices on clinical information exchange during transitions with other care facilities (admission, discharge, or transportation to outside diagnostic or therapeutic services). This will avoid loss of critical information such as pathogen exposure/colonized status, specific risk factors, and also avoid lapses, duplications and/or unnecessary changes in antimicrobial therapy.

- Hand Hygiene promotion and enforcement is a proven means of infection control, and presently still a low-hanging fruit, with compliance towards proper practices still below 50% overall. Consistent availability of alcohol-based hand-rubs improves compliance. Additionally, healthcare workers must be aware that some common non-clinical activities (such us dressing or transferring a patient) have a higher risk of transmission than generally perceived, and require protective equipment change.

- The burden of antimicrobial resistance organisms in NHs is now as high or higher than in acute care, posing frail NH residents at high risk of infection. This burden can be effectively reduced using active surveillance screening, either universal or for highest-risk individuals.

- Rehabilitation services involve a majority of NH residents, are an often overlooked means of pathogen spread. To minimize the burden of microorganism acquisition, dedicated infection prevention and control procedures should be established for individual rehabilitation settings, taking into account each settings' specific characteristics and risks.

- The Infection Preventionist, who has the central role in coordinating and evaluating all infection control measures for each facility, must follow and guide the many different aspects of day-to-day operations that may impact infection control, from ensuring that the most effective cleaning practices are adopted, to being able to recognize an emerging outbreak. This can only be accomplished when physicians and leadership provide all needed support in a timely fashion.

REFERENCES

1. Smith PW, Bennett G, Bradley SF, et al. Infection prevention and control in long-term care facilities. Infect Control Hosp Epidemiol 2008;29:785–814.

2. Friedman C, Barnette M, Buck AS, et al. Requirement for infrastructure and essential activities of infection control and epidemiology in out-of-hospital settings: a consensus panel report. Infect Control Hosp Epidemiol 1999;20:695–705.

3. Jarvis WR. Infection control and changing health-care delivery systems. Emerg Infect Dis 2001;7:170–3.

4. Graham NSN, Junghans C, Downes R, et al. SARS-CoV-2 infection, clinical features and outcome of COVID-19 in United Kingdom nursing homes. J Infect 2020;81(3):411–9.

5. Aronow WS. Clinical causes of death of 2372 older persons in a nursing home during 15-year follow-up. J Am Med Dir Assoc 2009;10(2):147.

6. Warren JW, Palumbo FB, Fitterman L, et al. Incidence and characteristics of antibiotic use in aged nursing home patients. J Am Geriatr Soc 1991;39:963–72.

7. Gurwitz JH, Field TS, Avorn J, et al. Incidence and preventability of adverse drug events in nursing homes. Am J Med 2000;109:87–94.

8. Stone ND, Ashraf MS, Calder J, et al. Surveillance definitions of infections in long-term care facilities: revisiting the McGeer criteria. Infect Control Hosp Epidemiol 2012;33:965–77.

9. Loeb M, Bentley DW, Bradley S, et al. Development of minimum criteria for the initiation of antibiotics in residents of long-term-care facilities: results of a consensus conference. Infect Control Hosp Epidemiol 2001;22:120–4.

10. Wang L, Lansing B, Symons K, et al. Infection rate and colonization with antibiotic-resistant organisms in skilled nursing facility residents with indwelling devices. Eur J Clin Microbiol Infect Dis 2012;31:1797–804.

11. Olsho LE, Bertrand RM, Edwards AS, et al. Does adherence to the Loeb minimum criteria reduce antibiotic prescribing rates in nursing homes? J Am Med Dir Assoc 2013;14:309.e1-e7.

12. Mody L, Krein SL, Saint S, et al. A targeted infection prevention intervention in nursing home residents with indwelling devices: a randomized clinical trial. JAMA Intern Med 2015;175:714–23.

13. Evans ME, Kralovic SM, Simbartl LA, et al. Nationwide reduction of health care-associated methicillin-resistant Staphylococcus aureus infections in Veterans Affairs long-term care facilities. Am J Infect Control 2014;42:60–2.

14. Schora DM, Boehm S, Das S, et al. Impact of detection, education, research and decolonization without isolation in long-term care (DERAIL) on methicillin-resistant Staphylococcus aureus colonization and transmission at 3 long-term care facilities. Am J Infect Control 2014;42:S269–73.

15. Ho ML, Seto WH, Wong LC, et al. Effectiveness of multifaceted hand hygiene interventions in long-term care facilities in Hong Kong: a cluster-randomized controlled trial. Infect Control Hosp Epidemiol 2012;33:761–7.

16. Ho SS, Tse MM, Boost MV. Effect of an infection control programme on bacterial contamination of enteral feed in nursing homes. J Hosp Infect 2012;82:49–55.

17. Temime L, Cohen N, Ait-Bouziad K, et al. Impact of a multicomponent hand hygiene-related intervention on the infectious risk in nursing homes: a cluster randomized trial. Am J Infect Control 2018;46(2):173–9.

18. Coleman EA. Falling through cracks: challenges and opportunities for improving transitional care for persons with continuous complex care needs. J Am Geriatr Soc 2003;51:549–55.

19. Montoya A, Mody L. Common infections in nursing homes: a review of current issues and challenges. Aging Health 2011;7(6):889–99.

20. Centers for Disease Control and Prevention. Guideline for hand hygiene in health-care settings: recommendations of the Healthcare Infection Control Practices

Advisory Committee and the HICPAC/SHEA/APIC/IDSA Hand Hygiene Task Force. MMWR Morb Mortal Wkly Rep 2002;51:S3–40.

21. Pittet D, Allegranzi B, Boyce J. The World Health Organization guidelines on hand hygiene in health care and their consensus recommendations. Infect Control Hosp Epidemiol 2009;30:611–22.

22. Aiello A, Malinis M, Knapp J, et al. Hand hygiene practices in nursing homes: does knowledge influence practice? Am J Infect Control 2009;37:164–7.

23. Mody L, McNeil SA, Sun R, et al. Introduction of a waterless alcohol-based hand rub in a long-term care facility. Infect Control Hosp Epidemiol 2003;24:165–71.

24. Pittet D, Sax H, Hugonnet S, et al. Cost implications of successful hand hygiene promotion. Infect Control Hosp Epidemiol 2004;25:264–6.

25. Mills JP, Zhu Z, Mantey J, et al. The devil is in the details: factors influencing hand hygiene adherence and contamination with antibiotic-resistant organisms among healthcare providers in nursing facilities. Infect Control Hosp Epidemiol 2019; 40(12):1394–9.

26. Hocine MN, Temime L. Impact of hand hygiene on the infectious risk in nursing home residents: a systematic review. Am J Infect Control 2015;43(9):e47–52.

27. Stone PW, Herzig CT, Pogorzelska-Maziarz M, et al. Understanding infection prevention and control in nursing homes: a qualitative study. Geriatr Nurs 2015;36(4): 267–72.

28. Schweizer ML, Reisinger HS, Ohl M, et al. Searching for an optimal hand hygiene bundle: a meta-analysis. Clin Infect Dis 2014;58(2):248–59.

29. Mody L, Saint S, Kaufman S, et al. Adoption of alcohol-based handrub by United States hospitals: a national survey. Infect Control Hosp Epidemiol 2008;29: 1177–80.

30. Pedersen LK, Held E, Johansen JD, et al. Less skin irritation from alcohol-based disinfectant than from detergent used for hand disinfection. Br J Dermatol 2005; 153:1142–6.

31. Roghmann MC, Johnson JK, Sorkin JD, et al. Transmission of Methicillin-Resistant Staphylococcus aureus (MRSA) to Healthcare Worker Gowns and Gloves During Care of Nursing Home Residents. Infect Control Hosp Epidemiol 2015;36(9): 1050–7.

32. Centers for Disease Control and Prevention Antibiotic Resistance Threats. 2019. Available at: https://www.cdc.gov/drugresistance/pdf/threats-report/2019-ar-threats-report-508.pdf.

33. Dommeti P, Wang L, Flannery EL, et al. Patterns of ciprofloxacin-resistant gram-negative bacteria colonization in nursing home residents. Infect Control Hosp Epidemiol 2011;32:177–80.

34. Spencer RC. The emergence of epidemic, multiple-antibiotic-resistant Stenotrophomonas (Xanthomonas) maltophilia and Burkholderia (Pseudomonas) cepacia. J Hosp Infect 1995;30(Suppl):453–64.

35. Hayakawa K, Marchaim D, Bathina P, et al. Independent risk factors for the co-colonization of vancomycin-resistant Enterococcus faecalis and methicillin-resistant Staphylococcus aureus in the region most endemic for vancomycin-resistant Staphylococcus aureus isolation. EurJ Clin Microbiol Infect Dis 2013;32(6):815–20.

36. Daneman N, Bronskill SE, Gruneir A, et al. Variability in antibiotic use across nursing homes and the risk of antibiotic-related adverse outcomes for individual residents. JAMA Intern Med 2015;175:1331–9.

37. Min L, Galecki A, Mody L. Functional disability and nursing resource use are predictive of antimicrobial resistance in nursing homes. J Am Geriatr Soc 2015;63: 659–66.
38. Bradley SF. Issues in management of resistant bacteria in long-term care facilities. Infect Control Hosp Epidemiol 1999;20:362–6.
39. Hujer AM, Bether CR, Hujer KM, et al. Antibiotic resistance in the institutionalized elderly. Clin Lab Med 2004;24:343–61.
40. Goldrick BA. MRSA, VRE and VRSA: how do we control them in nursing homes? Am J Nurs 2004;104:50–1.
41. Muto CA, Jernigan JA, Ostrowsky BE, et al. SHEA guideline for preventing nosocomial transmission of multidrug-resistant strains of Staphylococcus aureus and enterococcus. Infect Control Hosp Epidemiol 2003;24:362–86.
42. Siegel JD, Rhinehart E, Jackson M, et al. Management of multi-drug resistant organisms in healthcare settings. 2006. Available at: https://www.cdc.gov/infectioncontrol/pdf/guidelines/mdro-guidelines.pdf. Accessed on December 15, 2020.
43. Bowler WA, Bresnahan J, Bradfish A, et al. An integrated approach to methicillin-resistant Staphylococcus aureus control in a rural, regional-referral healthcare setting. Infect Control Hosp Epidemiol 2010;31(3):269–75.
44. Siegel JD, Rhinehart E, Jackson M, et al. 2007 guideline for isolation precautions: preventing transmission of infectious agents in healthcare settings. Available at: https://www.cdc.gov/niosh/docket/archive/pdfs/NIOSH-219/0219-010107-siegel.pdf.
45. Mody L, Crnich C. Effects of excessive antibiotic use in nursing homes. JAMA Intern Med 2015;175:1339–41.
46. McKinnell JA, Miller LG, Eells SJ, et al. A systematic literature review and meta-analysis of factors associated with methicillin-resistant Staphylococcus aureus colonization at time of hospital or intensive care unit admission. Infect Control Hosp Epidemiol 2013;34:1077–86.
47. Kindschuh W, Russo D, Kariolis I, et al. Comparison of a hospital-wide antibiogram with that of an associated long-term care facility. J Am Geriatr Soc 2012; 60:798–800.
48. Troillet N, Carmeli Y, Samore MH, et al. Carriage of methicillin-resistant Staphylococcus aureus at hospital admission. Infect Control Hosp Epidemiol 1998;19: 181–5.
49. Latour K, Catry B, Broex E, et al. Indications for antimicrobial prescribing in European nursing homes: results from a point prevalence survey. Pharmacoepidemiol Drug Saf 2012;21:937–44.
50. Horan TC, Gaynes RP. Surveillance of nosocomial infections. In: Mayhall CG, editor. Hospital epidemiology and infection control. 3rd edition. Philadelphia: Lippincott Williams & Wilkins; 2004. p. 1661–702.
51. McGeer A, Campbell B, Emori TG, et al. Definitions of infection for surveillance in long-term care facilities. Am J Infect Control 1991;19:1–7.
52. Stevenson KB, Moore J, Colwell H, et al. Standardized infection surveillance in long-term care: interfacility comparisons from a regional cohort of facilities. Infect Control Hosp Epidemiol 2005;26:231–8.
53. Mody L, Bradley SF, Galecki A, et al. Conceptual model for reducing infections and antimicrobial resistance in skilled nursing facilities: focusing on residents with indwelling devices. Clin Infect Dis 2011;52:654–61.
54. Jones M, Nielson C, Gupta K, et al. Collateral benefit of screening patients for methicillin-resistant Staphylococcus aureus at hospital admission: isolation of

patients with multidrug-resistant gram-negative bacteria. Am J Infect Control 2015;43(1):31–4.

55. Gibson KE, McNamara SE, Cassone M, et al. Methicillin-resistant Staphylococcus aureus: site of acquisition and strain variation in high-risk nursing home residents with indwelling devices. Infect Control Hosp Epidemiol 2014;35(12): 1458–65.

56. Cassone M, McNamara SE, Perri MB, et al. Impact of intervention measures on MRSA clonal type and carriage site prevalence. mBio 2016;7(2):e00218.

57. Muder RR, Brennen C, Wagener MM, et al. Methicillin-resistant staphylococcal colonization and infection in a long-term care facility. Ann Intern Med 1991;114: 107–12.

58. Ramsey AH, Skonieczny P, Coolidge DT, et al. Burkholderia cepacia lower respiratory tract infection associated with exposure to a respiratory therapist. Infect Control Hosp Epidemiol 2001;22(7):423–6.

59. Embril JM, McLeod JA, AL-Barrak AM, et al. An outbreak of methicillin-resistant Staphylococcus aureus on a burn unit: potential role of contaminated hydrotherapy equipment. Burns 2001;27:681–8.

60. Gontjes KJ, Gibson KE, Lansing B, et al. Contamination of common area and rehabilitation gym environment with multidrug-resistant organisms. J Am Geriatr Soc 2020;68(3):478–85.

61. Centers for Disease Control and Prevention. Guideline for Disinfection and Sterilization in Healthcare Facilities, 2008. W, Rutala, D. Weber Infection Control Practices Advisory Committee (HICPAC).

62. Bardenheier BH, Shefer AM, Lu PJ, et al. Are standing order programs associated with influenza vaccination? - NNHS, 2004. J Am Med Dir Assoc 2010; 11(9):654–61.

63. Centers for Disease Control and Prevention. Influenza Vaccination Information for Health Care Workers. 2016. Available at: www.cdc.gov/flu/professionals/.

64. Murti M, Otterstatter M, Orth A, et al. Measuring the impact of influenza vaccination on healthcare worker absenteeism in the context of a province-wide mandatory vaccinate-or-mask policy. Vaccine 2019;37(30):4001–7.

65. Advisory Committee on Immunization Practices, Centers for Disease Control and Prevention (CDC). Immunization of health-care personnel: recommendations of the Advisory Committee on Immunization Practices (ACIP). MMWR Recomm Rep 2011;60(RR-7):1–45.

66. Roup BJ, Scaletta JM. How Maryland increased infection prevention and control activity in long-term care facilities, 2003-2008. Am J Infect Control 2011;39(4): 292–5.

67. Available at: https://www.cms.gov/Medicare/Provider-Enrollment-and-Certification/GuidanceforLawsAndRegulations/Downloads/Appendix-PP-State-Operations-Manual.pdf.

68. Smith PW, Bennett G, Bradley S, et al, Society for Healthcare Epidemiology of America (SHEA), Association for Professionals in Infection Control and Epidemiology (APIC). SHEA/APIC guideline: infection prevention and control in the long-term care facility. Am J Infect Control 2008;36(7):504–35.

69. Cohen CC, Pogorzelska-Maziarz M, Herzig CT, et al. Infection prevention and control in nursing homes: a qualitative study of decision-making regarding isolation-based practices. BMJ Qual Saf 2015;24(10):630–6.

70. Travers J, Herzig CT, Pogorzelska-Maziarz M, et al. Perceived barriers to infection prevention and control for nursing home certified nursing assistants: a qualitative study. Geriatr Nurs 2015;36(5):355–60.

71. Centers for Disease Control & Prevention. Guide to infection prevention for outpatient settings: minimum expectations for safe care. Available at: https://www.cdc.gov/HAI/settings/outpatient/outpatient-care-guidelines.html.   Accessed December 20, 2020.

72. Koonin LM, Hoots B, Tsang CA, et al. Trends in the Use of Telehealth During the Emergence of the COVID-19 Pandemic — United States, January–March 2020. MMWR Morb Mortal Wkly Rep 2020;69(43):1595–9.

73. Jensen PA, Lambert LA, Iademarco MF, et al. Guidelines for Preventing the Transmission of Mycobacterium tuberculosis in Health-Care Settings, 2005 Recommendations and Reports, December 30, 2005 / 54(RR17);1–141.

74. Conner R, Spry C. Comprehensive guide to steam sterilization and sterility assurance in health care facilities. ANSI/AAMI ST79; 2017. Arlington (VA): AAMI, 2017. American National Standard.

75. Association for the Advancement of Medical Instrumentation. Flexible and Semirigid Endoscope Processing in Health Care Facilities. ANSI/AAMI ST91; 2015. Arlington (VA): AAMI, 2015. American National Standard.

76. Medicare Payment Advisory Commission (MEDPAC). Report to the Congress: Medicare Payment Policy. 2017. Available at: http://www.medpac.gov/-documents-/reports. Accessed March 22, 2017.

77. The Joint Commission Ambulatory Health Care: 2021 National Patient Safety Goals. Available at: https://www.jointcommission.org/standards/national-patient-safety-goals/ambulatory-health-care-national-patient-safety-goals/.   Accessed December 20, 2020.

78. Berríos-Torres SI, Umscheid CA, Bratzler DW, et al, Healthcare Infection Control Practices Advisory Committee. Centers for Disease Control and Prevention guideline for the prevention of surgical site infection, 2017. JAMA Surg 2017. https://doi.org/10.1001/jamasurg.2017.0904.

79. Centers for Disease Control and Prevention, National Healthcare Safety Network. The outpatient procedure component. 2020. Available at: https://www.cdc.gov/nhsn/ambulatory-surgery/index.html. Accessed December 20, 2020.

80. Spaulding EH. Chemical disinfection of medical and surgical materials. In: Lawrence C, Block SS, editors. Disinfection sterilization and preservation. Philadelphia: Lea & Febiger; 1968. p. 517–31.

81. Needlestick Safety and Prevention Act (PL 106-430), Nov. 6, 2000. Available at: https://www.osha.gov/pls/oshaweb/owadisp.show_document?p_id=16265&p_table=FEDERAL_REGISTER. Accessed December 14, 2020.

82. Centers for Disease Control and Prevention National Center for Emerging and Zoonotic Infectious Diseases. Division of healthcare quality promotion single-dose/single-use vial position and messages. Atlanta, GA: CDC Website; 2012. Available at: https://www.cdc.gov/injectionsafety/cdcposition-singleusevial.html. Accessed December 15, 2020.

83. Centers for Disease Control and Prevention (CDC). Transmission of Hepatitis B and C Viruses in Outpatient Settings-New York, Oklahoma, and Nebraska, 2000-2002. MMWR Morb Mortal Wkly Rep 2003;52(38):901–6.

84. Hepatitis B outbreak in New York City, 2001. Infect Control Hosp Epidemiol 2005; 26:745–60.

85. Centers for Disease Control and Prevention (CDC). Acute Hepatitis C Virus Infections Attributed to Unsafe Injection Practices at an Endoscopy Clinic-Nevada, 2007. MMWR Morb Mortal Wkly Rep 2008;57(19):513–7.

86. Centers for Disease Prevention and Control. Injection safety. Available at: https://www.cdc.gov/injectionsafety/index.html. Accessed December 23, 2020.

87. U.S. Food and Drug Administration Alert. FDA: insulin pens and insulin cartridges must not be shared. Spring (MD): US Food and Drug Administration; 2009. Available at: https://www.fda.gov/drugs/drug-safety-and-availability/fda-advises-health-care-professionals-and-patients-about-insulin-pen-packaging-and-dispensing. Accessed December 10, 2020.

88. APIC Text of Infection Control and Epidemiology On Line. 2020. Community Based Infection Prevention Practices: Emergency Management, Chapter 121 and Infectious Disease Disasters: Bioterrorism, Emerging Infections, and Pandemicsp. 1-63. Available at: https://apic.org/resources/apic-text/?utm_campaign=Homepage&utm_medium=webad&utm_source=Spotlight&utm_content=632021_ATO. Accessed December 10, 2020.

Health Care–Acquired Infections in Low- and Middle-Income Countries and the Role of Infection Prevention and Control

Gina Maki, DO[a],*, Marcus Zervos, MD[b]

KEYWORDS

- Hospital infections • Infection control • Antibiotic resistance • LMIC

KEY POINTS

- Health care–associated infections (HAIs) are a large cause of morbidity worldwide.
- Low- and middle-income countries have larger burdens of HAIs than high-income countries.
- Infection prevention and control plays a large role in decreasing the rate of HAIs and reducing antimicrobial resistance.

INTRODUCTION

Health care–associated infections (HAIs) account for many morbidity and mortality worldwide.[1] There are hundreds of millions of people affected by HAIs in all countries worldwide each year; however, low- and middle-income countries (LMIC) are disproportionately affected in adverse outcomes.[2] The total burden of HAIs is unknown especially in LMIC due to a lack of reported data, with LMIC studies reporting HAIs often being from individual centers or wards.[3] HAIs are infections that begin 48 hours or more after hospitalization or within 30 days after receiving health care.[1] Infection prevention and control (IPC) programs have been instituted in many settings in effort to decrease HAIs. They have the goal to reduce the risk of HAIs between patients, health care workers (HCW), and the environment, leading to a reduction in HAI-related morbidity, mortality, and avoidable costs.[2] Because of limited resources, LMIC face significant and often insurmountable challenges to accomplish this goal.

[a] Division of Infectious Diseases, Henry Ford Hospital, CFP-3, 2799 West Grand Boulevard, Detroit, MI 48202, USA; [b] Division of Infectious Diseases, Henry Ford Hospital, Wayne State University, CFP-3, 2799 West Grand Boulevard, Detroit, MI 48202, USA
* Corresponding author.
E-mail address: Gmaki1@hfhs.org

Infect Dis Clin N Am 35 (2021) 827–839
https://doi.org/10.1016/j.idc.2021.04.014
0891-5520/21/© 2021 Elsevier Inc. All rights reserved.

Therefore, optimal approaches must be tailored for LMIC and balance the feasibility, effectiveness, and cost.

RISK FACTORS TO ACQUIRE HEALTH CARE–ASSOCIATED INFECTIONS IN LOW- AND MIDDLE-INCOME COUNTRIES

Common types of HAI include central line–associated bloodstream infections (CLABSI), catheter-associated urinary tract infections, surgical site infections, hospital-acquired pneumonia, ventilator-associated pneumonia (VAP), clostridium difficile infections, and multidrug-resistant organisms (MDRO). Individual and system factors can contribute to the acquisition of HAIs, including increased length of health care facility stay, use of invasive devices, older patient age, patient comorbidities, mechanical ventilatory support, and stay in intensive care unit.[4] LMIC have additional risk factors contributing to HAI acquisition such as lack of resources and surveillance systems, lack of personnel and understaffing, lack of education in IPC and HAIs, overcrowding, and lack of supplies including cleaning supplies and soaps.

SURVEILLANCE AND RATES OF HEALTH CARE–ASSOCIATED INFECTIONS

Surveillance plays an important role in addressing rates of HAIs. By surveilling and monitoring specific HAIs problem areas can be identified; furthermore, gathering initial data and continued monitoring can assess areas of improvement and areas that continue to require improvement after program implementation. A study in India revealed an infection rate of 33 infections per 100 patients.[5] The most common HAIs in this study were urinary tract infections, followed by surgical site infections, wound infections, and nosocomial pneumonia.[5] A meta-analysis reviewing HAIs in Ethiopia reviewed 18 studies with 13,821 patients. This study found the pooled prevalence of HAIs among these studies to be 17.0%. The highest rates of HAIs were found to be surgical site infections, followed by urinary tract infections, bloodstream infections, then respiratory tract infections.[6]

How surveillance can be performed in low-resource settings should be addressed when starting a program within a facility.[7] Prospective clinical surveillance is often too resource intensive for low-resource settings. Automated surveillance is another recommended form for HAI surveillance that can also be difficult for resource-limited settings.[8] A study in South Africa looked at 3 various techniques including antimicrobial prescription surveillance, laboratory surveillance, and repeated point prevalence surveys. They found that the repeated point prevalence surveys were significantly less sensitive than the antimicrobial prescription and laboratory surveillance. Both laboratory and prescription-based surveillance had risk of false-positive identification of HAIs. The combination of antimicrobial prescription with laboratory surveillance reduced the false-positive rate. This combination also improved the estimates of HAI incidence, suggesting that this combination of surveillance may provide the most accurate estimate of the true HAI burden.[9] These methods can be considered as an alternative to more resource-intensive methods in resource-constrained settings. Although LMIC often face many challenges including limited human resources, diagnostics, and medical supplies, it is important to work around these barriers to find ways to best implement HAI surveillance.[10,11]

ANTIMICROBIAL RESISTANCE SURVEILLANCE

With an increase in MDRO and the limited antimicrobials to treat the many new resistant infections that are in circulation, it is important to be able to monitor the rates of antimicrobial resistance (AMR). Many MDRO originate in LMIC where the ability to control the spread can be limited due to a lack of resources. A major concern for AMR bacteria are the highly resistant carbapenemases. Two major examples are *Klebsiella pneumoniae* carbapenemase, which was identified in 2001, and New Delhi metallo-β-lactamase-1, identified in 2008[12,13]—2 highly resistant carbapenemases that have since been found to spread worldwide.[14,15]

Many health care facilities in LMIC lack the infrastructure and financial and human resources to create a robust program for AMR surveillance. With increasing resistance and the rapid spread among and between countries, it is of the utmost importance to monitor AMR.

In hospitals that are able to assess AMR, there are reports of high levels of HAI infections.[5] A study in India revealed a large percentage of nosocomial infections, with a high rate of resistance. More than 80% of isolates were gram-negative bacteria; common organisms isolated were *Pseudomonas aeruginosa*, *Escherichia coli*, *Acinetobacter baumannii*, as well as the gram-positive *Staphylococcus aureus*. Of these isolates, 69.9% of isolates were resistant to all antibiotics for which susceptibility testing was performed. *S aureus* isolates were found to be resistant to methicillin in 71.4% of isolates, and 88.2% were found to be sensitive to vancomycin, showing the concern for increasing glycopeptide resistance.[5] Another study in India revealed the most common organisms in VAP to be gram-negative organisms, with the most frequently isolated being *Acinetobacter* spp., followed by *Klebsiella* spp. and *Pseudomonas* spp.[16] In this study, 23% of the isolates causing VAP were multidrug resistant.

ANTIMICROBIAL STEWARDSHIP IN RELATION WITH INFECTION PREVENTION AND CONTROL

By the year 2050, global estimates of the impact of AMR will include more than 10 million annual deaths, making AMR the leading cause of death worldwide, surpassing deaths due to cancer, diabetes, and diarrheal diseases.[17] With limited antibiotics continuing to be produced as the rates of AMR increase, prevention plays a key role in tackling this major issue. Antimicrobial usage has seen exponential increase in LMIC over the last decade. The increase in antimicrobial use has been enabled by increasing incomes, availability of cheaper generic antimicrobials, unregulated over-the-counter pharmacy dispensation, indiscriminate antimicrobial use in livestock, and inappropriate antimicrobial use in health care; this is further aggravated by inadequate public health and infection control measures. Unfortunately, increased antimicrobial consumption has exerted selective pressure leading to emergence of resistant organisms. Because antimicrobial consumption is the driving factor for AMR, there needs to be a coordinated effort to optimize antimicrobial usage and prevent the transmission of resistant organisms. AMR poses a grave threat to the potential gain achieved in reducing mortality related to infections in the previous century by rendering all available antimicrobials ineffective against the resistant organisms. Because there are no newer antimicrobials in the pipeline for the foreseeable future, antimicrobial stewardship (AMS) programs have emerged as a key strategy in combating AMR. Both AMS and IPC programs are important in limiting the development and spread of MDRO.

In September 2016, the United Nations General Assembly held the first ever high-level meeting regarding AMR. The emphasis of the meeting focused on taking a One Health approach, recognizing the relation of health among humans, animals, and the environment. In response to this, many countries developed a national action plan for combating AMR. Although many countries developed a national action plan, few had started the process of program implementation to address AMR. The World Health Organization (WHO) created a practical toolkit for AMS programs in health care facilities in LMIC.[18] This toolkit was created to address the fourth strategic objective of the global action plan on AMR[19] by giving guidance on how to develop AMS programs or to strengthen programs that are already in place, including IPC programs. The toolkit begins with a checklist to be reviewed by the national leadership, hospital leadership, and hospital staff. This lends a point to begin assessment of what is in place and what the next steps are. The importance of the link between IPC and AMS is evident throughout the document when discussing the prevention of developing and spreading of AMR. Both programs have a goal of improving patient outcomes and patient safety and are used in the prevention of MDRO infections. In 2017 the Geneva IPC-think tank brought together 42 international experts to discuss strengthening of the global IPC network with the outcome of recognizing the importance of combining AMS and IPC under one umbrella.[20]

HEALTH CARE–ASSOCIATED TUBERCULOSIS

In 2018 there were an estimated 10 million new cases of tuberculosis (TB) worldwide, with 1.5 million TB deaths.[21] HCW remain at risk for contracting TB in the health care setting.[22] Risk seems particularly high when there is increased exposure combined with inadequate facilities for respiratory isolation and lack of rapid diagnostic tools.[23,24] In a review comparing the risk of TB infection and disease in high-income countries (HIC) and LMIC, the median prevalence of latent TB infection in HCW was 63% in LMIC and 24% in HIC.[24] The median annual incidence of TB infection that was considered to be caused by health care exposure was 5.8% in LMIC and 1.1% in the HIC studied.

The WHO guidelines recommend a prioritization of administrative controls as the most important measures, because engineering and personal controls do not work in the absence of solid administrative measures. Although engineering measures require resources, opening windows to increase natural ventilation and the use of fans to control the direction of airflow are examples of inexpensive measures that can be implemented. Personal measures are the most expensive and least effective measures and, therefore, should only be used in specialized settings and when all other IPC measures have been implemented.[25]

EMERGING INFECTIONS: CORONAVIRUS DISEASE 2019

The coronavirus disease 2019 (COVID-19) caused by the novel severe acute respiratory syndrome coronavirus (SARS-CoV-2) was declared a pandemic by the WHO on March 11, 2020. It has been important to note the nature of asymptomatic spread of the virus. Many of those infected with the SARS-CoV-2 do not develop symptoms, and in those that do become symptomatic there is a period of transmissibility before the onset of symptom development.[26,27]

COVID-19 has been found to affect certain vulnerable populations, which require additional focus and precautions. Many of the vulnerable populations that have been noted to be heavily affected in HIC make up much of the populations of LMIC. Indigenous populations often live outside of the large urban centers with limited access to medical care as well as may have language barriers and beliefs, which can lead to difficulties in seeking and obtaining medical care.[28] Many LMIC health care facilities function with an already limited supply of resources, which can be exacerbated by the pandemic. The workload of HCWs is increased by the pandemic, as there is often already limited human resources. Living in close quarters is a risk for increased transmission, and it is known that often large families that are financially limited live in poor housing conditions.[28] The elderly have been shown to have the highest risk of poor outcomes with COVID-19 infection. Nursing home residents were heavily affected by the COVID-19 pandemic, with multiple cities reporting outbreaks within the nursing homes.[29] In one study of nursing homes in Detroit, Michigan, USA, it was found that there was a 44% COVID-19 attack rate among the nursing home residents, with 37% of those requiring hospitalizations, and 24% died.[30] Another vulnerable population noted in the United States were nonwhite Americans, especially Black Americans. In Michigan, Black Americans make up 14% of the population; however, they made up 37% of COVID-19 cases and 42% of deaths.[31,32] It is important to be aware of these vulnerable populations in order to address prevention of adverse outcomes.

COVID-19 has played a role in the contribution to HAIs and AMR.[29,33] Multiple studies revealed the extensive use of antibiotic coverage in COVID-19 pneumonia despite the low evidence of confirmed bacterial coinfection.[34–36] This evidence shows the opportunity for AMS efforts to decrease the overuse of antimicrobials in COVID-19 infection. With COVID-19 hospital admissions comes increased hospital stays and increased duration of stay, which in turn leads to an increased risk for acquiring HAIs. Early in the pandemic, personal protective equipment became high in demand, and many settings worldwide developed a severe shortage. With a shortage in personal protective equipment, this decreased the comfort of HCW entering COVID-19 patient rooms and/or areas, which led to less time spent at the bedside, which in turn led to a decrease in infection prevention care, such as addressing of ventilator and lines bundles. With increased availability of personal protective equipment and increased learning of the disease, the comfort of caring for patients with COVID-19 disease increases and more attention can be paid to the details of prevention of HAIs.

Wearing masks was an early recommendation to stop the spread of the COVID-19 infection.[37] It is important for all people to wear a mask and not only COVID-19-positive patients due to the asymptomatic transmission of the virus. For HCWs working with COVID-19 positive and suspected patients, it was recommended to use both droplet and contact precautions, with the use of a mask, with N-95 or respirator use in the setting of an aerosol generating procedure, along with gown, gloves, and eye protection.[37]

During the COVID-19 outbreak the WHO created guidance that included IPC recommendations to implement strategies with the goal of preventing or limiting health care transmission of COVID-19.[38] These included ensuring triage, early recognition, and source control; applying standard precautions for all patients; implementing additional precautions such as droplet, contact, and airborne when applicable; implementing administrative controls; and using environmental and engineering controls.[38] Within this guidance, they reinforced the recommendation of standard precautions in all patients at all times within health care facilities (**Box 1**).[38–40] These practices can also inhibit the spread of other HAIs.

Recommended isolation precautions can be a challenge in LMIC settings. In addition to standard precautions as described earlier, contact and droplet precautions in all suspected or confirmed COVID-19 cases are recommended.[38] These recommendations include wearing a medical mask, eye protection such as goggles or a face shield, gown, and gloves when possible. Additional precautions can be implemented when feasible including cohorting, separation of patients by 1 m apart, and airborne precautions for aerosol-generating procedures such as tracheal intubation and noninvasive ventilation.

Box 1
Standard precautions for all patients

1. Hand hygiene
   a. Cleanse hands with an alcohol-based hand rub or with soap and water;
   b. Alcohol-based hand rubs are preferred if hands are not visibly soiled;
   c. Wash hands with soap and water when they are visibly soiled.

2. Respiratory hygiene
   a. Cover nose and mouth with a tissue or elbow when coughing or sneezing;
   b. Offer a medical mask to patients with suspected COVID-19 while they are in waiting/public areas or in cohorting rooms;
   c. Perform hand hygiene after contact with respiratory secretions.

3. Correct personal protective equipment according to risk
   a. Maintain adequate and regular supplies;
   b. Maintain staff training.

4. Safe injection practices, sharps management and injury prevention
   a. Using a clean workspace;
   b. Hand hygiene before and after;
   c. Use a sterile safety-engineered syringe;
   d. Use sterile vial of medication and diluent;
   e. Appropriate skin cleaning and antisepsis;
   f. Appropriate collection of sharps;
   g. Appropriate waste management.

5. Safe handling, cleaning, and disinfection of patient care equipment
   a. Clean patient care equipment between each patient use.

6. Appropriate environmental cleaning; safe handling and cleaning of soiled linen
   a. Clean and soiled linen should be stored and handled separately;
   b. Cleaning should occur on regular basis per standard protocols.

7. Appropriate waste management
   a. Ensure appropriate waste management protocols are followed.

Data from Refs.[38–40]

HEALTH AND ECONOMIC IMPACT

The cost of health care is an important factor for all problems and interventions in the health care setting. Associated factors such as prolonged hospital stay, disability, increased AMR, increased costs, and increased deaths are more pronounced in LMIC. VAP is a leading cause of HAI in patients within the intensive care unit. VAP has been found to occur at a higher rate in Asian countries than averages from the International Nosocomial Infection Control Consortium data.[41] The International Nosocomial Infection Control Consortium reported that device-associated infections increase length of stay by 10 days, costs between $5000 and $12,000 US dollars, and doubles the rate of mortality.[42–44] In LMIC, although the magnitude and impact of the problem is more remarkable, there are few objective data on the financial burden, and this burden varies from country to country.[43,44] The limitations in health care facilities, including infrastructure, patient load, and staff shortages, provide many challenges. Limitations in access to care, issues of sanitation, and poverty also complicate measures to control HAIs.

EXAMPLE OF SUCCESSFUL INFECTION CONTROL STRATEGY IN RESOURCE-LIMITED SETTINGS

The International Nosocomial Infection Control Consortium implemented a multidimensional approach on VAP in 11 hospitals in Argentina over a 4-year period. The baseline data of this study revealed that there were higher rates of VAP per 1000 mechanically ventilated days when compared with HIC including USA VAP rates from the Centers for Disease Control and Prevention and German data from the German Krankenhaus Infektions Surveillance System. Through interventions including a bundle of infection prevention practice interventions, education, outcome surveillance, process surveillance, feedback on VAP rates and consequences, and performance feedback of process surveillance there was a 52% rate reduction in VAP.[45] They found that for each VAP there was an extra length of stay of 16 days on average, 4-fold higher than patients without VAP, with a cost of $1000 US dollars per each bed-day; this led to a total savings of 176 days per each intensive care unit per year and a savings of $176,000 US dollars per year.

A consortium of 15 LMIC developed a successful strategy by focusing on education, performance feedback and outcome, and outcome and process surveillance. The study took place in 86 intensive care units and showed improved IPC adherence and reduced CLABSI incidence by 33% in the first 6 months of the program and by 54% over the first 24 months.[46] The number of deaths in patients with CLABSI decreased by 58%. Specific interventions in which improvement was noted included adherence to hand hygiene, use of maximal sterile barriers during line insertion, use of chlorhexidine for antisepsis measures, removal of unneeded catheters, and decreased duration of catheters.[46]

These studies reveal that with bundled IPC practices the rates of HAIs such as VAP and CLABSI can be drastically reduced.

DESIGNING AND SUSTAINING INFECTION CONTROL PROGRAMS AND INTERVENTIONS

Once the assessment of the need for IPC programs is evaluated, it is important to then address the implementation. It was noted by the WHO that implementation of the measures to address IPC and AMR are often the largest challenge. They recommend that in the development of any IPC or AMS curriculum implementation skills should be a priority.[47] A manual was published in 2017 by the WHO in an effort to be a practical manual to support the implementation of WHO guidelines on the core components of IPC programs with a focus on low-resource settings. The 3 aims of the manual include the following:

"(1) to provide clear direction and supporting resources to aid the development of a practical outcome-focused action plan, (2) to describe how to operationalize the plan based on evidence and national-level implementation experience informed by local examples and existing realities, and (3) to support sustainability of the plan with a focus on integrating and embedding IPC within relevant national policies and strategies."[48]

According to the WHO manual there are 8 core components relevant to the facility-level IPC programs, outlined in **Box 2**.

For those with an IPC program already started, it is important to also evaluate for sustainability and improvement. In the WHO guide for IPC, they recommend a 5-step approach for IPC program improvement (**Box 3**) with more in-depth guidance within the manual.[49]

CREATING AN ANTIMICROBIAL STEWARDSHIP PROGRAM

As AMS programs play a large role in the limiting of development of AMR and MDROs, it is important for health care facilities to develop an AMS program that is adjusted to fit within the current needs and resources. WHO created a toolkit that serves as a document describing how to begin and build a successful AMS

Box 2
Core components relevant to the facility-level infection prevention and control program

1. IPC programs

2. Evidence-based guidelines

3. Education and training

4. Health care–associated infection surveillance

5. Multimodal strategies

6. Monitoring and audit of IPC practices and feedback

7. Workload, staffing and bed occupancy

8. Built environment, materials, and equipment for IPC

Data from World Health Organization. Improving infection prevention and control at the health facility: Interim practical manual supporting implementation of the WHO Guidelines on Core Components of Infection Prevention and Control Programmes. Geneva: World Health Organization; 2018.(WHO/HIS/SDS/2018.10).

---

program within health care facilities in LMIC.[18] In creation of the toolkit, interviews were undertaken in order to evaluate the feasibility of the toolkit within LMIC.[50] Input was gathered from national leaders, health care facility leadership, and health care facility staff. This input was then incorporated into the toolkit to ensure the most

---

Box 3
Core components relevant to the facility-level infection prevention and control program

Step 1. Preparing for action: this step ensures that all of the prerequisites that need to be in place for success are addressed, including the necessary resources (human and financial), infrastructures, planning and coordination of activities, and the identification of roles and responsibilities (including key opinion leaders and champions). The facility senior managers/leaders play a critical role in this step.

Step 2. Baseline assessment: conducting an exploratory baseline assessment of the current situation, including the identification of existing strengths and weaknesses, is critical for developing a tailor-made action plan that addresses the reality of a health care facility. A ready-to-use assessment tool based on the WHO IPC core components is available for step 2 (WHO IPC Assessment Framework [IPCAF]). Ideally, additional IPC assessment tools (eg, the Hand Hygiene Self-assessment Framework [HHSAF] and/or observation-based tools to evaluate IPC practices) could be used.

Step 3. Developing and executing an action plan: the results of the baseline assessment support the development and execution of an action plan based around a multimodal improvement strategy.

Step 4. Assessing impact: conducting a follow-up assessment using the same tools as in step 2 is crucial to determine the effectiveness of the plan. The focus is on impact, acceptability, and cost-effectiveness.

Step 5. Sustaining the program over the long term: an important step in the cycle of improvement is to develop an ongoing action plan and review schedule to support the long-term impact and benefits of the IPC program, thus contributing to its overall impact and sustainability.

Data from World Health Organization. Improving infection prevention and control at the health facility: Interim practical manual supporting implementation of the WHO Guidelines on Core Components of Infection Prevention and Control Programmes. Geneva: World Health Organization; 2018 (WHO/HIS/SDS/2018.10).

usability. The WHO AMS toolkit is divided into 6 sections: (1) Structural Core Elements for AMS Implementation at the National Level; (2) Structural Core Elements for AMS Implementation at the Facility Level; (3) Planning AMS Programs; (4) Performing AMS Interventions; (5) Assessing AMS Programs; and (6) Education and Training. During the feasibility studies of the WHO AMS toolkit, it was noted that strong leadership support at the national and senior facility management levels was needed for successful implementation.[50] The WHO AMS toolkit is a resource for facilities within LMIC to create a strong AMS program and serves as a reference to continue to build on structures put in place, such as current IPC committees, in an effort to continue to control the development and spread of AMR.[18]

ADDRESSING GAPS WHILE PRIORITIZING RESOURCES

To prioritize resources, efforts should first focus on inexpensive yet high-impact IPC measures in order to increase success with limited resources and then later medium-term and long-term solutions. Low-cost measures, such as educational programs on hand hygiene and prevention of device-associated infections, have shown cost-effectiveness and should be the first items to be addressed. When considering IPC measures that are applicable to the setting and resources, it is best to first consider the available national guidelines or international guidelines that address the LMIC settings and resources. Examples are the WHO guidelines for injection safety,[51] hand hygiene,[52] and for the prevention of TB in health care facilities in resource-limited settings[25] or the use of checklists, such as the surgical safety checklist, to reduce morbidity and mortality in a global population.[53] Guidelines, recommendations, and interventions known to be effective in HIC settings can be a starting point to prioritize and plan how and where measures should be implemented.

SUMMARY

IPC programs are an important tool in the prevention of HAIs. In order to be practical, measures for IPC programs should be simple, cost-effective, and designed to suit the local needs and circumstances. Evidence-based measures should be used, along with achievable goals and a plan for short-term, medium-term, and long-term actions. More studies are necessary to evaluate the implementation of programs and policies that are possible in LMIC. HIC must have a shared interest in developing the capacity of neighboring countries and can serve an important role by providing training and resources.

As the health care environment continues to change, new challenges and risks arise for HAIs. It is important for continued education and awareness, as well as political engagement in the support of IPC programs to halt the progression of HAIs.

CLINICS CARE POINTS

- When developing infection control practices in a low resource setting, use a stepwise approach based on available resources.
- Strategies must start with simple and cost-effective measures and then expand to include more complicated measures.
- It is important to have administrative leadership input when developing infection control and antimicrobial stewardship programs.

DISCLOSURE

No disclosures related to present study. Disclosures of M. Zervos include grants to institution, Moderna, Johnson & Johnson, Merck, Pfizer, and consultant ContraFect.

REFERENCES

1. Revelas A. Healthcare - associated infections: a public health problem. Niger Med J 2012;53:59–64.
2. Vandijck D, Cleemput I, Hellings J, et al. Infection prevention and control strategies in the era of limited resources and quality improvement: a perspective paper. Aust Crit Care 2013;26:154–7.
3. World Health Organization. Report on the burden of endemic health care-associated infection worldwide. Geneva (Switzerland): World Health Organization; 2011. Available at: https://apps.who.int/iris/handle/10665/80135. Accessed December 22, 2020.
4. Monegro AF, Muppidi V, Regunath H. Hospital acquired infections. StatPearls. Treasure Island (FL): StatPearls Publishing; 2020. Available at: https://www. ncbi.nlm.nih.gov/books/NBK441857/. Accessed December 22, 2020.
5. Kamat U, Ferreira A, Savio R, et al. Antimicrobial resistance among nosocomial isolates in a teaching hospital in goa. Indian J Community Med 2008;33:89–92.
6. Alemu AY, Endalamaw A, Bayih WA. The burden of healthcare-associated infection in Ethiopia: a systematic review and meta-analysis. Trop Med Health 2020; 48:77.
7. Centers for Disease Control and Prevention. Outline for healthcare-associated infections surveillance. 2006. Available at: https://www.cdc.gov/nhsn/pdfs/ outlineforHAIsurveillance.pdf. Accessed December 28, 2020.
8. van Mourik MSM, Perencevich EN, Gastmeier P, et al. Designing surveillance of healthcare-associated infections in the era of automation and reporting mandates. Clin Infect Dis 2018;66:970–6.
9. Dramowski A, Cotton MF, Whitelaw A. Surveillance of healthcare-associated infection in hospitalised South African children: which method performs best? S Afr Med J 2016;107:56–63.
10. Allegranzi B, Bagheri Nejad S, Combescure C, et al. Burden of endemic healthcare-associated infection in developing countries: systematic review and meta-analysis. Lancet 2011;377:228–41.
11. Vilar-Compte D, Camacho-Ortiz A, Ponce-de-Leon S. Infection control in limited resources countries: challenges and priorities. Curr Infect Dis Rep 2017;19:20.
12. Castanheira M, Deshpande LM, Mathai D, et al. Early dissemination of NDM-1- and OXA-181-producing Enterobacteriaceae in Indian hospitals: report from the SENTRY Antimicrobial Surveillance Program, 2006-2007. Antimicrob Agents Chemother 2011;55:1274–8.
13. Linciano P, Cendron L, Gianquinto E, et al. Ten years with New Delhi Metallo-beta-lactamase-1 (NDM-1): from structural insights to inhibitor design. ACS Infect Dis 2019;5:9–34.
14. Szekely E, Damjanova I, Janvari L, et al. First description of bla(NDM-1), bla(OXA-48), bla(OXA-181) producing Enterobacteriaceae strains in Romania. Int J Med Microbiol 2013;303:697–700.
15. Liu Z, Gu Y, Li X, et al. Identification and Characterization of NDM-1-producing Hypervirulent (Hypermucoviscous) Klebsiella pneumoniae in China. Ann Lab Med 2019;39:167–75.

16. Mathai AS, Phillips A, Kaur P, et al. Incidence and attributable costs of ventilator-associated pneumonia (VAP) in a tertiary-level intensive care unit (ICU) in northern India. J Infect Public Health 2015;8:127–35.

17. Review on Antimicrobial Resistance. Tackling drug-resistant infections globally: final report and recommendations. 2016. Available at: https://www.biomerieuxconnection.com/wp-content/uploads/2018/04/Tackling-Drug-Resistant-Infections-Globally_-Final-Report-and-Recommendations.pdf. Accessed February 1, 2021.

18. World Health Organization. Antimicrobial stewardship programmes in health-care facilities in low- and middle-income countries: a WHO practical toolkit. Geneva (Switzerland): World Health Organization; 2019. Available at: https://apps.who.int/iris/handle/10665/329404. Accessed December 22, 2020.

19. World Health Organization. Global action plan on antimicrobial resistance. Geneva (Switzerland): World Health Organization; 2015. Available at: https://apps.who.int/iris/handle/10665/193736. Accessed December 22, 2020.

20. Zingg W, Storr J, Park BJ, et al. Broadening the infection prevention and control network globally; 2017 Geneva IPC-think tank (part 3). Antimicrob Resist Infect Control 2019;8:74.

21. World Health Organization. Global tuberculosis report 2020. Geneva (Switzerland): World Health Organization; 2020. Available at: https://apps.who.int/iris/bitstream/handle/10665/336069/9789240013131-eng.pdf. Accessed December 22, 2020.

22. Nathavitharana RR, Bond P, Dramowski A, et al. Agents of change: the role of healthcare workers in the prevention of nosocomial and occupational tuberculosis. Presse Med 2017;46:e53–62.

23. Agaya J, Nnadi CD, Odhiambo J, et al. Tuberculosis and latent tuberculosis infection among healthcare workers in Kisumu, Kenya. Trop Med Int Health 2015;20:1797–804.

24. Menzies D, Joshi R, Pai M. Risk of tuberculosis infection and disease associated with work in health care settings. Int J Tuberc Lung Dis 2007;11:593–605.

25. World Health Organization. Guidelines for the prevention of tuberculosis in health care facilities in resource-limited settings. Biella (Italy): World Health Organization; 1999. Available at: http://www.who.int/tb/publications/who_tb_99_269.pdf. Accessed January 3, 2021.

26. Li G, Li W, He X, et al. Asymptomatic and presymptomatic infectors: hidden sources of coronavirus disease 2019 (COVID-19). Clin Infect Dis 2020;71:2018.

27. Gandhi M, Yokoe DS, Havlir DV. Asymptomatic transmission, the Achilles' heel of current strategies to control Covid-19. N Engl J Med 2020;382:2158–60.

28. Mesa Vieira C, Franco OH, Gomez Restrepo C, et al. COVID-19: the forgotten priorities of the pandemic. Maturitas 2020;136:38–41.

29. Kimball A, Hatfield KM, Arons M, et al. Asymptomatic and presymptomatic SARS-CoV-2 infections in residents of a long-term care skilled nursing facility - King County, Washington, March 2020. MMWR Morb Mortal Wkly Rep 2020;69:377–81.

30. Sanchez GV, Biedron C, Fink LR, et al. Initial and repeated point prevalence surveys to inform SARS-CoV-2 infection prevention in 26 skilled nursing facilities - Detroit, Michigan, March-May 2020. MMWR Morb Mortal Wkly Rep 2020;69:882–6.

31. Byrne P, McNamara B, Todd B, et al. Michigan coronavirus cases: tracking the pandemic. Detroit Free Press 2020. Available at: https://www.freep.com/in-depth/news/nation/coronavirus/2020/04/11/michigan-coronavirus-cases-tracking-covid-19-pandemic/5121186002/. Accessed December 23, 2020.

32. Whitmer G. Whitmer: virus trains harsh spotlight on racial health disparities. Detroit Free Press 2020. Available at: https://www.freep.com/story/opinion/contributors/2020/04/12/whitmer-coronavirus-racial-health-disparities-michigan/5134653002. Accessed December 23, 2020.

33. Arons MM, Hatfield KM, Reddy SC, et al. Presymptomatic SARS-CoV-2 infections and transmission in a skilled nursing facility. N Engl J Med 2020;382:2081–90.

34. Rawson TM, Moore LSP, Zhu N, et al. Bacterial and fungal coinfection in individuals with coronavirus: a rapid review to support COVID-19 antimicrobial prescribing. Clin Infect Dis 2020;71:2459–68.

35. Townsend L, Hughes G, Kerr C, et al. Bacterial pneumonia coinfection and antimicrobial therapy duration in SARS-CoV-2 (COVID-19) infection. JAC Antimicrob Resist 2020;2:dlaa071.

36. Hughes S, Troise O, Donaldson H, et al. Bacterial and fungal coinfection among hospitalized patients with COVID-19: a retrospective cohort study in a UK secondary-care setting. Clin Microbiol Infect 2020;26:1395–9.

37. World Health Organization. Mask use in the context of COVID-19: interim guidance. 2020. Available at: https://apps.who.int/iris/bitstream/handle/10665/337199/WHO-2019-nCov-IPC_Masks-2020.5-eng.pdf?sequence=1&isAllowed=y. Accessed February 1, 2021.

38. World Health Organization. Infection prevention and control during health care when novel coronavirus (nCoV) infection is suspected: interim guidance. 2020. Available at: https://www.who.int/publications/i/item/10665-331495. Accessed December 22, 2020.

39. World Health Organization. Injection safety tools and resources. 2020. Available at: https://www.who.int/infection-prevention/tools/injections/training-education/en/. Accessed December 22, 2020.

40. World Health Organization, Pan American Health Organization. Decontamination and reprocessing of medical devices for health-care facilities. Geneva (Switzerland): World Health Organization; 2016. Available at: https://www.who.int/infection-prevention/publications/decontamination/en/. Accessed December 22, 2020.

41. Rosenthal VD. International Nosocomial Infection Control Consortium (INICC) resources: INICC multidimensional approach and INICC surveillance online system. Am J Infect Control 2016;44:e81–90.

42. Rosenthal VD. Device-associated nosocomial infections in limited-resources countries: findings of the International Nosocomial Infection Control Consortium (INICC). Am J Infect Control 2008;36:S171.e7-12.

43. World Health Organization. The burden of health care-associated infection worldwide. A summary. 2010. Available at: https://www.who.int/gpsc/country_work/summary_20100430_en.pdf. Accessed December 22, 2020.

44. Pittet D, Allegranzi B, Storr J, et al. Infection control as a major World Health Organization priority for developing countries. J Hosp Infect 2008;68:285–92.

45. Rosenthal VD, Desse J, Maurizi DM, et al. Impact of the International Nosocomial Infection Control Consortium's multidimensional approach on rates of ventilator-associated pneumonia in 14 intensive care units in 11 hospitals of 5 cities within Argentina. Am J Infect Control 2018;46:674–9.

46. Rosenthal VD, Maki DG, Rodrigues C, et al. Impact of International Nosocomial Infection Control Consortium (INICC) strategy on central line-associated bloodstream infection rates in the intensive care units of 15 developing countries. Infect Control Hosp Epidemiol 2010;31:1264–72.

47. Zingg W, Storr J, Park BJ, et al. Implementation research for the prevention of antimicrobial resistance and healthcare-associated infections; 2017 Geneva infection prevention and control (IPC)-think tank (part 1). Antimicrob Resist Infect Control 2019;8:87.
48. World Health Organization. Interim practical manual supporting national implementation of the WHO guidelines on core components of infection prevention and control programmes. Geneva (Switzerland): World Health Organization; 2017. Available at: https://www.who.int/infection-prevention/tools/core-components/cc-implementation-guideline.pdf?ua=1. Accessed January 2, 2021.
49. World Health Organization. Improving infection prevention and control at the health facility: Interim practical manual supporting implementation of the WHO Guidelines on Core Components of Infection Prevention and Control Programmes. Geneva (Switzerland): World Health Organization; 2018. Available at: https://apps.who.int/iris/handle/10665/279788. Accessed December 22, 2020.
50. Maki G, Smith I, Paulin S, et al. Feasibility study of the World Health Organization health care facility-based antimicrobial stewardship toolkit for low- and middle-income countries. Antibiotics (Basel) 2020;9:556.
51. World Health Organization. WHO best practices for injections and related procedures toolkit. Geneva (Switzerland): World Health Organization; 2010. Available at: http://apps.who.int/iris/bitstream/10665/44298/1/9789241599252_eng.pdf. Accessed January 3, 2021.
52. World Health Organization. WHO guidelines on hand hygiene in health care. First global patient safety challenge clean care is safer care. Geneva (Switzerland): World Health Organization; 2009. Available at: http://apps.who.int/iris/bitstream/10665/44102/1/9789241597906_eng.pdf. Accessed January 2, 2021.
53. Haynes AB, Weiser TG, Berry WR, et al. A surgical safety checklist to reduce morbidity and mortality in a global population. N Engl J Med 2009;360:491–9.

Moving?

Make sure your subscription moves with you!

To notify us of your new address, find your **Clinics Account Number** (located on your mailing label above your name), and contact customer service at:

Email: journalscustomerservice-usa@elsevier.com

800-654-2452 (subscribers in the U.S. & Canada)
314-447-8871 (subscribers outside of the U.S. & Canada)

Fax number: 314-447-8029

Elsevier Health Sciences Division
Subscription Customer Service
3251 Riverport Lane
Maryland Heights, MO 63043

*To ensure uninterrupted delivery of your subscription, please notify us at least 4 weeks in advance of move.